P9-CDB-573

Nutrition for the Recreational Athlete

CRC SERIES ON NUTRITION IN EXERCISE AND SPORT

Editors, Ira Wolinsky and James F. Hickson, Jr.

Published Titles

Luke Bucci
Nutrients as Ergogenic Aids for Sports and Exercise

Ira Wolinsky & James F. Hickson, Jr.
Nutrition in Exercise and Sport, 2/E

Ronald R. Watson & Marianne Eisinger
Exercise and Disease

Luke Bucci
Nutrition Applied to Injury Rehabilitation and Sports Medicine

Catherine G. R. Jackson
Nutrition for the Recreational Athlete

James F. Hickson, Jr.
Sports Nutrition

Editor, Ira Wolinsky

Published Titles

Constance V. Kies and Judy A. Driskell
Sports Nutrition: Minerals and Electrolytes

Forthcoming Titles

Jaime S. Ruud
Nutrition and the Female Athlete

E. R. Buskirk & S. Puhl
Body Fluid Balance: Exercise and Sport

Jana Parizkova
Nutrition, Physical Activity and Health in Early Life

Nutrition for the Recreational Athlete

Catherine G. Ratzin Jackson
School of Kinesiology and Physical Education
University of Northern Colorado
Greeley, Colorado

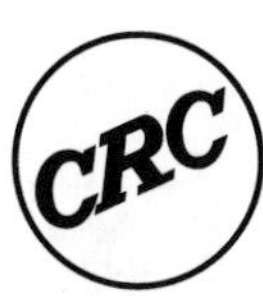

CRC Press
Boca Raton Ann Arbor London Tokyo

Library of Congress Cataloging-in-Publication Data

Nutrition for the recreational athlete / edited by Catherine G. Ratzin Jackson.
p. cm. -- (Nutrition in exercise and sport)
Includes bibliographical references and index.
ISBN 0-8493-7914-8
1. Athletes--Nutrition. I. Ratzin Jackson, Catherine G. II. Series.
TX361.A8N873 1994
613.2′024796--dc20 94-19402
CIP

Direct all inquiries to CRC Press, Inc., 2000 Corporate Blvd., N.W., Boca Raton, Florida 33431.

International Standard Book Number 0-8493-7914-8
Library of Congress Card Number 94-19402
Printed in the United States of America 1 2 3 4 5 6 7 8 9 0
Printed on acid-free paper

SERIES PREFACE

The CRC series on Nutrition in Exercise and Sport provides a setting for in-depth exploration of the many and varied aspects of nutrition and exercise, including sports. The topic of exercise and sports nutrition has been a focus of research among scientists since the 1960s, and the healthful benefits of good nutrition and exercise have been appreciated. As our knowledge expands, it will be necessary to remember that there must be a range of diets and exercise regimes that will support excellent physical condition and performance. There is not a single diet-exercise treatment that can be the common denominator, or the single formula for health, or panacea for performance.

This series is dedicated to providing a stage to explore these issues. Each volume provides a detailed and scholarly examination of some aspect of the topic.

Contributors from any bona fide area of nutrition and physical activity, including sports and the controversial, are welcome.

Ira Wolinsky, Ph.D.
Series Editor

PREFACE

The majority of books that have been written about nutrition in the immediate past have focused on the high-performance athlete. Additionally, much of the scientific literature profiles this population. As a result, information presented to recreational athletes is often based on a very unique and select segment of the population of exercisers. While it can be argued that the information is the same for all people, it sometimes presents problems in interpretation and, in some respects, has created heightened concern over nutrition for the recreational execiser that is often unwarranted. It is the intent of this volume to meet the needs of this vast group of people with sound advice for their well-being, so that dietary practices will support the activities chosen, and compliance with exercise will not be a chore but will continue for a lifetime.

Each chapter of this volume was chosen to give information to fulfill a specific need of the recreational athlete. Chapter 1, as an introduction to the book, explores the cultural issues and the definition of a recreational athlete. The point is clearly made that this group of exercisers is vast and varied. Chapter 2 details the reasons recreational athletes should understand the relationship between the type of activity and how energy is delivered within the cells of the body. It is this knowledge that will help identify the specific chapters of interest that follow (Chapters 3 to 7). Chapter 3 gives information for recreational athletes who determine that their activity would be categorized as aerobic or endurance. Chapter 4 specifically discusses the nutritional recommendations for activities that are identified as strength or resistance. Chapter 5 details the needs of cross-training, an area about which there is very little current information. Chapter 6 discusses the special category of vegetarian athletes and includes the latest advice for them. Chapter 7 has all of the major recommendations from a variety of sources for reducing the risk of cardiovascular diseases by following appropriate dietary modifications. Although geared to the individual who has just had a heart attack, it should be read by all individuals who wish to avoid them. Lastly, Chapter 8 covers the area of fluids and hydration, which should be a concern for all recreational athletes.

Finally, the editor would like to acknowledge the assistance of several key individuals. A thank you is due to Ira Wolinsky whose advice and persistence guided this book through to completion. Kevin Taylor, who helped with computer program conversions, and Shawn Simonson, who labored with the manuscript preparation, should also be acknowledged. Jim Pagliasotti was instrumental in rechecking the editing and found more spacing errors than I did. Finally, as many have done before me, I thank my family for being willing, albeit at times reluctantly, to do without my presence for long periods of time. Because of the help thus mentioned and the effort of the contributing authors of the book, enjoy!

Catherine G. Ratzin Jackson, Ph.D.
Editor

THE EDITOR

Catherine G. Ratzin Jackson, Ph.D., is Professor of Kinesiology in the School of Kinesiology and Physical Education, College of Health and Human Sciences at the University of Northern Colorado, Greeley, Colorado. She has held positions as Department Chair and Coordinator of Kinesiology Programs.

Dr. Jackson received undergraduate and Master's degrees in chemistry from Montclair State University, Upper Montclair, New Jersey. She completed her doctorate in exercise physiology at the University of Colorado, Boulder, which included work and a subsequent research associateship at the University of Colorado Health Sciences Center School of Medicine, Denver, Colorado. She has been at the University of Northern Colorado since 1985.

Dr. Jackson is a Fellow of the American College of Sports Medicine and is current President of the Rocky Mountain Chapter of the American College of Sports Medicine. She is also a member of the American Society for Gravitational and Space Biology and is current Executive Director of Western States Association of Faculty Governance. Past associations have included the American Heart Association and the U.S. Fencing Association. As an active competitor in the sport of fencing over a period of 18 years, which included being the State of Colorado Women's Champion two times in foil, she has a unique understanding of the nutritional needs of the recreational athlete.

Dr. Jackson has been awarded a NASA Joint Venture and spent two fellowships at Stanford University and NASA Ames Research Center, Moffett Field, California, where the hydration and nutritional needs of astronauts continues to be investigated. She has taught exercise nutrition and body composition classes at both the undergraduate and graduate level for many years. A sought-after speaker, she has made close to 100 professional juried and nonjuried presentations. She has published over 30 papers dealing with a variety of topics that fundamentally study the influence of exercise on the human body under the stress of environment or injury.

CONTRIBUTORS

Jennifer Anderson, Ph.D., R.D.
Department of Food Science and Human Nutrition, Colorado State University, Fort Collins, Colorado

Jacqueline R. Berning, Ph.D., R.D.
University of Colorado & The Olympic Training Center, Colorado Springs, Colorado

Sherrie L. Frye, Ph.D., R.D.
Department of Community Health and Nutrition, College of Health and Human Services, University of Northern Colorado, Greeley, Colorado

Robert J. Hanisch, M.A.
Diabetes Treatment Center, Columbia Hospital, Milwaukee, Wisconsin

Catherine G. Ratzin Jackson, Ph.D., F.A.C.S.M.
School of Kinesiology and Physical Education, University of Northern Colorado, Greeley, Colorado

Rosemary A. Ratzin, Ed.D.
Department of Health, Physical Education, and Recreation, Frostburg State University, Frostburg, Maryland

Jaime S. Ruud, M.S., R.D.
Sports Nutrition Consultant, Lincoln, Nebraska

Shawn Simonson, Ed.D.
School of Kinesiology and Physical Education, University of Northern Colorado, Greeley, Colorado

Ann C. Snyder, Ph.D., F.A.C.S.M.
Exercise Physiology Laboratory, Department of Human Kinetics, University of Wisconsin, Milwaukee, Wisconsin

Norbert R. Van Dinter, Ed.D., C.L.P.
Department of Human Services, College of Health and Human Services University of Northern Colorado, Greeley, Colorado

Ralph S. Welsh, B.S.
Exercise Physiology Laboratory, Department of Human Kinetics, University of Wisconsin, Milwaukee, Wisconsin

Ira Wolinsky, Ph.D.
Department of Human Development, University of Houston, Houston, Texas

CONTENTS

DEDICATION

With respect for the past, entirely through Ellis Island, this is dedicated to Grandmother Anna and my first-generation American parents, Mary and Theodozy, who all taught me high carbohydrate ethnic cooking. Their toast was always "Na zdróvja!" (To your health).

Chapter 1

INTRODUCTION COMPETITIVE VS. RECREATIONAL ATHLETES: AN AMERICAN RECREATIONAL AND CULTURAL PERSPECTIVE

N. R. Van Dinter

CONTENTS

0-8493-7914-8/95/$0.00+$.50

I. OVERVIEW OF SPORTS IN AMERICAN CULTURE

Since the conclusion of World War II, American culture has gone through a great many changes that have influenced and been influenced by the sport subculture. Some of these changes included the impact of the Cold War struggle between democracy and communism; a growing awareness of discrimination toward minorities, women, the aged, and handicapped; an electronic revolution that impacted every segment of society; and the burgeoning effect of sports on the American leisure culture.

A. COLD WAR

The evolution of the political struggle between democracy and communism, beginning with the Korean conflict in 1950 and continuing through the eventual collapse of the Soviet Union in 1990, caused a growing sense of anxiety among the American public. The battle for dominance between conflicting political philosophies, one that championed the individual vs. one that argued for the State, greatly affected the course of world events, including athletic competition.

At the height of the conflict, the boycotts of the 1980 Olympics by the U.S. and the 1984 Olympics by the Soviet Union highlighted the intrusion of politics into sports, which previously had witnessed the exclusion from the games for political reasons of South Africa in 1972 and nationalist China in 1976. Still, the voluntary withdrawal of world superpowers from successive games placed the Olympics in a precarious position and brought about significant changes in long-held concepts of Olympic competition, such as the recent entry of professional tennis and basketball athletes into the "amateur" games.

B. MINORITIES, WOMEN, DISABLED

In the affluent years following World War II, the plight of previously ignored and underserved segments of the American society, namely minorities, women, and the disabled, came to the public's attention. Slowly, but systematically, barriers to full participation in the American way of life were removed for these populations. As they moved into the social mainstream, certain role models emerged who fed the growing aspirations of these newly empowered groups.

Although every field of endeavor was represented, the greatest impact on society, at least in terms of recognition, arguably was made by sports. The happy marriage of a burgeoning mass media with the public's appetite for spectator sports created national attention for the sports heroes, and among them suddenly were African Americans, women, and even the disabled.

When Jackie Robinson broke the color barrier in major league baseball, the other professional leagues grudgingly followed suit. Soon, the media were filled with images of black Americans who excelled in their particular field of dreams, whether Jimmy Brown in football, Wilt Chamberlain in basketball, Arthur Ashe in tennis, or any of the hundreds who followed them. Not only were they becoming famous, they were becoming rich. Few Americans of any color could match the income of basketball's Michael Jordan, whose athletic salary was exceeded tenfold by his lucrative endorsement contracts. Who could have imagined some few years earlier that millions of young people would come to covet the chance to "be like Mike". Together with the desegregation of the nation's universities, the breaking of the color line in sports brought ever-increasing numbers of black Americans into high visibility positions, mirroring their less visible but equally impressive progress in other endeavors.

Similarly, the post-War era was a time of emancipation for women, who demanded and received greater access to roles other than those tradition had assigned them. They too profited from media exposure of their invasion into the sports world. Despite successes in politics, business, religion, and a host of other arenas, the watershed moment in the women's movement was a nationally televised and much ballyhooed tennis match between Billie Jean King and Bobby Riggs, which saw the woman beat the man in straight sets, forever changing the face of sports and answering emphatically the question of women's abilities to succeed in a "man's world". Although women's sports lag behind men's in attendance, they have made steady progress in attracting attention and respect. The success of the professional women's golf and tennis tours, in particular, is evidence of the narrowing gap between the genders as popular athletes.

The disabled population came to the fore, as well, when physical barriers to their unique needs were removed. Public awareness was heightened after the return of veterans from Vietnam, many of whom had, at a young age, suffered disabling injuries. Their courage in reordering their lives and seeking a full measure of access to the American lifestyle won the admiration of the public. The involvement of the Kennedy family in initiating the Special Olympics, and the participation of celebrities in publicizing them, created an empathetic understanding of the physically and mentally challenged citizens of our country. Role models such as major league pitcher Jim Abbott engendered a focus on the capabilities, rather than the limitations, of handicapped athletes. Legislation in the form of the Americans with Disabilities Act further removed limitations on their lifestyle, and the disabled continue to expand their participation in every facet of life, including recreational athletics.

C. BABY BOOMERS AND WELLNESS

Based on sheer numbers alone, the most notable population of the post-World War era, and one that includes all of the above-mentioned groups, is known as the Baby Boomers. So massive was the birth rate between 1946 and 1964 that American culture forever after was altered. The "pig in the python" of the country's demographic profile was born into relative affluence, with a surfeit of leisure time and discretionary income at its disposal. So numerous were this generation's choices that they came to see leisure as a birthright.[1] This attitude has had a profound impact on sport at every level, from the attendance at major sporting events to participation in recreational sports on a regular basis.

One of the offshoots of this demographic upheaval was the introduction of the concept of "wellness".[2] Wellness is the relationship of total lifestyle to one's physical, mental, and emotional development.[2] This concept has been one of the most important influences on sport and exercise during the past two decades, the time during which the "boomers" came into adulthood. Wellness includes the appropriate exercise, nutrition, labor, and rest so that the individual may derive the best experiences from and for life.[2] Appropriate exercise comes from any of the variety of sport in its broadest physical sense, as an individual participant or team member, amateur or professional. It serves several attributes of wellness, including stress reduction.

D. ELECTRONICS

Another profound impact on American society in the post-World War years was the mass availability of affordable electronic equipment, particularly televisions and computers. Television and its companion technologies, cable vision and video cassette recorders, have created a public interest in media that filled leisure hours with a vast and sometimes bountiful menu of news, entertainment, and sporting events. The ability to witness real time broadcasts of events from beyond one's immediate environment, the creation of the so-called "global village," has affected American culture in fundamental ways. The increased access to information and image greatly expanded the available role models of individual and social aspirations, providing a visually enhanced interpretation of the parameters of existence and endeavor. Television provided society a view of what in life was possible.

Although television is constantly accused of fostering and encouraging a variety of social ills because of its reliance on sensationalism, its pandering to the lowest common denominator of taste, and its engendering of passivity in its audience, it can also be stated that, in the world of sport particularly, television has elevated the public's standard of excellence. There is little question that without the dynamics of this medium we would not have seen the explosion of professional and major college sports, nor would but a few of us had the opportunity to witness the achievements of the world's best athletes engaged in their highest levels of competition. Not only has television created great wealth for the individuals and institutions that excelled at sport, it has illustrated an image of accomplishment that draws more participants with greater expectations into the arena.

The other electronic device that has strongly affected the role of sport within American society is the computer, which over the past four decades has continued to become smaller, cheaper, and more commonly available. Today there are computer programs that aid in the study of proper motion in various sport actions to assist the athlete in improving performance. The computer also has been very instrumental in the development of outstanding athletic facilities, the refinement of scheduling and implementing of events, and the research and development of better sports equipment such as clubs, bats, racquets, shoes, protective gear, and clothing, all of which has improved performance and increased participation in recreational athletics.

E. SPORTS: THE AMERICAN PHENOMENON

Concurrent with the aforementioned changes in American society, there has been a massive evolution in the sociophysical phenomenon of sport. Few segments of our culture have experienced greater growth or had more impact on the total culture than has sports. Its growth has profoundly influenced two elements of the public: the athlete and the spectator. Our best athletes have been deified, and the image of excellence they have impressed upon the American society has grown both the legion of avid spectators and the recreational participants who enthusiastically emerged in their wake.

II. COMPETITIVE ATHLETE

To properly address the topic of the athlete, one first must differentiate between two categories: the competitive and recreational athlete. The competitive athlete participates in one of two manners, professionally or on a college/university varsity or other type of formal, highly organized team. The difference between these athletes and the recreational athlete primarily is one of contractual obligation, a commitment to participate under certain predetermined conditions during a specified period of time for some form of remuneration, be it wages, scholarship, free products, or even a job in a sponsoring organization. The competitive athlete accepts a lifestyle that is rigorous, time-demanding, and energy consuming, one that is largely determined by a commitment to sport.

A. TEAM SPORTS

At the professional level, football, basketball, and baseball are regarded as home-grown sports and therefore are warmly embraced by the American public. Hockey, in the past two decades, has gained wider acceptance while soccer still lacks the status accorded it internationally.

Major league sports in America is big business, with many of the characteristics common to any other industry subset, including the adversarial relationship between workers and management. Players and owners negotiate contracts aided by a phalanx of agents, lawyers, and accountants. Professional athletes belong to players' associations, which are unions for the nation's highest paid laborers, representing their members in grievance proceedings, pension arrangements, and other such labor issues.

Nothing, however, has so impacted the fate of professional sports as has the thorough insinuation of television into the fabric of American life. Profitability of the clubs and salaries of the players has escalated in direct proportion to the growth of the television market, and the impact of product endorsements on the income of celebrated players is far greater in television than any other medium.

The downside to the average professional sports career is longevity, which is governed by a number of factors, including injury, skill deterioration, contract disputes, and the yearly infusion of fresh talent to the team. The National Football League Players' Association estimates the average span of professional sport participation to be 3.5 years.[3] There are some very notable exceptions to that average such as George Blanda, who retired from professional football at age 48; Nolan Ryan, who pitched in professional baseball until the age of 46; and Dave Winfield, who has passed the age of 42 and is still playing very well.[4] Minnie Minoso set the longevity record by playing professional baseball in 5 decades, finally retiring at the age of 53.[5]

B. INDIVIDUAL SPORT PROFESSIONALS

The professional who engages in individual, nonteam, sport faces different demands than those of the team athlete. The two major sports in this category are golf and tennis, which differ in play format but are similar in the year-round schedules of competition.

Tennis players tend to begin competing at an earlier age than golfers and play in seeded brackets, meaning that the lowest ranked meet the top ranked players in the early rounds. Because the novice players are unlikely to earn enough prize money to support their efforts, sponsors are needed to nurture their development and pay for the coaching, equipment, travel, and other needs of the touring professional.

Although some tennis players attend college while participating in the professional tour, there are numerous top-ten ranked players, both male and female, who have not completed high school before they win a major tournament. Gabriela Sabatini reached the semi-finals of the French Open at age 14, while Steffi Graf won the Gland Slam of tennis at age 18.[6] Michael Chang at age 15 was the youngest competitor to play center court at Wimbledon and, at age 17, the youngest to win the French Open.[7] Andre Agassi is now in his 20s and has yet to finish high school.[8] Tennis players peak in their late 20s to early 30s and have few opportunities to continue competing professionally due to the lack of a senior circuit.

The professional golfer competes in events that usually have second-day cuts which eliminate half the field. While they do not necessarily employ coaches, they do have travel, equipment, and other expenses that cause them to seek sponsorship. Golfers tend to have much longer careers than tennis players due to the less physically demanding nature of the sport and a thriving senior circuit that offers substantial prize money. However, in both sports, the prize money and endorsements, if wisely invested, offer the chance for comfortable retirement at relatively early ages.

C. WOMEN'S PROFESSIONAL SPORTS

Opportunities for women in professional sports continue to be limited in comparison to men, except for tennis and golf, where the evolution of professional associations, the emergence of superstars, and the securing of major commercial sponsorship during the past two decades has greatly enhanced the professions. Prize money in women's tennis has been the most improved due to the long term commitment of sponsor Virginia Slims and the growing popularity of the Grand Slam events, which include Wimbledon and the U.S., French, and Australian Opens. In fact, the U.S. and Australian Open tournaments pay women prize money equal to men, which in 1993 amounted to $535,000 for winners. These tournaments are longer than the average professional tennis event, extending over 2 weeks compared to the usual 5- or 6-day event.[9] Women's professional golf, on the other hand, has advanced greatly over the years, but still is far from parity with the men's tour.

Attempts to promote women's professional basketball have failed to attract public support and committed sponsorship. The key to the success of any major professional sport is directly dependent on national television coverage. Without it, public interest of sufficient scale cannot be generated, salaries are suppressed, and the cost of supporting a team cannot be maintained. Women basketball players have not been able to capture the level of public support necessary for television coverage. However, the commitment on the part of the female athlete in terms of time and effort is equally demanding to that of her male counterpart. And it is worth noting that the level of competition among women basketball players in collegiate and high school has improved dramatically over the past two decades, with corresponding increases in fan interest, indicating that the possibility for a successful professional league is growing.

D. COLLEGIATE SPORTS

College/university varsity sports comprise the other segment of competitive sports. The primary enticements, in addition to the chance for fame and a professional contract, are scholarships or tuition waivers, room, board, and expense money. The propriety and parameters of these enticements are constantly debated by the National Collegiate Athletic Association (NCAA), which regulates college sports. Recent demands by the NCAA that the athlete achieve and sustain an acceptable minimum grade point average in order to compete has made it more difficult for some athletes to gain entry to college and maintain their scholarships via eligibility once they are accepted. From a purely athletic perspective, however, the commitment of time and energy that the successful college athlete expends is obvious. Most sports demand year-round physical conditioning in order to participate, and the hectic schedule during the season of practice, travel, and playing extracts an extraordinary demand on the student-athlete.

E. MALE INTERCOLLEGIATE SPORTS

The two major college sports for men are football and basketball, which are funded by the media, particularly television, and support from alumni. The completely self-supported programs tend to be those of the NCAA Division I schools—the Big Ten, PAC Ten, Southwest, and Big Eight (now Big Twelve) conferences, among others. The Division II teams and other smaller sized schools tend to require other assistance and support, especially in football.

The major collegiate football and basketball programs serve the professional leagues as training programs that produce a steady crop of talented prospects at little or no cost to the big league clubs. The schools with consistently strong programs attract the best athletes, especially those with hopes of entering the professional athletic ranks.

Other collegiate sports are viewed as "minor" because of the absence of a direct relationship with professional franchises. Baseball, tennis, golf, wrestling, track, soccer, gymnastics, fencing, swimming, and the other "lesser" sports receive far less financial commitment from the schools in terms of scholarships for athletes, although certain colleges and universities have eliminated football in order to concentrate more resources on these sports.

F. FEMALE INTERCOLLEGIATE SPORTS

Women have made great strides toward parity with their male counterparts in intercollegiate sports since the passage by the federal government in 1972 of Title IX; however, there remains a large gap both in philosophical and financial commitment to equality of the genders.[10] Generally, colleges offer three major sports for women—volleyball, basketball, and softball. They receive adequate support from athletic departments and alumni, but of a sum that is vastly inferior to the major sports offered men. Because television revenues are virtually nil, the inequity is excused on the basis of the relative earning powers to the universities of men's and women's sports. Women also are provided opportunities to participate in minor sports such as tennis, golf, track and field, soccer, gymnastics, swimming, field hockey, and fencing.

III. RECREATIONAL ATHLETES

A. DEFINITION

The presently accepted definition of recreation was developed in the early 1970s by David Gray, who eliminated the concepts of "constructive" and "socially acceptable" after decades of very rigid terminology. Gray proposed that only two elements need be considered: is the experience enjoyable (fun), and did the person take part voluntarily?[11]

The traditional concept of an athlete implies involvement in competitive sports by one who likely possesses pertinent natural abilities. The current understanding of an athlete is of one who may train to compete in some form of competition, or exercise, or may use a competitive sport for recreation. An individual's participation in a given sport will be in direct relationship to an anticipated result. Therefore, the term "recreational athlete" must be studied in the context of "motivation". Why does that person train or condition in the sport?

B. MOTIVATION

Martindale and Kerr studied certain motivational aspects of sports among high level competitors and recreational athletes and logically found that the higher the level, the more competitive and committed the person is, and that the recreational athlete exhibited a lower level of competitive expectation.[12,13] Interestingly, Martindale found that the competitive athlete also possessed higher social goals than did the recreational athlete.

The question certainly must be asked—if one engages in a sport activity for something other than fun, why does he/she do it? Even though the individual may fully enjoy the experience, an additional four possible reasons may be considered.

Social contact, the desire to be around others of similar interest, is one of the primary reasons that people play a sport. The activity may well require more than one to play, i.e., team sports, and the one-on-one sports such as tennis, racquetball, boxing, and wrestling. Very few sports allow the player to participate alone—bowling, golf, and certain exercises.

Competition in and of itself is a major attraction to people who have learned or played in a competitive environment earlier in their lives. Even the very best professional athletes find satisfaction in recreational sports outside their particular profession. Michael Jordan and tennis pro Ivan Lendal, for instance, both love golf; the list of such examples is endless.[4] The thrill of winning and the personal satisfaction of achievement attracts people to sports.

The growing appreciation for wellness as an achievable state of being, which came into vogue during the 1980s and 90s, has had a tremendous influence on the increased participation in both competitive sports and the noncompetitive activities of aerobics, weight training, biking, running, and hiking. The relentless portrayal in the media of thin and active as the ideal, together with the recognition of many corporations that healthy employees are cost-effective, has increasingly made people more aware of the need for a commitment to a healthier lifestyle. Dramatic growth in the sales of exercise equipment during the past decade and the proliferation of fitness clubs throughout America illustrates the desire of the public to condition themselves for a better life and to associate with people of similar disposition.[1]

The fourth reason beyond enjoyment as a prime factor for participating in sport is occupational advancement. Some people use sport to enhance their employment or advancement opportunities, while others may feel compelled to play on the company sports team, join in company-sponsored recreational activities, or engage in their superior's favorite pastime, simply to show that they literally are "on the team". The above-cited motivations for team and individual sport and noncompetitive sport participation are illustrated in Tables 1 and 5 of Appendix A. Another measure of the motivation of the recreational athlete can be observed in the physical aspects of the various sports, which are illustrated in Tables 2 and 6 of Appendix A.

One aspect of motivation that has not been researched to any great extent is the "obsessive". Some people become so involved in a recreational experience that their lives are out of balance, businesses or jobs are lost, and family relationships are destroyed, due to an excessive investment of time and money in attempting to achieve some recreational goal. However, this phenomenon, which appears not only in sports but in all aspects of life, is outside the context of the treatment of this chapter.

C. OPPORTUNITIES TO PARTICIPATE

One of the likely reasons for the great increase in recreational athletics is the growth in opportunities for the average American to participate. Without digressing into the chicken-or-egg argument, it is notable that numerous agencies, foremost among them being municipal governments that are charged with enhancing the citizens' quality of life, find recreational activities to be enriching. There also is a leisure profession with accreditation and certification processes. The National Recreation and Park Association lists approximately 23,000 members and 12,000 practicing professionals.[14]

Public facilities often include multipurpose centers, indoor and outdoor swimming pools, athletic complexes with a variety of ball fields, golf courses, tennis courts, and parks that house a variety of recreational opportunities. Costs run from $3.5 million in cities of 10,000 population to some in larger cities that run to more than $10 million. User fees often are necessary to cover construction, maintenance, and staffing costs. Many cities also utilize local school facilities when not in use by the school district. Public facilities compete with the commercial/private sector sports facilities for members.[15]

Municipal facilities usually are designed for multipurpose use. Most neighborhood parks have a baseball/softball diamond, tennis courts, and basketball courts that are available free on a first-come basis, although popular centers sometimes have instituted a reservation system and/or a time limit system. They usually feature both spontaneous play and organized tournaments, and, in the case of the fields, are adapted for seasonal use by football and soccer players as well as baseball/softball.[16]

The commercial recreation industry has increased the availability of fitness, racquetball, tennis, and swimming facilities. There are both nationally franchised and locally owned clubs that depend solely on membership fees to cover construction costs, operation expense, and profit. Additional facilities are provided by the YMCAs, the military, industry, churches, and colleges. In total, they have greatly enhanced recreational opportunities for the American public.

Much of the increased demand for recreational facilities, as previously stated, has been fostered by the acceptance of wellness as a lifestyle. Fundamental to the concept is the individual's acceptance of responsibility for his/her own health and well-being, and the belief that maintaining health is preferable to restoring it; hence, there is a lowered reliance on the health care system. An opposing view cites athletic injuries as the downside, but studies support the contention that time and money invested in wellness via recreational activities results in a healthier, happier, and more productive populace.

D. PROGRAMS

The previously cited organizations provide recreational experiences in a variety of ways. The most typical are leagues and tournaments, which attract both team and individual sports participants.

The commitment to league play by members of a team means that the players will be available as often as several times a week throughout the season, depending on the level of competition. Some highly competitive teams practice several times per week and then play in tournaments on weekends, especially in softball. Adult softball is by far the most popular recreational team sport, with communities of 50,000 having as many as 200 teams each season at different levels of competition. Leagues usually are structured in round robin formats with teams playing one or two nights per week. Tournaments are of shorter duration, usually one weekend or throughout a week, than the season-long league schedule. Any sport that uses the league format for its schedule also can be played in tournament form. Tournaments usually are formatted with the opportunity to play more than one game, rather than single elimination, especially when contestants have had to travel to the site from another town.

Most recreational agencies also offer lessons, specialized facilities, and special events. Recently, the state-wide senior citizen games developed into a national extravaganza, growing from 2500 athletes at the national games in St. Louis in 1987 to 7100 participants in the U.S. National Senior Sports Classic at Baton Rouge in 1993.[17]

E. TYPES OF COMPETITION

Various sports, by the nature of the time commitment, talent, and age appropriateness they require, have developed levels of competition that the participant can select. Many states have developed recreational athletic organizations to program and promote recreational sport on a state level. For many years, the Texas Amateur Athletic Federation and, since 1970, the Colorado Association of Recreational Athletics have offered adult team competition at the state level to provide the recreational athlete an additional level of competition beyond the local community level. Local teams must qualify to move up to the state level. Additionally, some sports such as track, swimming, and tennis include a masters category for athletes who wish to compete in middle and senior age groups.

For various reasons, some recreational athletes are unsatisfied by play that is limited to the local level and desire more intense competition at state and national levels. Organizations such as the Amateur Softball Association and the United States Slo-Pitch Softball Association have developed classification systems for abilities and upper-level tournaments for those athletes who desire that outlet for their talents.

These types of organizations have developed their own systems of competitive classification to better serve their members. The three classes are "competitive", whose players are at the highest skill and commitment level of recreational athletics; "recreation", who are similar to "competitive" except that they do not travel to compete; and "leisure", who often participate only once a week, often for purely social reasons. Golf and bowling also have traditionally used a handicap system to equalize competition in the sport.

Adults usually play team sports with little or no instruction, but may practice and play under the supervision of a coach or manager. Basketball, volleyball, and softball are the three major adult sports and Tables 3 and 7 of Appendix A show the relationship between adult participation and the manner in which the sports usually are played.

Age is a factor in the type of recreational sport chosen by the participant. Although there are senior leagues for most team sports, the average senior citizen prefers individual to team sports. Tables 4 and 8 of Appendix A illustrate age group participation in individual and team sports.

Age groupings tend to follow those in the individual and dual player sports. Seniors tend to participate less in activities with extreme physical requirements. The four most used sports are running, biking, aerobics, and exercise machines. It is interesting that the first two are nonprogram/facility activities, while aerobics and exercise machines most often are organization/facility offerings that can involve substantial expense.

F. MANUFACTURING AND MEDICINE

The impact of the recreational athlete on the sports equipment industry has been profound, particularly in the past 25 years. In recognition of a high-growth market, manufacturers constantly improve athletic equipment and accessories, employing the latest technologies and styles to stimulate sales. Golf clubs that once were made of wood now are fashioned from steel or graphite, tennis racquets from composites, softball bats from aluminum, and bicycles from metals and fabrics unknown two decades ago. Uniforms have incorporated changes that enhance safety, but the primary driver of change is style. Moreover, apparel has been created for new sports, such as aerobics and racquetball, and existing clothing lines have changed in response to the growing demands of recreational athletes for higher performance and higher style wares.[18] Athletic shoes, once exemplified by the canvas "tennis" shoe, is now an industry of explosive growth, having become a mandatory fashion accessory even for the nonathlete.

The field of sports medicine, which in the past was fairly restricted to professional and varsity use, has begun to recognize the need for a number of recreational sport applications both in the treatment of injuries and in the research aspects of the conditioning process. Recreational athletes who take their physical leisure interests very seriously are unwilling to suspend or end their enjoyment because of an injury; so, they seek medical treatment to prolong their "careers" and accurate information for training and nutrition. Many company insurance policies now allow for treatment of sports related injuries, making it easier for the recreational athlete to continue to exercise.

G. CHANGES TOWARD LESS COMPETITIVE ACTIVITIES

Profound changes have taken place in the athletic world since the end of World War II, and particularly in the past two or three decades. Sports that always had been the domain of only the better players trended toward the democratic. More people wanted access to athletics, and various organizations and systems emerged to meet their needs.

The first, and possibly the most dramatic, was the creation of Slo-Pitch Softball in the 1960s. As it began throughout the country, recreation professionals and players alike greeted it with skepticism. However, its popularity quickly grew and it is now firmly in place in communities of every size and place. The leagues include three to five levels of competition for men, women, and co-ed teams. National organizations have been created to promote and present tournaments, for which the right to participate is fiercely contested. The popularity of Slo-Pitch Softball lies in the all-inclusiveness of the game, which greatly enhanced the involvement of players of every ability by making the ball easier to hit.

Other sports that have undergone alterations toward less competition and greater availability to the masses are 2-on-2 volleyball, played primarily on sand, and 3-on-3 basketball. The changes in volleyball have been made for the young adult while the changes in basketball have been utilized even in the National Senior Sports Classic. An offshoot of volleyball was created by using racquetball courts to work a variation on the theme, partly in response to the availability of courts freed up by a leveling off of the racquetball craze. In each case, the environment was altered to meet and respond to increased demand for sports.

In the mid-1970s the fun run developed as an enhancement of the running/fitness phenomenon. Using the 5 or 10 kilometer measurement, it became very popular and was immediately adapted for a variety of fund-raising purposes. Although awards often were made to certain winners, every runner received a t-shirt or some such logo-bearing symbol of participation, which served to strengthen interest.

The running craze developed into major events such as full marathons, which were altered in some areas to accommodate the more casual recreational runner.

These new forms included half-marathons and, eventually, mini-triathlons of biking, running, and swimming. The Volkssport of Europe added walking. Volkswalks of 6 to 12 miles allow walkers to enter at any stage of the event.[19] The event usually takes place in a scenic area and the goals involve exercise and aesthetic appreciation. International organizations promote international participation and some walkers keep a certified book on the events they have entered. Biking, swimming, and skiing also are included in the international offering.

Two major changes have occurred in the area of exercise. While free weight systems still are very popular with those who wish to develop certain muscle characteristics, the growing market is in exercise machines—bikes, rowing machines, treadmills, cross-country skiing machines, and stairmasters. Commercial clubs and community centers include a variety of these devices to accommodate their clients. Clubs also employ exercise trainers to assist in the proper use of the equipment and to guide the user toward a particular fitness goal. There are more than a dozen major equipment companies that produce the popular exercise machines. In a busy world where time is increasingly precious, some clubs have installed televisions so the exercisers can watch their favorite "soaps" or athletic events while simultaneously improving their physical condition.

The evolution of aerobics probably has been the most notable change in the way Americans engage in sports. Aerobics officially began in 1968,[20] and by 1986 the word was included in dictionaries. Clubs and recreation centers, as well as the physical education departments of colleges and high schools, have taken advantage of the demand by offering a wide variety of instructors and types of exercises. Although these activities can be done at home, there is in aerobics, like exercise machines and most other forms of exercise, a highly social involvement that is intrinsic in its rise to popularity. Clubs and centers have specific aerobics rooms featuring special floors, mirrored walls, colors, and sound systems, which apparently provide crucial stimulation. Colorful clothing has been an important attraction to this activity because it adds an element of personal expression for the individual within the group.

The latest addition to the exercise is step aerobics, in which the exerciser steps up and down during the session. All aerobic activity is based on increasing the heart rate to a recommended level and sustaining it for a specific period in order to improve the cardiovascular system of the individual. Exercise physiologists have been hard at work supplying this new industry with healthful information to assist in the overall process. Adding to the craze are the numerous celebrities who have produced video cassettes for home use. Some are very helpful, while others have been questioned by critics who doubt their actual benefit or even suspect the possibility of real harm that may result from poorly researched techniques.

A number of new games also have been created in the past few decades. Racquetball is less than 30 years old, evolving from and largely replacing handball, and few are the clubs built in the past 10 or 15 years that do not include at least a couple of racquetball courts. Frisbee has impacted recreation nearly as much as aerobics and Slo-Pitch Softball. The variety of uses for the disc, ranging from simple games of catch and throw to Frisbee golf, soccer, and other social activities, include even the exercising of dogs. The Hacky Sack, skateboards, and roller blades are other new and exciting forms of exercise and opportunities for competition.

The growing popularity of cross-country skiing has impacted the ski industry. Although downhill, or alpine, skiing still is more popular and certainly more profitable to the ski companies, cross-country, or Nordic, skiing in its many variations is far less dangerous and considerably less expensive.

Finally, another alteration in the world of sport is the leisure swimming pool. The time when pools were primarily constructed for competitive swim meets has given way to the European influence on swim facility design. Pools now are constructed with an "O" base for entry, which better serves the very young, the very old, and other less physically adept users. Pools have ladders, ropes, even fountains and other scenic devices. Elaborating on the diving board, a less demanding and more exhilarating form of entering pools is via a slide. Major water parks have successfully enticed the public with lengthy, elaborately twisting chutes and slides, as well as wave machines and other "non-swimming" attractions. Many newly constructed indoor facilities have replaced diving boards with slides.

The factors of competition and occupation associated with recreational athletics, while still important, are dramatically less pervasive in the matrix of American sport culture. Instruction, wellness, fun, and social contact increasingly are major motivations to participation. The physical demands of noncompetitive and less competitive sports are oriented toward strength and endurance, with less dependence on speed and agility. Those changes place different demands as well on the requirements for conditioning and nutrition. Tables 2 and 6 of Appendix A provide further illustration.

IV. WHAT IS A RECREATIONAL ATHLETE?

The construct of what constitutes today's recreational athlete is very complex and involves many variables. Nearly every American could in some sense be considered a recreational athlete, since nearly everyone engages in some form of physical activity for enjoyment, but that may paint too general of a picture. From the person who plays golf a few times each summer to the person who plays in two leagues per season so that he/she is engaged every day of the week, the recreational athlete covers a broad spectrum of participation. Simply defined, the athlete must freely choose to participate on a regular basis for the purpose of fun. If other elements intervene, such as employment or financial compensation, the true recreational experience is diluted.

The term "athlete" is much more diverse in this setting. It does not exclude the individual who bowls a few lines with friends on the occasional Friday night in favor of the enthusiast who belongs to two leagues, practices twice a week, and bowls in two tournaments a month. Commitment to regular participation is required, but the degree of commitment varies widely. The recreational athlete must be distinguished from the person who partakes of an activity randomly and then only because a spouse or friend would like to fill some spare time. In other words, one chooses to participate on a regular basis for a certain purpose rather than engaging in the activity only for want of something better to do.

Each of the sports in our culture has its ardent player who is fully involved in every aspect of the endeavor, playing it regularly and intensely, watching the professionals, studying it, always seeking an edge to his/her game. And each of these sports rewards certain types of physical abilities over the efforts of the less able. But the serious student recognizes that talent alone cannot ensure victory. It demands practice, stamina, proper exercise and diet, and psychological preparation, as well. And, to a greater or lesser degree, the recreational athlete draws on these elements of success to find his/her personal level of enjoyment in the activity.

While all sports require a high degree of concentration to succeed, different sports demand different levels of physical activity. Some are nearly constant in their physical output, while others are comprised of short bursts of activity between periods of relative inactivity. Basketball involves far more constant action than does softball. Bowling and golf are similar in their regular intervals of inaction, whereas tennis and racquetball share a much higher degree of constant action. These activities can be placed on an energy continuum with relative physiological and nutritional demands. Although team sports may allow substitutions and other periods of rest, the continuous-action team sports such as basketball and soccer require more endurance and short bursts of high energy delivery, and therefore a different training and diet regimen, than does volleyball, softball, or the other increments on the action scale.

Similarly, individual sports such as tennis, boxing, golf, and bowling have different requirements for strength and endurance capacity. The first two involve the most constant body movement while the latter two are less demanding. Swinging a golf club 80 or 90 times over a 4-h period is not very demanding on the cardiovascular system, but it will increase the need for strong tendons and bones. The so-called noncompetitive sports, or those perhaps more accurately described as competing solely with oneself, also have a wide variety of physical needs. Biking, swimming, walking, running, cross-country skiing, and aerobics have constant energy demands and, depending on the length of involvement and the terrain, the relevant endurance capacity definitely is a consideration.

Recreational sport instructors tend to be more concerned with the technique or skills training than the overall physical condition of the athlete in relation to the sport. The former is more oriented to tradition whereas the latter is subject to ongoing revelations of scientific inquiry. Comparing the physical needs of the competitive athlete with those of the recreational athlete is difficult. The recreational athlete, unlike his compensated counterpart, is usually not required by a coach or manager to devote his/her time and energy exclusively to a sport. It is a question, then, of defining the level of commitment to the endeavor if one is to define a recreational athlete. Only then can we assess the athlete's needs.

How motivated is the athlete? To what extent is the recreational athlete willing to commit? Motivation and commitment define the athlete's needs. If the athlete engages in a sport for the fun of it and worries about no other outcome but enjoyment, the physical demand is far less than the need of the athlete whose physical and psychological condition must be optimum to obtain results that will satisfy personal goals. To succeed, even if the goal merely is enjoyment, it is important that the recreational athlete no less than the competitive athlete understands the physiological demands of the sport and the nutritional demands required to meet them. It is the intent of the specific chapters of this book to fill this need.

V. ACKNOWLEDGMENT

Thanks to James Pagliasotti, B.A., for editing of this chapter

REFERENCES

1. **O'Sullivan, E.,** Baby boomers—the new marketing challenge, *Parks Recreation,* February, 38, 1988.
2. **Kraus, R. and Curtis, J.,** *Creative Management in Recreation,* 3rd ed., C.V. Mosby, St. Louis, 1982, 190.
3. National Football League Player's Association, personal communication, September 8, 1993.
4. *Great Athletes of the Twentieth Century,* Salem Press, Pasadena, CA, 1992, 2, 247; 10, 2193; 15, 1440; 20, 2786.
5. **Porter, D. L., Ed.,** *Biographical Dictionary of American Sport, 1989–92 Supplement,* Greenwood Press, New York, 1992, 140.
6. **Newman, B.,** Talk about net gains, *Sports Illustrated,* 68 (18) 52, May 2, 1988.
7. **Lidz, F.,** Tennis is chemistry, *Sports Illustrated,* 69 (17), 62, October 17, 1988.
8. **Kirkpatrick, C.,** Born to serve, *Sports Illustrated,* 70 (11), 66, 1989.
9. **Evert, C.,** It's a whole new game, *USA Weekly, The Denver Post,* August 27–29, 5, 1993.
10. "After Grove City," *Athletic Business,* p. 10, May 1985.
11. **Gray, D.,** Exploring inner space, *Parks Recreation,* p. 19, December 1972.
12. **Martindale, E., Sloan, A., and Vise, S.,** Participation in college sports: motivational differences, *Perceptual Motor Skills,* 71, 1139, 1990.
13. **Kerr, J.,** Differences in the motivational characteristics of 'Professional,' 'Serious Amateur,' and 'Recreational' sports performers, *Perceptual Motor Skills,* 64, 379, 1987.
14. Mid Year Report, *Natl. Recreation Park Assoc.,* Arlington, VA, 1993.
15. Colorado Senate Bill 76, State of Colorado Legislature, April 18, 1989.
16. **Van Dinter, N. R., Ed.,** *Recreation Facilities Design and Management School Handbook* (unpublished), Colorado Park and Recreation Association, Wheat Ridge, CO, 1993.
17. **Cordman, D. G.,** President's corner, *United States National Senior Olympics Newsletter,* Chesterfield, MO, p. 2, Summer 1993.
18. Fascinating facts, *University of California, Berkeley Wellness Letter,* June 1989, July 1989, March 1990.
19. **Landes, C.,** Volkssporting—the sport for everyone, *Parks Recreation,* p. 38, August 1989.
20. **Fishwick, L. and Hays, D.,** Sport for whom? — Differential participation patterns of recreational athletes in leisure-time physical activities, *Sociol Sport J.,* 6, 269, 1989.

Chapter 2

THE RELATIONSHIPS BETWEEN HUMAN ENERGY TRANSFER AND NUTRITION

Catherine G. Ratzin Jackson
Shawn Simonson

CONTENTS

0-8493-7914-8/95/$0.00+$.50

I. INTRODUCTION

A. EARLY VIEWS OF HUMAN NUTRITION

The concept that diet can impart specific qualities to the human is not new. There is a reference in the Old Testament in the Book of Daniel to what may be called one of the first observations relating nutrition to performance.[1] As the tale goes, the chief of eunuchs who supervised the training of youths in the Court was requested by Daniel to be excused from wine and the King's delicacies. This diet,which was high in fat and protein and which was also dehydrating due to the alcohol, had been prescribed by the King for the past 3 years. Daniel and 3 of his friends wished to consume only "pulses" (vegetables) and water for 10 days. It was noted that they improved in appearance and performance at the end of this time. We now know that they consumed a high complex carbohydrate diet that significantly enhanced their glycogen stores and provided important vitamins and minerals missing in the previous dietary practice. They probably lost some body fat and improved endurance performance. The water would have hydrated them. However, it took science several thousand years and the introduction of elaborate techniques of sampling muscle to understand what had happened.

There abounds much mythology which associates food with performance and many concepts are steeped in myth and magic. From the offerings of food to vengeful ancestors to the acquisition of characteristics of animals whose flesh was consumed, we have long traditions suggesting that protein contributes greatly to energy production which to this day is difficult to dispel. If it is considered that it has only been for approximately 30 years that we have studied protein as a source of energy to the cell and that its contribution to exercise is still not clearly understood,[2] we can see why this particular myth is still promulgated today. The scientific study of nutrition related to human performance has evolved in relatively recent times.

B. NUTRITION AND PERFORMANCE INVESTIGATION

The science of nutrition has not necessarily been considered a major area for investigation unless it has been of necessity and was often related to military pursuits. In World War II, German scientists were compelled to investigate the number of calories needed for survival of people working in industry for food rationing, and thus was developed a portable apparatus (spirometer) to measure oxygen consumption and energy expenditure.[3] Not only was this a convenient method to use, it has prevailed to this day and is now used extensively for athletic performance investigations rather than survival studies. The protocols for assessing aerobic power and caloric expenditure, the most widely used technique to measure aerobic fitness today, were developed by Bruno Balke when he needed to find a method to measure the progress made by German pilots who trained at altitude in order to fly.[4] Pressurized cabins were not yet a reality. The assessment of body composition did not matter much until nitrogen narcosis became a problem with divers in World War II and was thought to be worse in those with higher percentage of body fat.[5] This has developed into an area which is extensively investigated today for human performance and nutrition, not military, purposes. The fundamental work in human hydration was done so that soldiers could march for long periods of time in full gear.[6] Today these principles are applied to rehydration drinks used by almost everyone who exercises and now includes special formulations for astronauts in microgravity.[7] Much of the work on vitamins was originally done to investigate disease states induced by deprivation of these nutrients under extreme circumstances as found in war time food rationing.[8] This information is now extrapolated to human nutrition at all levels.

When the eras of investigation into human nutrition are viewed, it becomes apparent that the science is relatively new. The real beginning was the measurement of heat by Lavosier in 1750 and measurement of calories and nitrogen balance which followed in the 19th century. From 1900 until 1940 the trace elements, vitamins, and amino acids were initially identified. The disease links to nutrition occurred after 1945, World War II having influenced this endeavor. The first studies linking human performance, not disease, to nutrition began in the 1950s. However, many of the old myths are periodically repackaged for the contemporary consumer.

II. HUMAN ENERGY TRANSFER

A. ENERGY CYCLE

The human organism produces energy in a way which is similar to most animals on the planet. Carbon dioxide, a by-product of animal energy production, is cycled through the plant kingdom while oxygen, a by-product of plant energy metabolism, is cycled through the animal kingdom; both processes use the by-products of the other to generate energy. While the global scope of interaction is of interest to some, the particular way the human transitions through the different pathways which phosphorylate (add phosphate groups to) adenosine diphosphate (ADP) to form adenosine triphosphate (ATP), the universal carrier of energy, is the object of much study with many questions remaining to be answered. The general principles have been meticulously elucidated in the past,[9] but there emerges the concept of a specificity of diet related to performance just as there has emerged the concept of specificity of exercise related to performance.

B. ATP

Many excellent book chapters have been written outlining human energy metabolism;[10-13] therefore, only the salient points will be reviewed. Ultimately all of the substrates for utilization which are consumed (fats, carbohydrates, protein) are potentially useful in producing the ATP molecule. ATP is the only energy carrier molecule that can directly supply the potential energy to the cellular

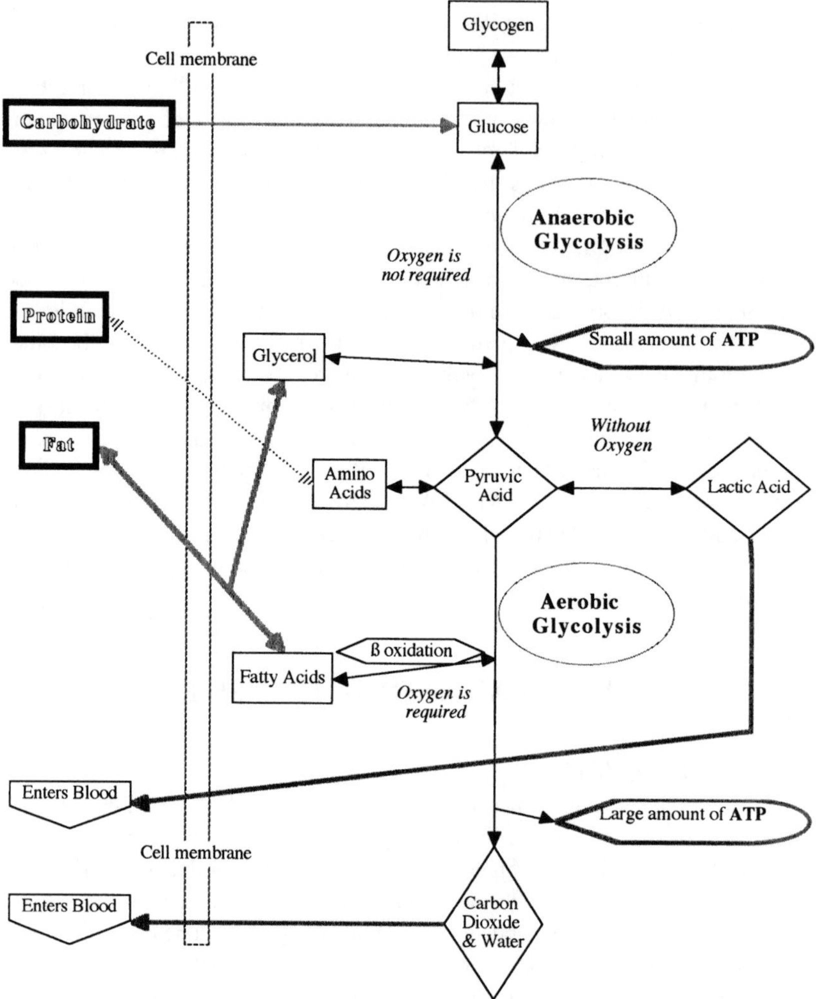

Figure 1. Interaction of substrates to produce energy.

machinery necessary for all functions. All other energy reservoirs must first transfer their energy to ATP before use by the cell. This transfer of energy is often the limiting factor in physical activity.

As the ATP molecule releases its phosphate groups, energy is released to perform biological work. In terms of physical performance, it is the work of mechanical contraction of the muscles which is of greatest interest. The phosphate groups liberated from ATP to produce energy must be replaced to allow continuous energy transfer. The process where a phosphate is attached to ADP to form ATP is of greatest importance in understanding human energy metabolism. Figure 1 illustrates the concepts which will be discussed in the subsequent sections on energy transfer.

C. PHOSPHAGEN SYSTEM

The phosphagen system is named for the two high energy phosphate compounds, ATP and creatine phosphate (CP), which couple energy transfer reactions. At rest the body is in primarily aerobic metabolism since all of the needs of the cell for oxygen can be met by blood flow related to functioning of the cardiovascular system. During this time the phosphagen system functions, but it is not overly stressed. When an activity is begun, however, this balance cannot be maintained and the phosphagen system is immediately used to a very high degree or intensity.

During exercise or activity of any type, the immediate source of ATP is that which is already stored and is coupled for acquisition of the phosphate group with CP. This particular system can provide energy only for brief periods of intense activity such as golf or tennis swings, sprints, or jumps. Under these circumstances the phosphate groups needed to replenish the ADP are easily supplied in the exercise recovery period. Creatine phosphate is the immediate source of the phosphates and energy used to restore ADP to ATP. All humans seem to possess approximately the same ratio of CP to ATP, which is 5 to 1, respectively, and is related to muscle mass. While highly intense activity such as sprinting can deplete phosphate groups within 10 seconds, a lower intensity activity can allow one to remain at this stage for a longer time. The ATP is located in specific places in muscle and tends to increase proportionately when the amount of muscle is increased. Thus, there is little that can be done to effectively enhance access to this system nor are there many nutritional practices which will allow these reactions to occur more rapidly.

D. LACTIC ACID SYSTEM

If exercise continues in duration beyond the capability of the phosphagen system to supply the ATP needed, either glucose or glycogen (which degrades to glucose) are mobilized for phosphate replacement, and thus, energy production. When this occurs lactic acid is formed. The lactic acid system, the second system activated to supply ATP, is named after one of the by-products which is always formed to some degree, but the title is somewhat misleading. Lactic acid is always formed in the cell to a certain degree and this is considered normal at rest. When activity ensues, there are times when the amount of lactic acid (lactate) in the system is rapidly cleared and thus the levels of this substance are minimal. At other times, particularly if one does not proceed to the aerobic system, the lactic acid accumulation will be high enough to terminate activity. The lactic acid system tends to predominate in activities lasting from 1 to 3 min.

The first stages of glucose degradation are always anaerobic (without oxygen) and this is named anaerobic glycolysis. Anaerobic glycolysis progresses to the formation of energy-rich pyruvic acid. If oxygen delivery cannot be or is not increased sufficiently, the process remains anaerobic, and pyruvic acid is converted to lactic acid. If this conversion of pyruvic acid to lactic acid occurs, anaerobic glycolysis results in very little energy transfer to produce ATP because the majority of the potential energy is left in the lactic acid. Lactic acid is thought to quickly cross the cell membrane into the blood where it can be initially cleared or taken out of the blood. Much of this lactic acid is used by other cells in the body to form ATP. However, the rate of clearance can be exceeded by the rate of production with the result that high levels of blood lactate accumulate. Under these circumstances exercise cannot continue for long periods because muscular contraction will soon be hindered.

Fueling this system is the exclusive use of either glycogen stored in muscle or glucose brought into the cell and the subsequent degradation of glucose for energy. It is known that carbohydrate stores in muscle (glycogen) can be enhanced by dietary practices that favor a high carbohydrate diet (carbohydrate loading)which will in turn affect the length of performance.[14] However, not all activities benefit from this practice. The greatest benefit is derived when the activity is categorized as aerobic.

In activities where one remains in anaerobic glycolysis, glycogen is not completely degraded aerobically to water and results in the accumulation of precursors that can reassemble back to glycogen. This eliminates the need for much additional carbohydrate in the diet after activities of this type.[15] This would include bodybuilding, weightlifting, and resistance exercises. A more fundamental concern in activities of this type would be that glycogen or carbohydrate loading would make the muscle feel tight and it will be more prone to injury since glycogen is stored with water, which is not compressible.

E. AEROBIC (OXYGEN) SYSTEM

If oxygen delivery can be increased, then glycolysis proceeds to the aerobic system and results in much more ATP production. The pyruvic acid formed during anaerobic glycolysis is then further degraded to water and carbon dioxide when oxygen delivery increases, rather than converting to lactic acid and being exported from the cell. This produces approximately 18 times more ATP than would have been produced through anaerobic glycolysis. Additionally, the aerobic process will more efficiently clear the lactic acid previously produced and concurrently formed.

At the end of aerobic glycolysis, the glycogen or glucose is degraded to water and is thus not recoverable as glucose within the cell. Few precursors remain and glycogen cannot be reformed except through intake of carbohydrate (glucose) in the diet. This would be the case with rhythmic aerobics, running, and other endurance exercises. Carbohydrate or glycogen loading may be considered by recreational athletes in these activities, but a better practice would be to convert the diet permanently to higher carbohydrate intake. Thus, a specificity of diet with respect to carbohydrate intake is suggested, based upon the metabolic pathway stressed in the activity. This is an important concept for recreational athletes to understand if they are to use nutrition effectively to enhance the enjoyment of their activity.

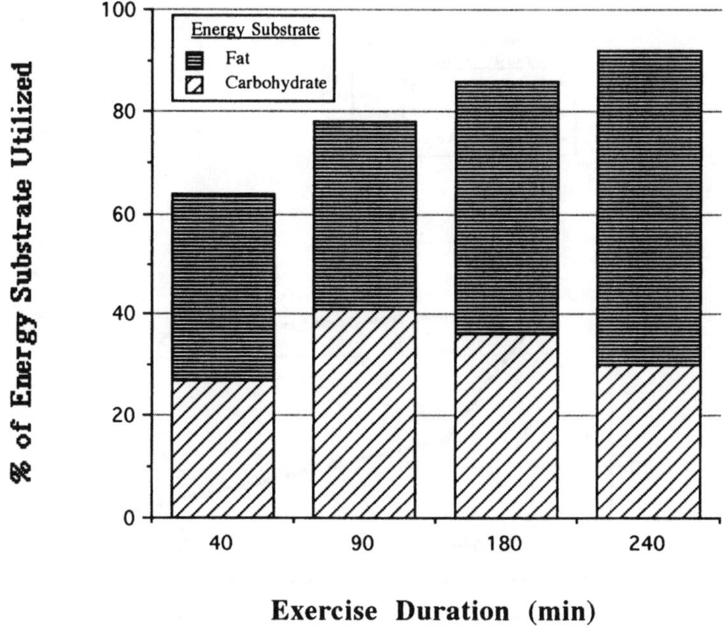

Figure 2. Interaction of carbohydrate and fat utilization during long duration exercise.[11]

If the exercise duration allows the aerobic system to predominate, ATP is formed in great quantities. This system does not rely heavily on carbohydrate, although it is still used and cannot function without it, but can now use fats (fatty acids) and protein (amino acids) for ATP production. By far the greatest amount of ATP can be produced from the degradation of fat (Figure 2). The difficulty usually encountered is that the aerobic system must first be overloaded and then stressed for long periods of time to produce the enzyme levels necessary to use this system to a high degree at the cellular level.

The aerobic system requires that oxygen be delivered in greater quantities than were previously necessary, which takes a complex series of reactions in the body to match cardiac output and capillary blood flow to the needs of the cell. In terms of cellular metabolism, the aerobic system is slow to become initiated and predominate during activity, and is probably not used to a great degree until at least 5 min of continuous activity have elapsed. While the general principles of these energy transitions have been known for some time, they are still not completely understood and it takes many years of painstaking research to clearly understand even simple relationships in a single activity. Commonly misunderstood is the fact that energy production is not a question of the three systems taking turns. Rather it is a fact that all systems function at all times and while one predominates, the others begin to function in greater degrees in order to be ready when needed. Figure 3 illustrates the interaction of the 3 systems of energy delivery in the first 2 min of exercise. Figure 4 shows the systems as they are

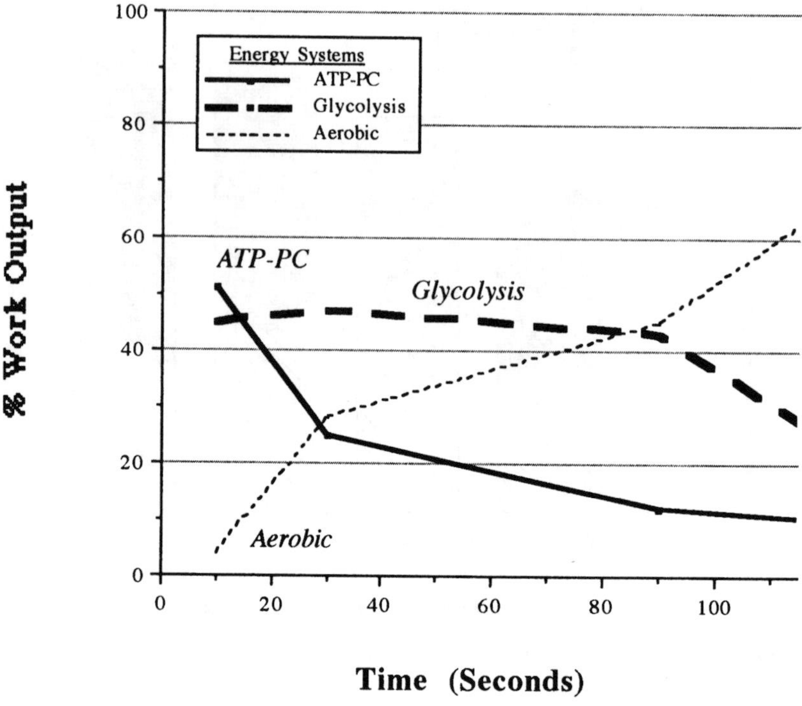

Figure 3. Interaction of energy systems in short duration, high intensity work.[11]

related in long term activity. Thus, it is important for recreational athletes to understand which energy system predominates in their activity and to follow the specific dietary practices which enhance performance.

F. SUBSTRATES FOR ENERGY PRODUCTION: PROTEIN, CARBOHYDRATE, FAT

The three dietary sources of energy are protein, carbohydrate, and fat. At rest and during normal daily activities, fats are the primary energy source, providing 80 to 90% of the energy.[11] Carbohydrates and protein provide 5 to 18% and 2 to 5%, respectively.[11] During exercise these proportions change.

Highly intense anaerobic activities that stress the phosphagen system do not directly use any of the three substrates during the activity. However, post-activity, this system can be restored using the glucose stored as glycogen in the muscle cells. Anaerobic glycolysis does degrade muscle glycogen; however, in this case it is used to generate additional ATP to sustain the intense anaerobic activities. Post-exercise, the muscle glycogen must be restored, much of it from glycogen precursors.

Whenever glycogen is degraded to water it must be replaced through the diet. All ingested carbohydrates degrade in the digestive system to glucose, galactose

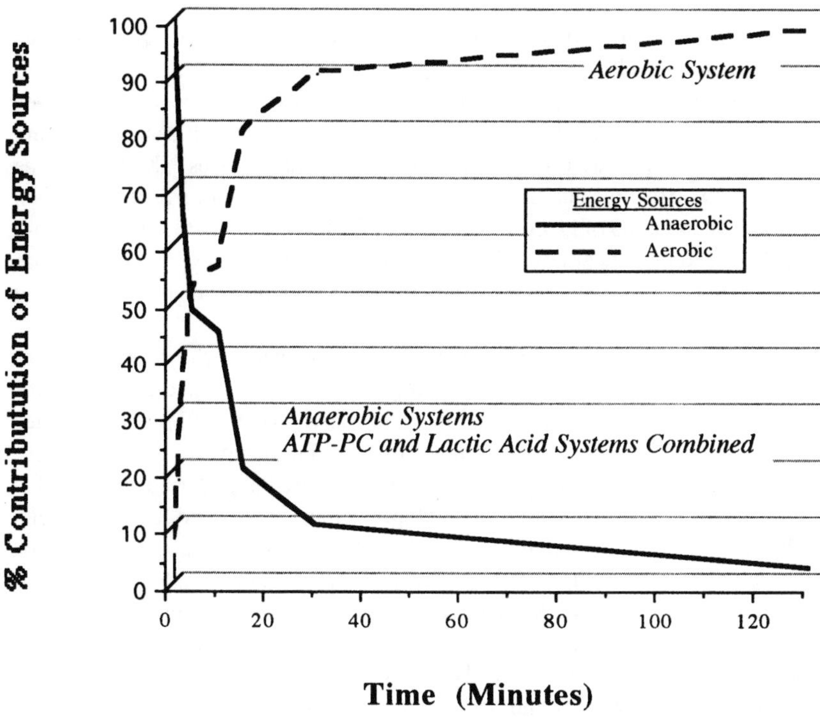

Figure 4. Primary energy sources for long duration activity.[10]

(milk sugar), and fructose (fruit sugar), with glucose being predominant. The majority of galactose and fructose are converted to glucose in the cells lining the small intestine and most of the remainder is converted in the liver. Glucose is absorbed into the blood and transported to the body tissues for use or storage in the liver and muscles as glycogen.[16] Glycogen is composed of hundreds of glucose molecules which are linked together within the cells. Therefore, glucose must be brought into the cell and then strung together as glycogen. The process of storage or replacement of glycogen is not rapid, however, and could take up to 2 days to complete.[17]

The situation may arise where there is insufficient carbohydrate to provide glucose to regenerate muscle glycogen. If glucose supplies are low, the muscle glycogen will not be restored.[18] The available glucose in the blood will be spared for use by the brain and the muscle will be left wanting for a carbohydrate energy supply. If glucose levels fall below the levels necessary for proper brain function, other sources of glucose exist. Protein in the body can be degraded to its amino acid building blocks which can then be converted to pyruvic acid in the liver.[11] Two pyruvic acids can be combined to form one glucose molecule which enters the blood. The primary source of protein for this process is the breakdown of muscle tissue; thus, glucose may be generated at the expense of protein. This reaction also occurs when the body is in starvation or when the individual consumes low levels of calories.

Fats, composed of glycerol and three fatty acids, can also be used to provide glucose. The glycerol can be converted to glucose; the fatty acids cannot. The fatty acids must either be used aerobically or they become ketones.[16] Ketones in the blood are toxic in large quantities and are undesirable. Therefore, depending upon fat for the generation of glucose is not desirable. It is clear that the alternative use of protein and fat rather than carbohydrate for glucose or glycogen restoration has negative implications. An adequate amount of carbohydrate needs to be ingested for successful participation in any activity.

When aerobic glycolysis becomes the principle pathway of energy production, the situation changes. Muscle glycogen is the initial source of glucose for aerobic energy; however, the duration of the activity often outlasts the supplies stored within the muscle cell and other substrates, fats and protein, must be used.

During lower intensity aerobic activities, fats are the preferred substrate for utilization (Figure 5). Fats are stored within the muscle cells and fat storage cells (adipocytes); they also circulate in the blood. Blood-borne fat is available for muscle use as fatty acids and fat is easily liberated from the adipocytes to the circulation for muscle use. As mentioned earlier, fats can be degraded to glycerol and three fatty acids. The glycerol can enter the glycolysis pathway in the anaerobic portion and eventually becomes pyruvic acid to be used in aerobic glycolysis. The fatty acids undergo a process called β oxidation which converts them to a compound that can be used in aerobic glycolysis to produce energy. The use of fatty acids in aerobic metabolism results in far greater ATP production than the use of carbohydrates. Even when fats are the predominant energy source, carbohydrates must still be available. Carbohydrates are necessary to continuously prime the breakdown of fatty acids to provide ATP. Thus, fats are never the sole energy source. Even if there is an abundance of fat available, but no carbohydrates to prime their breakdown, aerobic degradation of fat will stop. Other inhibitors of fat utilization are high insulin levels, such as those found after a large intake of simple sugars, and high lactic acid levels.[20]

As mentioned earlier, proteins can be converted to pyruvate and can be used for energy production during aerobic activities. There is some disagreement among researchers as to how much energy can be provided by protein. Ranges from 5 to 15% of the total energy during aerobic activity have been reported. Greater amounts of protein appear to be used as the duration of exercise increases.[21] However, it is generally agreed that the amount is relatively insignificant compared to fat and carbohydrate.

It has been established that all three substrates (fat, carbohydrate, protein) can be utilized for energy production during physical activity. It is possible, and not uncommon, for the supply to outweigh the demand. Protein is utilized for cellular structure, enzymes (the molecules that govern the breakdown and buildup of other chemicals), hormones (chemical messengers), blood-borne carriers, and energy. Excess protein is not stored at any site in the human body but will be converted to fats to be stored in the adipocytes.

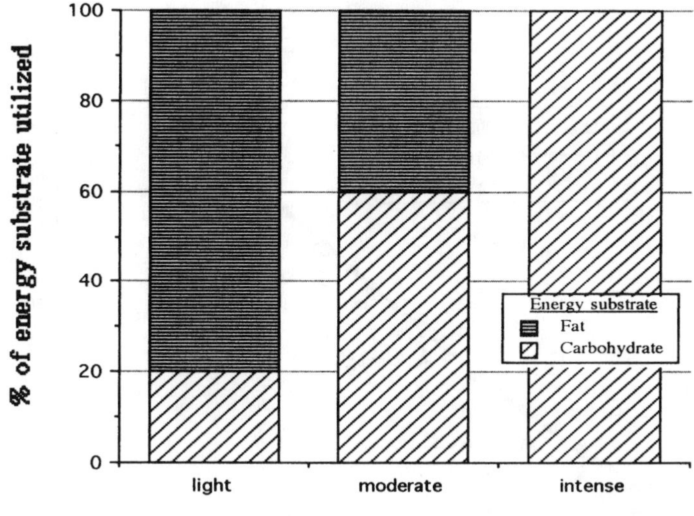

Figure 5. Interaction of carbohydrate and fat utilization during different intensities of exercise.[19]

Carbohydrates are utilized for cellular structure, hormones, and energy. Excess carbohydrates are stored in the muscles and the liver as glycogen. These stores can be increased by a combination of a high carbohydrate diet and regular, activity-induced, depletion. However, these stores are limited. When the glycogen storage capacity is exceeded, carbohydrates are converted to fats and stored in adipocytes.

Fats are utilized for cellular structure, hormones, blood-borne carriers, insulation, organ protection, and energy. Fats are the highest energy source available and the most easily stored. Fats are not usually converted to either protein or carbohydrate for storage. Fat storage occurs within muscle cells, for use during aerobic activity, and within adipocytes. Excess fats can also be found circulating in the blood and lining the walls of blood vessels. High levels of fat within the circulatory system are highly correlated with cardiovascular disease. It is clear that an excess of any one energy source results in an increase in fat storage.

G. POWER

While the previous discussion focused on energy transitions which can be viewed as a sliding scale forwards and back, there is another concept which must be viewed. Because the work produced is the product of force times distance, the power of these transitions is determined by work divided by time. Thus, more power is generated as the duration of work is shortened; nutritional practices should also reflect this relationship. Calculation of energy expenditure and calories needed for good nutrition depends on these measurements. Walking, though viewed as a simple activity, may place different demands upon the ability to deliver oxygen and the number of calories needed. As the speed of walking is increased the time is shortened and the activity generates more power (Figure 6).

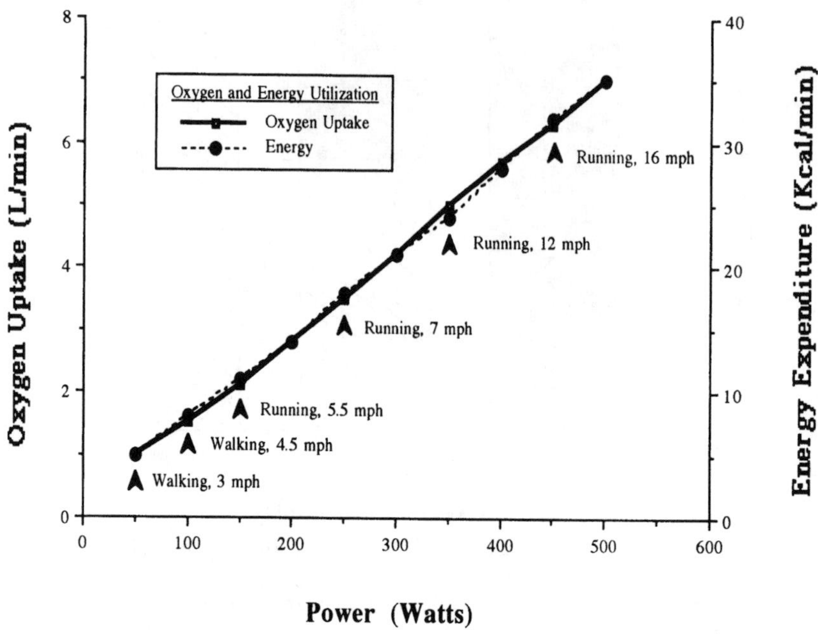

Figure 6. Energy expenditure related to exercise intensity.[2]

This results in an increased need for oxygen and additional calories are used.[2] All activity can be characterized by its frequency, intensity, and duration; understanding these relationships is fundamental to understanding the specificity of diet related to a particular activity. Figure 5 illustrates the influence of intensity of exercise on the substrate used to produce energy. Low intensity activities will rely more upon fat for the generation of energy while carbohydrate is utilized as power and intensity increases. Figure 2 illustrates the relationship between duration of activity and substrate utilization. It becomes clear that if the desire is to diminish fat stores in the body, low intensity and long duration activities should be chosen. Conversely, if hypertrophy of muscle is desired, activities should be chosen which generate more power.

III. CELLULAR RELATIONSHIPS

A. HUMAN MUSCLE

There is a direct relationship between nutritional concerns for energy production and specific characteristics of human muscle. Normal human muscle is a mosaic of fiber types which can be viewed as having properties along a spectrum from highly aerobic to highly anaerobic.[22] However, it is usually viewed in simpler relationships, and three major groups of fibers (I, IIa, IIb) are classified according to their histochemical, physiological, anatomical, or biochemical properties. The fibers identified using one property are not necessarily the same when viewed with another.[23]

Type I (slow twitch [ST], slow twitch oxidative [SO], red, dark) fibers are those that possess maximum capabilities for aerobic energy production. These are the fibers stressed in endurance activities such as running, cycling, and swimming. All of the biochemical parameters that support aerobic metabolism are at high levels in these fibers; we find elevated amounts of carbohydrate (glycogen, glucose) and fat (neutral lipids, triglycerides), which are the substrates for aerobic energy production. Aerobic conditioning enhances the ability of this particular fiber type to use energy substrates by increasing the amount and activity of enzymes which allow their use. It has been reported that persons participating for long periods of time in endurance activities such as marathons have higher than normal percentages of type I fibers.[24] The type I fiber, however, does not have the capability to hypertrophy to a great degree, even if it is overloaded due to the need to get oxygen to the center of the fiber.[24] Thus, the individuals who stress endurance activities stress the type I fiber and will find, with time, that the muscles will not enlarge greatly and that body fat stores tend to diminish. There is also a need to keep glycogen stores high through diet. Although it has long been accepted that muscle glycogen stores are the most important factor in successful endurance performance, the adaptations to fat metabolism have been recently investigated with conflicting results.[2,26]

Type II fibers (fast twitch, white, light) have two major subgroups, fast-twitch-oxidative-glycolytic (IIa, FTa, FOG) and fast-twitch-glycolytic (IIb, FTb, FG). These fibers possess maximum capabilities for anaerobic energy delivery; however, the IIa also has a high capacity for aerobic energy production, and, therefore, it is sometimes called "super fiber" in terms of performance. These are the fibers stressed in resistance activities such as weightlifting and bodybuilding. All of the biochemical parameters that support anaerobic metabolism are at high levels in these fibers. Consequently, high amounts of glycogen are found in the IIa fiber.[27] Conditioning enhances the ability of these particular fiber types to use energy substrates by increasing the amount and activity of enzymes which allow their use. It has not, however, been shown that individuals who participate in resistance activities over long periods of time have greater than normal percentages of these fibers.[28] Rather, transitions between the percentages of IIa and the IIb have been shown to occur with exercise along with changes in their size, thereby either enhancing either the aerobic (IIa) or the anaerobic (IIb) capacity of the muscle as a whole.[24] The type II fiber will significantly hypertrophy with use and is responsible for the great increases in muscle mass seen in strength conditioning and bodybuilding. There is a consideration for speed of movement, as slower movements show more rapid increases in power,[29] thereby increasing tension and hypertrophy to a greater degree than fast movements. It has even been suggested that these fibers can split and increase their numbers (hyperplasia); however, this has not been conclusively proved.[30] Thus, the individuals who stress the use of these fibers will find that their muscles will enlarge and that they have a need for carbohydrate in their diet in order to produce energy through anaerobic glycolysis. There is evidence, however, that the amount of fat in the diet may directly affect testosterone production, which is known to in turn affect increases in muscle mass, whereas low fat diets show decreases in testosterone production.[31]

B. HUMAN FAT CELLS

Human fat cells, whose only function is to store fat, are called adipocytes. They are found in stores which are superficial (directly beneath the skin) and deep (surrounding organs). The latter type of storage is termed essential fat. Adipocytes are known to significantly increase in number (hyperplasia) during the last 3 months of fetal development, the first year of life, and the prepubertal adolescent growth spurt.[32] They may also increase in number in pregnancy, but this has not yet been proved. These are the only times when the cells increase in number in an individual who is not obese.

The adipocytes are known to fill with a particular amount of lipid (triglycerides, fat) which is under control of the brain. It is thought that a normal person increases fat stores by increasing the amount of triglycerides in each cell, rather than by increasing fat cell numbers (Figure 7). Fat loss occurs by a decrease in the stores in each cell, rather than by losing fat cells. The amount of filling will be the same for all in the body, thereby suggesting that one cannot "spot reduce" a particular area without reducing stores in the entire body first.[32] Obese individuals have been shown to have greater numbers of adipocytes, which have greater lipid volumes than nonobese individuals. Thus, it is postulated that hyperplasia may also be induced when the existing adipocytes can no longer accommodate filling.[33]

Not all human adipocytes are of equal size, and the metabolic characteristics of adipose tissue vary in different locations.[34] Although the percent filling may be similar, the adipocytes themselves tend to be larger in the gluteo-femoral (buttocks) and femoral (thigh) region than in the abdominal region of young women as compared to young men.[35] These differences are not seen in middle-aged females and males. Gender hormones may influence the regional influx of triglyceride in and out of the cells in these regions. It is clear that the way the body stores fat is complex and is related to both the number, size, and filling of adipocytes.

Recreational athletes often comprise a large portion of the millions of individuals who wish to modify or diminish the fat stores in the body through the use of the thousands of diets and hundreds of weight loss programs available to them. Considering the fact that there are over 30,000 published diets alone, it cannot help but be noticed that if one of them worked successfully over the long term there would not be a need for the other 29,999. Caloric restriction must be coupled with

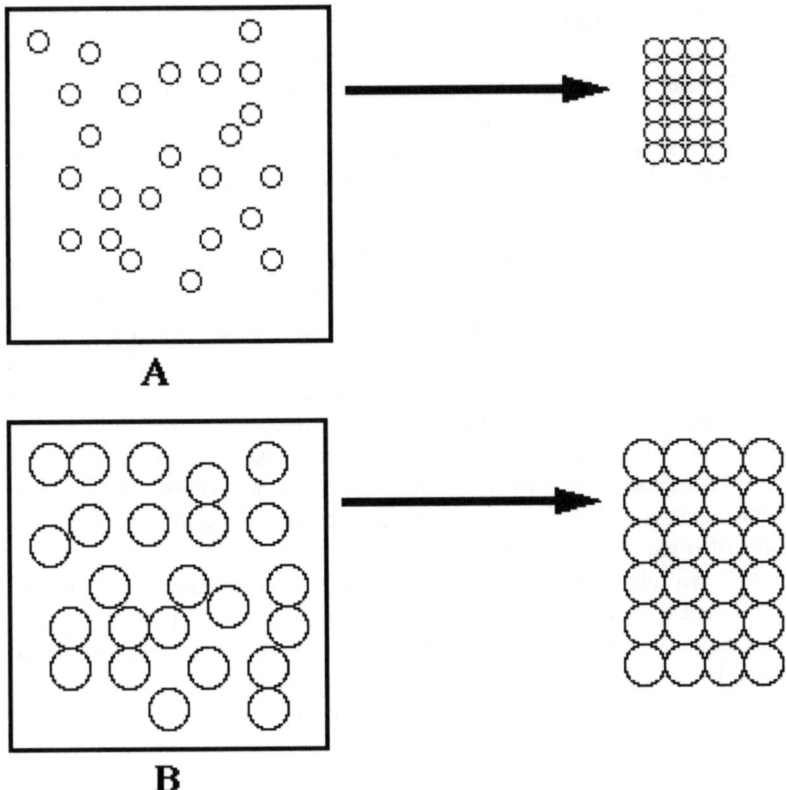

Figure 7. Human adipocyte filling. The filling and appearance of adipocyte volume is illustrated in Panel A for lean individuals and Panel B for obese individuals. Note that the number of cells is the same.

exercise as the two practices are synergistic. Individuals are directed to review the proper and improper weight loss programs position stand of the American College of Sports Medicine (Appendix B) for sound, scientifically based advice. However, it is recommended that manipulation of body fat stores not be done unless necessary and the individual has had their percentage body fat assessed by someone trained in the appropriate methods and in how to interpret the results.

Body fat stores are assessed by numerous methods[36] with hydrostatic weighing considered the "gold standard" and skinfold caliper measurements considered the most practical. Considerable misinterpretation of results abounds in the popular literature. The assessment of body composition where the percentage of body fat is determined is most appropriately used as a tool to monitor progress rather than as an absolute number or criteria for performance. There is heightened awareness of these measurements in the population but little understanding of what the percentages mean or how to apply the knowledge. The percentage body fat range for healthy adult males is 10 to 25% for optimal health, 12 to 20% for optimal fitness, and over 25% is considered obese.[37] The percentage body fat range for healthy adult females is 18 to 33% for optimal health, 16 to 25% for ideal fitness, and over 35% is considered obese.[37] Fitness requires not only a range of body fat within acceptable limits but includes proper nutrition and the appropriate combination of activities known to produce "total fitness"(Appendix C).

C. CELLS OF THE IMMUNE SYSTEM

The immune system, which is the surveillance system that protects the human from disease and illness, is affected by diet and exercise practices. Although there remains yet much controversy, a review of the literature has shown certain trends.[38] Moderate exercise appears to enhance the ability of the system to function and seems to reduce the incidence of disease.[39] Severe exercise and overtraining tends to depress the immune response and illnesses are more common.[39] There also appears to be a relationship between exercise and the type of infection; bacterial infections may be less severe and viral infections[40,41] may be exacerbated with exercise during the illness.[41-43]

Diet will also affect the immune system because vitamins, minerals, and protein intake are crucial. Since antibodies are protein structures, low protein intake can lead to low antibody production and decreased surveillance and response. Proteins are also used by immune cells for an energy source and low intake may lead to decreased function and an increase in illness.

IV. SUMMARY

Recreational athletes should understand energy requirements and cellular consequences of their activities and should choose the nutritional regimens which support this choice. However, regardless of the choice, health should be a major concern. There is a direct relationship between the effects of aging and the effects of inactivity as one reflects the other. With the current difficulties encountered in the American health care system it seems more prudent to assume responsibility for one's health in order to enjoy a better quality of life and to reduce health care costs. We now know that lower levels of activity than previously thought are sufficient to diminish the risk of several degenerative diseases (Appendix D). This may not be the level of activity necessary for measurable increments in fitness, and recreational athletes may determine that their goals exceed concerns for health. Recommendations of the American College of Sports Medicine address the quality and quantity training issues related to the development and maintenance of cardiorespiratory fitness, body composition, and muscular strength and endurance in healthy adults (Appendix C). The rest of the chapters of this book provide the information necessary to support the exercise choices with sound nutritional advice.

REFERENCES

1. The Book of Daniel, *The Holy Bible,* The World Publishing Co., New York, 1:1–21.
2. **Hagerman, F. C.,** Energy metabolism and fuel utilization, *Med. Sci. Sports Exerc.,* 24, S309, 1992.
3. **McArdle, W. D., Katch, F. I., and Katch, V. L.,** *Exercise Physiology: Energy, Nutrition, and Human Performance,* 3rd ed., Lea & Febiger, Philadelphia, 1991, chap. 8.
4. **Balke, B.,** personal communication, 1994.
5. **Behnke, A. R., Green, B. G., and Welham, W. C.,** The specific gravity of healthy man, *JAMA,* 118, 495, 1942.
6. **Consolazio, C. F., Johnson, R. E., and Pecora, L. J.,** *Physiological Measurements of Metabolic Function in Man,* McGraw-Hill, New York, 1963.
7. **Greenleaf, J. E., Geelen, G., Jackson, C. G. R., Saumet, J.-L., Juhos, L. T., Keil, L. C., Fegan-Meyer, D., Dearborn, A., Hinghofer-Szalkay, H., and Whittam, J. H.,** Vascular uptake of rehydration fluids in hypohydrated men at rest and exercise, *NASA Technical Memorandum 103942,* Moffett Field, 1992.
8. **Lozy, M., Herrera, M. G., Latham, M. C., McGandy, R. B., McCann, M. B., and Stare, F. J.,** *Nutrition,* Upjohn, Kalamazoo, MI, 1980.
9. **Gollnick, P. D.,** Free fatty acid turnover and the availability of substrates as a limiting factor in prolonged exercise, in *The Marathon: Physiological, Medical, Epidemiological, and Psychological Studies,* Milvey, P., Ed., The New York Academy of Sciences, New York, 1977, 64.
10. **Fox, E. L., Bowers, R. W., and Foss, M. L.,** *The Physiological Basis for Exercise and Sport,* 5th ed., Brown & Benchmark, Dubuque, IA, 1989, chap. 2.
11. **McArdle, W. D., Katch, F. I., and Katch, V. L.,** *Exercise Physiology: Energy, Nutrition, and Human Performance,* 3rd ed., Lea & Febiger, Philadelphia, 1991, chap. 1, 6, 11.
12. **Williams, M. H.,** *Nutrition for Fitness and Sport,* 3rd ed., Wm. C. Brown Publishers, Dubuque, IA, 1992.
13. **Wolinsky, I. and Hickson, J. F.,** *Nutrition in Exercise and Sport,* 2nd ed., CRC Press, Boca Raton, FL, 1993.
14. **Bergstrom, J., Hermansen, L., Hultman, E., and Saltin, B.,** Diet, muscle glycogen and physical performance, *Acta Physiol. Scand.,* 71, 140, 1967.
15. **Hermansen, L. and Vaage, O.,** Lactate disappearance and glycogen synthesis in human muscle after maximal exercise, *Am. J. Physiol.,* 233(5), E422, 1977.
16. **Guyton, A. C.,** *Textbook of Medical Physiology,* 8th ed., W. B. Saunders, Philadelphia, 1991, chap. 67 and 68.
17. **Piehl, K.,** Time course for refilling of glycogen stores in human muscle fibers following exercise-induced glycogen depletion., *Acta Physiol. Scand.,* 90, 297, 1974.
18. **Hultman, E. and Bergstrom, J.,** Muscle glycogen synthesis in relation to diet studied in normal subjects, *Acta Med. Scand.,* 182, 109, 1967.
19. **Sharkey, B. J.,** *Coaches Guide to Sport Physiology,* Human Kinetics Pub., Champaign, IL, 1986, chap. 5.
20. **Steinberg, D.,** Metabolism, in *Best and Taylor's Physiological Basis of Medical Practice,* West, J. B., Ed., Williams & Wilkins, Philadelphia, 1990, 728.
21. **Powers, S. K. and Howley, E. T.,** *Exercise Physiology: Theory and Application of Fitness and Performance,* 2nd ed., Brown and Benchmark, Dubuque, IA, 1994, chap 4.
22. **Romanul, F. C. A., Streter, F. A., Salmons, S., and Gergely, J.,** The effects of a changed pattern of activity on histochemical characteristics of muscle fibres, in *Exploratory Concepts in Muscular Dystrophy II,* Milhorat, E. A. T., Ed., Excerpta Medica, Amsterdam, 1974.
23. **Dubowitz, V.,** *Muscle Biopsy, A Practical Approach,* 2nd. ed., Balliere Tindall, Philadelphia, 1988.

24. **Costill, D., Daniels, J., Evans, W., Fink, W., Krahenbuhl, G., and Saltin, B.,** Skeletal muscle enzymes and fiber composition in male and female track athletes, *J. Appl. Physiol.,* 40, 149, 1976.
25. **Jackson, C. G. R., Dickinson, A. L., and Ringel, S. P.,** Skeletal muscle fiber area alterations in two opposing modes of resistance-exercise training in the same individual, *Eur. J. Appl. Physiol.,* 61, 37, 1990.
26. **Hagenfeldt, L.,** Turnover of individual free fatty acids in man, *Fed. Proc.,* 34, 2236, 1975.
27. **Jackson, C. G. R., Dickinson, A. W., Ringel S. P., and Barden, M. T.,** Histochemical profile of muscular cellular alterations following two modes of training in the same individual, unpublished data, 1994.
28. **Jackson, C. G. R. and Dickinson, A. L.,** Adaptations of skeletal muscle to strength or endurance training, in *Advances in Sports Medicine and Fitness,* Vol. 1, Grana, W. A., Lombardo, J. A., Sharkey, B. J., and Stone, J. A., Eds., Year Book Medical Publishers, Chicago, 1988, 45.
29. **Coyle, E. F., Costill, D. L., and Lesmes, G. R.,** Leg extension power and muscle fiber composition, *Med. Sci. Sports.,* 11(1), 12, 1979.
30. **Gollnick, P. D., Timson, B. F., Moore, R. L., and Riedy, M.,** Muscular enlargement and number of fibers in skeletal muscles of rats, *J. Appl. Physiol.,* 50(5), 936, 1981.
31. **Ratzin, R. A.,** Effect of aerobic conditioning on resting serum testosterone levels and muscle fiber types in vegetarian and nonvegetarian sedentary males, Doctoral dissertation, University of Northern Colorado, Greeley, 1990.
32. **Katch F. I. and McArdle, W. D.,** *Nutrition, Weight Control, and Exercise,* Lea & Febiger, Philadelphia, 1988, chap. 6.
33. **Hirsch, J. and Knittle, J. L.,** Cellularity of obese and nonobese human adipose tissue, *Fed. Proc.,* 29(4), 1516, 1970.
34. **Rebuffe-Scrive, M.,** Adipose tissue metabolism and fat distribution, in *Human Body Composition and Fat Distribution,* Norgan, N. G., Ed., Euro-Nut, Wageningen, The Netherlands, 1985, 212.
35. **Sjostrom, L., Smith, U., Krotkiewski, M., and Bjorntorp, P.,** Cellularity in different regions of adipose tissue in young men and women, *Metabolism,* 21, 1143, 1972.
36. **Lohman T. G., Roche, A. F., and Martorell, R.,** *Anthropometric Standardization Reference Manual,* Human Kinetics Books, Champaign, IL, 1988.
37. **Lohman, T. G.,** ACSM tutorial: body composition assessment, presented at American College of Sports Medicine Annual Meeting, Baltimore, June 1, 1989.
38. **Hardesty, A. J., Greenleaf, J. E., Simonson, S., Hu, A., and Jackson, C. G. R.,** *Exercise, Exercise Training, and the Immune System: A Compendium of Research (1902–1991),* NASA Technical Memorandum 108778, Moffett Field, 1993.
39. **Nash, M.S.,** Exercise and immunology, *Med. Sci. Sports Exerc.,* 26(2), 125, 1994.
40. **Cannon, J. G. and Kluger, M. J.,** Exercise enhances survival rate in mice infected with *Salmonella typhimurium, Proc. Soc. Exp. Biol. Med.,* 175, 518, 1984.
41. **Ilback, N.-G., Friman, G., and Beisel, W.R.,** Response of the mouse myocardium to physical exercise during infection with *F. tularensis* or influenza and modifying effects of physical preconditioning, *Clin. Res.,* 30, 369A, 1982.
42. **Russel, W. R.,** Poliomyelitis: the paralytic stage, and the effect of physical activity on the severity of paralysis, *Br. Med. J.,* 2, 1023, 1947.
43. **Russel, W. R.,** Paralytic poliomyelitis. The early symptoms and the effect of physical activity on the course of the disease, *Br. Med. J.,* 1, 465, 1949.

Chapter 3

NUTRITIONAL CONCERNS OF RECREATIONAL ENDURANCE ATHLETES WITH AN EMPHASIS ON SWIMMING

Jacqueline R. Berning

CONTENTS

0-8493-7914-8/95/$0.00+$.50

I. INTRODUCTION

Many factors, including genetics, training, and motivation, influence aerobic or endurance performance. Endurance activities are those that require sustained muscular contractions with high numbers of repetitions against low resistance or are continuous for long periods of time. Examples are swimming, running, jogging, walking, cycling, and aerobic dance. Just how fast an endurance athlete is able to race or move depends on how scientifically based their training program is and how wise they are in selecting food items that are nutritionally sound. Like all athletes, recreational endurance athletes require a nutritionally balanced diet that contains nutrients to sustain not only normal daily activities but also those associated with conditioning, training, and competition. By making wise food choices, exercising muscles are provided with the proper fuels that allow them to be trained harder.

To clarify how nutrition can improve aerobic performance, it is important to thoroughly understand and practice the following points:

- A well-balanced diet, high in carbohydrates, is essential during intense conditioning or training periods, tapers, and after competition.
- Dehydration as well as losses in muscle strength and endurance must be prevented during workouts and competitions.
- High fat diets tend to increase the chances of gaining unwanted weight and can pose other potential health problems.
- Good nutrition and proper weight control methods are vital to achieving peak performance.

These major aspects of sports nutrition will be covered. It is the premise of this chapter that, by making wise food choices, performance and health can be maximized.

TABLE 1 Approximate Calorie Expenditure per Minute (kcal/min) of Swimming Each Stroke at Endurance-Based Training Paces (Values Presented by Competition Level)

	Freestyle (kcal/min)	Backstroke (kcal/min)	Butterfly (kcal/min)	Breastroke (kcal/min)
Age group 11–15 years	7.0	7.5	7.5	8.5
High school 16–18 years	8.0	8.5	8.5	9.5
College 17–22 years	9.0	9.0	9.0	10.0
National caliber	7.0	7.5	7.5	8.0

II. CALCULATION OF ENERGY COST WITH THE EXAMPLE OF SWIMMING

The energy provided by foods and the energy required for all body functions including conditioning and training is measured in calories. Using swimming as an example, whether you are an age group swimmer or a masters swimmer, energy is needed to propel you through the water. Determining how many calories you use during a swimming workout will depend on many factors, some of which are your height, your weight, your gender, your age, and how efficient you are in the water. All aerobic performance is affected by these same parameters. Recent research completed at the U.S. Swimming's International Center for Aquatic Research has determined the number of calories needed per minute of swimming for various swimming events. You can determine the total number of calories needed in training by multiplying the time it takes you to swim the stroke in minutes by the caloric cost of each stroke (Table 1).

Once you have determined the number of calories utilized in swimming, you can then determine the total number of calories metabolized each day. To do this, add the number of calories used in swimming to the number of calories expended per day for your age group shown in Table 2. Table 2 shows the estimated daily caloric requirements for competitive swimmers. It is important to note that your caloric needs may differ from those given in the tables since efficient swimmers use fewer calories than inefficient swimmers when they swim the same distance at the same speed. The same calculations can be done for any endurance activity and there are many sources available that provide caloric expenditure data by activity (see Chapter 4, Table 2).

TABLE 2 Estimated Daily Calorie Requirement for Competitive Swimmers in kcals

Age Range	Basic Daily Caloric Needs	Training Daily Caloric Needs Based on Training Time/Day (Hours)
Males		
10 and under	2000	2200–2900
11–14	2500	2700–3600
15–18	3000	3200–4000
19–22	2900	3100–4200
Females		
10 and under	1800	2000–2800
11–14	2200	2400–3200
15–18	2200	2400–3500
19–22	2000	2200–3700

III. TRAINING DIET

A. PROTEIN

The principle role of protein in the body is to build and repair body tissues, including muscles, ligaments, and tendons.[1] Contrary to popular belief, protein is not a primary source of energy, except when recreational athletes do not consume enough calories or carbohydrates. The impact of energy intake, the amount of calories consumed, on protein utilization is well documented.[2] For any given protein intake, increasing energy intake will improve nitrogen balance, implying that protein requirements decrease as energy intake increases. It is the measurement of nitrogen balance that indicates if protein is catabolized, used for synthesis, growth or repair, or is excreted by the body. Conversely, for any given energy intake, there is an optimum protein intake beyond which the efficiency of nitrogen utilization falls off markedly. If a diet is not balanced, or if total daily caloric intake is insufficient, protein will be broken down and used as an energy source instead of being used for its intended job of tissue building. When an individual consumes more protein than the body can use, the excess amino acids are stored as fat. Concerns regarding excessive protein intake also include a monetary perspective, as protein supplements cost in excess of $50.00 per pound of protein.

Protein is composed of amino acids. When protein foods are eaten, these amino acids are absorbed and used to form muscle, hemoglobin, enzymes, and hormones. Most research on actual protein intakes of athletes in developed countries reveals that the average athlete already consumes protein in the highest recommended ranges. The suggested range of protein requirement for athletes is 1.0 to 2.0 g of protein per kilogram of body weight.[3] Thus, a 17-year-old male endurance athlete who weighs 145 pounds needs from 66 to 132 g of protein per day. Endurance activity or aerobic conditioning may promote a loss of muscle protein via reduced protein synthesis and increased protein breakdown during the

TABLE 3 Calculation of Daily Protein Requirement for Endurance Athletes

(Your weight in pounds)______ lbs/2.2 kg/lb = ______ kg (Your weight in kilograms)
(Your weight in kilograms) ______ kg × 1.5 g protein/kg =_______ **g protein/day**

exercise itself.[3] Therefore, the need for an adequate amount of protein in the diet is highest if the activity is aerobic in nature, contrary to the popular belief that it is the strength athlete who has the highest need for protein in the diet.

The typical American diet supplies about 1.5 g of protein per kg of body weight, which is adequate for recreational athletes to support growth and muscle development. However, recreational athletes tend to eat more protein than their sedentary counterparts because they eat more food. So while protein needs may be higher for endurance athletes, it is not difficult for them to meet their protein requirement. To determine your own protein requirement use the equations in Table 3.

To determine the amount of protein in common foods use the following as a guide:

- 8 g of protein per cup of milk, yogurt, or other dairy products
- 8 g of protein per ounce of cheese
- 7 g of protein per ounce of meat (beef, chicken, fish)
- 3 g of protein per serving of bread or grains (1 slice of bread, 1/2 cup of rice, 1/2 cup of pasta)

Additional gram weights of protein in common foods can be found in Table 4.

B. FAT

All macronutrients (fat, carbohydrate, and protein) are available as energy sources during exercise and at rest.[4] The proportion of energy contributed by each depends on the rate at which energy must be supplied. When the body needs energy at a rapid rate, blood glucose and muscle and liver glycogen are the primary fuels. As the stores of fuels that produce energy rapidly deplete, energy production becomes more dependent on fat. Thus, the intensity and duration of exercise become determinants of fuel sources used during an exercise bout.

Americans typically eat about 38% of their calories as fat, an amount that has been linked to numerous diseases and obesity.[5] Currently, many nonathletes attempt to reduce their fat intakes, and there is a heightened awareness of fat consumption in general within the American population. Recreational athletes need to be concerned about this as well.

Fat is a major energy source for endurance athletes. However, even though fat provides a significant energy contribution during prolonged workouts, no attempt should be made to store fat, since more fat is already stored in the body than is ever needed during an exercise workout.

Fats are the source of fatty acids, which are divided into two categories: saturated and unsaturated (including monounsaturated and polyunsaturated fatty acids). Saturated fat is solid at room temperature and is derived mainly from

TABLE 4 Protein Gram Weights of Common Foods

Food	Portion Size	Protein (g)
Milk (skim, 2%, whole)	1 cup	8
Yogurt (nonfat, low fat)	1 cup	8
Cheese (any variety)	1 oz	8
Lean hamburger patty	3 oz	26
Egg/egg white	1	7
Lean steak	3 oz	21
Chicken breast	3.5 oz	30
Taco	1	11
Pizza	2 slices	32
Tuna	3 oz	24
Peanut butter	1 tbsp	4
Whole wheat bread	1 slice	2
Pasta	1 cup	4

animal sources; unsaturated fat is liquid at room temperature and is found mainly in plants. A diet rich in polyunsaturated fats is the most healthful, for it tends to lower blood cholesterol levels, while saturated fats tend to raise blood levels of cholesterol. A high fat diet increases the risk of cardiovascular disease and cancer.[5] Eating too much fat generally decreases carbohydrate intake. Consequently, muscle glycogen stores cannot be adequately maintained on a high fat diet.

Fat has its place in the diet, but it should not exceed more than 30% of the total calories.[5] Some important points to keep in mind about fat are

- Fat exits the stomach slowly and can cause cramping; so, fat consumption should be held to a minimum prior to and during exercise.
- By consuming a high fat diet you have compromised carbohydrate intake and thus may have chronic fatigue.
- In order to use fat effectively as an energy source, sufficient carbohydrate must be consumed.

Obvious sources of fat are butter, margarine, shortening, and oils. Hidden fats are found in marbled meats, poultry skins, whole milk, cheese, ice cream, nuts, peanut butter, salad dressing, and many snack foods and most bakery products. Fried foods are also high in fats.

Foods that are low in fat include starchy or complex carbohydrate foods such as breads, rice, pasta, potatoes, and beans. Other low fat foods include fruits, vegetables, skim milk, low fat yogurt, and fish. Lowering the fat content of your favorite recipes and eating lower fat meals and snacks can be a real challenge. Some suggestions for lowering dietary fat are found in Table 5.

C. CARBOHYDRATE

Carbohydrate is the most important, and least abundant, nutrient for working muscles. Essential for any form of endurance performance, the principle functions of carbohydrate are to:

TABLE 5 Guidelines To Reduce Dietary Fat

Instead Of	Try
Whole milk	Skim milk
Cheddar, Jack, or Swiss cheese	Part-skim mozzarella, string or low fat cottage cheese, other cheese that contains less than 5 g of fat per oz
Ice cream	Ice milk or low fat/nonfat frozen yogurt
Butter or margarine	Jam, yogurt, ricotta cheese, light or nonfat cream cheese
Sour cream	Low fat yogurt, light sour cream, blender whipped cottage cheese dressing
Bacon	Canadian bacon or bacon bits
Ground beef	Extra lean ground beef or ground turkey
Fried chicken	Baked chicken without the skin
Doughnuts and pastries	Bagels, whole-grain breads, homemade low fat muffins and quick breads
Apple pie	Baked or raw apple
Chocolate candy or bars	Jelly beans, hard candy, licorice
Cookies, cakes, brownies	Vanilla wafers, ginger snaps, graham crackers, fig bars

- Serve as a primary energy source for working muscles
- Ensure that the brain and nervous system function properly
- Help the body use fat more efficiently

Stored carbohydrates (glycogen), the initial primary fuel for endurance activity which must be present to metabolize fat, can become depleted during prolonged aerobic exercise such as runs and distance swimming events, or can deplete gradually over several days of intense conditioning or training.[6] If a swimmer or other endurance athlete has a difficult time maintaining a normal workout intensity, they may be experiencing muscle glycogen depletion over several days of activity because there is not enough time for glycogen stores to become normalized. Since it takes approximately 48 h for this to occur, continued days of exercise may worsen the depletion. Performance gradually deteriorates and even light workouts may cause fatigue under these circumstances. The risk of injury also increases.

IV. TRAINING NUTRITION

A. TRAINING GLYCOGEN DEPLETION

Glycogen depletion can occur during exercise which requires repeated, near maximal bursts of effort as well as during endurance exercise. A certain sign of training glycogen depletion is when the athlete has difficulty maintaining a normal exercise intensity. A sudden weight loss of several pounds due to glycogen and water loss can accompany this depletion.[7] Athletes who do not consume enough carbohydrate and/or do not take rest days are prime candidates.

Training glycogen depletion can be prevented by consuming a carbohydrate-rich diet and incorporating periodic rest days into the training schedule to give the muscles time to rebuild their glycogen stores. Recreational endurance athlete's diets should consist of at least 60% carbohydrate.[8] Consumption of at least 500 g of carbohydrate per day or 8 to 10 g of carbohydrate per kg of body weight will replenish body carbohydrate reserves and maintain optimal performance capabilities.[8] The best way to increase carbohydrate intake is to increase amounts of fruits, vegetables, and grains in the diet. Table 14 in Chapter 7 lists foods that are good sources of complex carbohydrates.

Some endurance athletes participate in workouts twice daily in addition to other daily activities and may find it difficult to consume adequate calories and carbohydrates. Consequently, many exercisers tend to snack throughout the day and do not consume adequate amounts of carbohydrates. Those who have difficulty consuming enough carbohydrate can use a commercial, high carbohydrate supplement. These products do not replace regular food but are designed to supply supplemental calories and carbohydrate when needed.

B. SIMPLE VS. COMPLEX CARBOHYDRATE

The question is often asked if the type of carbohydrate, simple or complex, has an effect on muscle glycogen storage. The research is not clear on this issue. One study compared the effects of simple and complex carbohydrates during a 48-h period after a glycogen-depleting exercise. During the first 24 h, no differences were found in muscle glycogen synthesis between the two types of carbohydrates. However, after 48 h, the starch or complex carbohydrate diet resulted in significantly greater muscle glycogen synthesis than did the glucose or simple carbohydrate diet.[9] However, in a similar comparison study of simple and complex carbohydrate intake during both glycogen depleted and nondepleted states, others found that significant increases in muscle glycogen could be achieved with a diet high in either simple or complex carbohydrates.[10] The general recommendation is that athletes should consume 60 to 70% of their calories from carbohydrates and that 48% should be complex and 8 to 12% should be simple carbohydrates.

C. NUTRITION DURING A WORKOUT

During periods of intense conditioning or all-day competitions, energy stores deplete very rapidly. The best way to replenish these energy stores is to consume a good source of carbohydrates. In most cases, it is beneficial to consume a carbohydrate/electrolyte sport drink during workouts that last longer than 60 min. This type of beverage provides carbohydrates to the muscle as it replaces lost body fluids. A growing body of evidence suggests that a sport drink taken during a workout or competition improves performance by maintaining blood glucose levels at a time when energy stores are low.[11] This allows energy production to continue, thus delaying fatigue.

D. POST-WORKOUT/COMPETITION NUTRITION

Consumption of a high carbohydrate meal should begin as soon as possible after a workout. The exerciser should consume approximately 100 g of carbohydrate within 30 min after exercise, followed by an additional 100-gram serving every 2 to 4 h thereafter.[12] Examples of foods or combinations of foods that contain 100 g of carbohydrate or more include: a bagel with peanut butter and 2/3 of a cup raisins, a turkey sandwich on whole wheat bread with a cup of applesauce, or spaghetti with meat sauce and garlic bread. If an individual has difficulty consuming solid food immediately after a workout, a commercial carbohydrate beverage, such as GatorLode®, can be used as a carbohydrate replacement source. The practice of consuming a high carbohydrate meal immediately after aerobic conditioning also applies after competing. For example, many swim meets last more than 1 day; so, it is important that swimmers rebuild their glycogen stores immediately after competition in preparation for the next day's events. This applies to all endurance activities which continue for consecutive days.

E. DIET DURING SWIMMING TAPER

Swimmers often use a taper or decrease in training activity prior to major competitive events, a practice which would be wisely adopted in other endurance activities. The primary purpose of the taper is to give the swimmer's body a rest and allow it to adapt to the previous training period, in preparation for competition. Part of this preparation is to enhance and increase the muscle glycogen stores. To accomplish this, there is a gradual reduction in exercise duration in the weeks prior to competition. At the same time, there is a gradual increase in the amount of carbohydrate in the diet until it contains at least 70% total calories from carbohydrate (500 to 700 g of carbohydrate) during the 3 days to 3 weeks prior to competition. However, total caloric intake should decrease during a taper to match the decreased workload of exercise in order to avoid weight gain. This procedure results in carbohydrate loading or super compensation. While it is important for swimmers to maximize the amount of glycogen stored in the muscles during the taper, it should be remembered that a diet high in carbohydrate should be permanently maintained by all endurance or aerobic athletes during all phases of training. The same pattern described for swimmers may be followed by other recreational endurance athletes.

The food pyramid can be used as a guide to increasing carbohydrate intake during the taper (see Chapter 7, Figure 1). During the first 3 days the individual can follow the normal high carbohydrate diet: 2 servings from the meat group, 4 servings from the dairy group, 3 to 4 servings from the fruit group and 5 to 6 servings from the vegetable group, and 6 to 11 servings from the grain group. During the last 3 days, the number of servings of the grain group should be increased to 11 or more servings per day. Fruits and vegetables, particularly starch vegetables like corn, peas, and potatoes, are also high sources of carbohydrate and can help make up the grain group deficiencies after fruit and vegetable needs are met. If an exerciser has difficulty obtaining enough carbohydrates from food, he/she can consider adding a high-carbohydrate liquid supplement as 12 oz usually contain 70 g of carbohydrate. Again, these recommendations apply to all endurance activities.

F. PRE-EVENT NUTRITION

Since there are endurance events available to the recreational athlete that can last all day or sometimes longer, exercisers need to be concerned about what they consume before they participate. The type of food eaten may influence performance. Fatty foods such as potato chips, doughnuts, french fries, and Danishes take the longest to digest. Protein foods which also contain fat, such as peanut butter, cheese, and high fat meats like ribs and bacon may take longer to digest. If these types of foods are consumed prior to exercise, the blood diverts to the stomach to begin digestion, while at the same time there is a great need to provide oxygen to the exercising muscle. Unfortunately, the cardiovascular system cannot do both very well and it may result in an upset stomach or a poor performance.

Carbohydrate foods like pasta, cereals, bagels, and fruits and vegetables are digested quickly. These types of food can be processed and leave the stomach in approximately 2 h. Therefore, the pre-event or preconditioning meal should be composed primarily of carbohydrates. Recent research has found that the consumption of a carbohydrate-rich meal or food at least 3 h prior to the start of a workout may improve performance by maintaining blood glucose levels during the exercise bout.[13]

The same principle used to time pre-event or preconditioning meals also applies to all-day exercise bouts. If one exercises at 10:00 a.m. and again 2 h later, a meal high in fat and protein will more than likely still be in the stomach for the 2nd training session. The general rule is that one should consume 1 to 4 g of carbohydrate per kilogram of body weight 1 to 4 h prior to the exercise. To avoid potential gastrointestinal distress, the carbohydrate content of the meal should be reduced the closer to the exercise it is consumed. For example, a carbohydrate feeding of 1 g per kilogram is appropriate immediately within an hour before exercise, whereas 4 g per kg can be safely consumed 4 h before exercise.

G. GUIDELINES FOR ALL-DAY WORKOUTS OR EVENTS

Good examples of solid high carbohydrate foods for pre-exercise meals include fruit, bread products (adding jam or jelly increases carbohydrate content), and low fat or nonfat yogurt. Fruit juices and nonfat milk are good high carbohydrate beverages. The exerciser could also incorporate a commercial sport drink or high carbohydrate supplement into the pre-exercise meal. The timing of the workout or event then dictates the nutritional practice:

- If it is an hour or less between workouts or events, the exerciser should consume carbohydrate foods like fruit juices, or solid carbohydrates like bananas, crackers, or plain toast, or a sport drink like Gatorade®. The amount of food eaten should be limited.

- If it is 2 to 4 hours in between workouts or events, athletes should add more carbohydrate foods such as bagels, hot cereal like oatmeal, or English muffins along with some type of fruit juice or a sport drink.
- If it is 4 h or more in between workouts or events, athletes can add small amounts of protein with the carbohydrate foods. For example, a light spread of peanut butter on a bagel with fruit juice or a turkey sandwich on 2 slices of bread with a sport drink would be appropriate.

H. FLUID REPLACEMENT

Chapter 8 outlines greater detail for fluid consumption during exercise. However, some general principles will be discussed. As one trains or competes, fluid is lost through the skin and lungs, particularly in swimming. If this fluid loss is not replaced at regular intervals during exercise, it will lead to dehydration. Consequently, the amount of blood the heart pumps with each beat decreases, the muscles do not receive enough oxygen, exhaustion sets in, and the performance suffers. The best way to prevent dehydration is to maintain body fluid levels by consuming fluids before, during, or after a workout or race. Thirst is not an accurate indicator of how much fluid has been lost. If recreational athletes wait until they experience thirst to replenish body fluids, then they are already dehydrated. To maintain hydration levels, a water bottle should be carried during workouts or kept by the side of the pool, and the athlete should drink as often as desired, ideally in between intense bouts of exercise.

To prevent dehydration, recreational endurance athletes should follow these guidelines:

- Weigh in before and after training to monitor fluid losses. Drink 2 cups of water or a sports beverage for every pound of body weight lost.
- Drink 1 to 2 cups of fluid (8 to 16 oz) prior to working out or competing.
- Drink 4 to 10 oz of fluid every 15 to 20 min during training or competition.
- Check the color of urine. Dark colored urine may indicate the onset of dehydration and the need to replenish fluids.
- Avoid carbonated drinks, which can cause gastrointestinal distress and may decrease the volume of fluids consumed.
- Avoid beverages containing alcohol or caffeine. They are diuretics and contribute to fluid loss.
- An optimal fluid replacement beverage should taste good, stimulate fluid absorption, maintain proper fluid balance in the body, and provide energy to working muscles.
- Water is a good source of replenishment for exercise lasting less than 1 h. Sports beverages, which are formulated to encourage voluntary fluid consumption and replace carbohydrates, are also an effective fluid replacement, particularly for exercise that lasts greater than 1 h.[7]

V. TRAVELING

Where and what one eats are major concerns for the recreational endurance athlete who travels. To ensure that wise food choices are made while traveling, decisions about where to eat need to be made before the mealtime. Too often, exercisers who travel will eat at a fast food restaurant because it is convenient and affordable. While the meals at these restaurants can provide certain nutrients, careful selection is important because some fast foods are high in fat and low in carbohydrates, calcium, and vitamins A and C. Use the following guidelines for choosing meals while traveling and exercising or competing:

- General traveling tips
  - Order only the basics at the drive-through window and bring fresh fruits or vegetables, small containers of juice, or small boxes of dried fruit from home or purchased at a nearby supermarket.
  - Choose low fat milk or juices rather than soft drinks.
  - Avoid high fat foods like fried foods and gravies.
- Breakfast items to order
  - Pancakes/waffles with syrup, french toast, bagels/toast, cereal (hot or cold), fruit, fruit juice, jelly/jam, low fat or skim milk, low fat or nonfat yogurt.
  - Avoid bacon, breakfast sausage, eggs, croissants/sweet rolls, or doughnuts.
- Lunch items to order
  - Sandwiches (turkey, ham, roast beef, without butter or mayonnaise), mustard, lettuce, sprouts, tomato, salad bar (use low-calorie dressing), soup, rolls, crackers, plain baked potato, corn on the cob (unbuttered), fruit (fresh or canned), fruit juice, milk (low fat or skim), or low fat yogurt (fruited or plain).
  - Avoid hamburgers, fried foods, high fat milkshakes, coleslaw, cream soups, or mayonnaise-based salads.
- Dinner items to order
  - Baked chicken, turkey, fish, spaghetti with tomato sauce, thick-crust vegetarian pizza, plain potatoes, rice or pasta, bread, rolls, crackers, or bread sticks, steamed vegetables (unbuttered), salad (low-calorie dressing), fruit, fruit juice, fruit sorbet, sherbet, milk (low fat or skim), low fat or nonfat frozen yogurt.
  - Avoid steaks, hamburgers, sauces, gravies, fried or sautéed foods, ice cream, rich desserts, butter, sour cream, and regular salad dressings.

If the recreational athlete cannot afford restaurant meals or just has 1-day trips, nearby grocery stores can offer a great variety of foods. Many grocery stores now have soup and salad bars; fresh fruits and vegetables and low fat dairy products are almost always available. When traveling, remember to bring nutrient-dense snacks on the trip as well. Many exercisers prefer high fat, high calorie snack foods. To curb consumption of these foods, bring along fresh fruit, fruit juice, cut-up vegetables, bagels, muffins, raisins, crackers, and low fat string cheese.

VI. SPECIAL NUTRITION CONCERNS

A. FEMALE RECREATIONAL ENDURANCE ATHLETES

Because the number of women participating in sports and exercise has increased dramatically in the past decade, female athletes need to be aware of the nutritional requirements of women. By consuming a wide variety of foods that provide the calories needed to support conditioning and training, females should be able to meet their requirements for most nutrients. However, there are certain nutrients, particularly calcium and iron, that may be more difficult for females to obtain in adequate amounts. Female athletes can increase their intake of calcium by following these guidelines:

- Prepare canned soups with skim milk instead of water.
- Add nonfat dry milk to soups, stew, casseroles, and even cookie recipes.
- Add grated low fat mozzarella cheese to salads, tacos, or pasta recipes.
- Have yogurt as a snack, or use it to make low-calorie salad dressings and vegetable dip.
- Choose calcium-rich desserts such as low fat cheese and fruit, frozen or low fat or nonfat yogurt, and puddings made with skim milk.
- Drink hot chocolate with skim milk.

To ensure an adequate intake of iron, the following is recommended:

- At each meal, eat foods that are high in Vitamin C to help the body absorb iron.
- Include meat in the diet, preferably lean red meat, and the dark meat of chicken and turkey as they contain the form of iron that is more readily absorbed by the body.
- To increase iron content in the diet and add more carbohydrates, eat cereals, breads, and pastas that have the word enriched or fortified on the labels.

B. VEGETARIAN DIETS

Chapter 6 comprehensively covers vegetarian diet, but certain general recommendations will be made. Many recreational endurance athletes, especially those who wish to improve their carbohydrate intake, incorporate vegetarian eating styles into their diets. Because animal products are low in carbohydrate and are usually higher in fat, some athletes perceive them as having a negative effect on performance. While it is true that animal products are low in carbohydrate, this does not mean that they negatively affect performance. Animal products are an important source of protein and other nutrients. However, athletes can train and compete successfully on a vegetarian diet. A diet that derives its protein from vegetable sources can provide the protein, vitamins, and minerals, as well as high

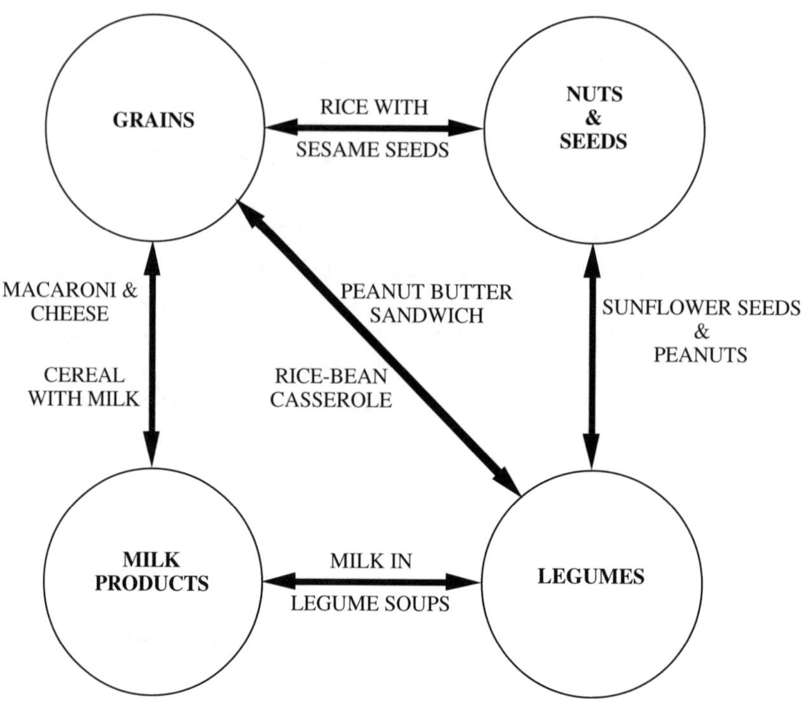

Figure 1. Complementation of protein to improve amino acid content in diets for vegetarians.

carbohydrate intake, needed to sustain heavy, prolonged workouts. Obtaining needed protein may be difficult if one is vegan and does not consume a wide variety of foods (see Chapter 6). Plant proteins are "incomplete" because they lack one or more of the nutritionally essential amino acids. It was previously recommended that this be corrected by complementing foods to improve amino acid content of the meal. Examples of protein complementation are shown in Figure 1. However, it may not be necessary to consume the complements at the same meal or within a short time of each other.

While there have been no controlled studies to determine the long-term effects of vegetarian eating, improperly planned vegetarian diets have been associated with iron deficiency anemia, irregular menstrual cycles, bone mineral loss, and protein malnutrition. However, athletes can expect to perform well on a properly planned vegetarian diet.

VII. EVALUATING RELIABLE NUTRITION INFORMATION

There are many individuals and organizations that can provide a recreational athlete with nutrition information. However, it is sometimes difficult to separate fact from fallacy.

A. SELECTING A RELIABLE NUTRITION BOOK

It is easy to find books about nutrition. However, it is not that simple to evaluate them for accuracy and reliability. The following is a list of questions to ask in order to provide direction for evaluation.

- What credentials does the author or editor have? What degrees does the author or editor legitimately have, in what field, and from what institution?
- Is the author or editor a member of a recognized, reputable organization and are they affiliated with reputable nutrition organizations?
- Are life-long, gradual changes encouraged?
- Does the diet or program include eating a wide variety of foods without eliminating certain food groups?
- Is the information factual, specific, and referenced or is it vague and presented in an emotional manner?
- Are recommendations based on scientific evidence or personal testimonials and anecdotes?
- Does the author or editor seem to agree with recommendations from recognized medical and health professionals?

B. SELECTING A RELIABLE SPORTS NUTRITIONIST

The decision is sometimes made by recreational athletes to seek further information and consultation from persons with expertise in nutrition. A reputable sports nutritionist should:

- Individualize a diet plan for each athlete's unique need that is based on lifestyle, training, food preferences, and medical history
- Consult with the exerciser's physician if they are under medical care
- Encourage meeting dietary requirements by eating a wide variety of foods instead of relying on vitamin and mineral supplements
- Advise that performance and health depends on many factors, nutrition being only one

A responsible, qualified sports nutritionist should not:

- Promise miraculous improvements in performance or muscular strength
- Claim that everyone needs nutrient supplements or health foods
- Use pseudo-medical jargon such as "detoxifying your body", "oxygenating your blood", or "strengthening your immune system"
- Promise quick, easy, or dramatic weight loss or cures
- Sell nutrient supplements after recommending that an athlete take them

VIII. SUMMARY

The objective of this chapter was to give sound nutritional advice to the recreational aerobic or endurance athlete. This unique group of individuals should consider dietary changes that favor reduction of fat and increased complex carbohydrate in the diet. The goal of the practices outlined and the advice given is to allow the individual to exercise in a healthful and enjoyable way throughout his/her life-span.

IX. FURTHER READING

The following is a list of books and various references that recreational athletes can use for additional nutrition information:

- The *Nutrition in Exercise* Series of CRC Press, in particular: *Nutrition in Exercise and Sport,* 2nd ed., Wolinsky, I. and Hickson, J. F., Eds., CRC Press, Boca Raton, FL, 1993.
- Gatorade Sports Science Institute, P.O. Box 81740, Chicago, IL 60681-0740.
- *Eating for Endurance,* Coleman, E., Bull Publishing Company, Palo Alto, CA.
- *Nancy Clark's Sports Nutrition Guide Book,* Clark, N., Leisure Press, Champaign, IL.
- *Sports Nutrition for the 90's: The Health Professional's Handbook,* Berning, J. R. and Steen S. N., Eds., Aspen Publishers, Gaithersburg, MD.
- *Swimming World,* Sport Publications, Inc., 116 W. Hazel, Inglewood, CA 90302.
- *Food Power,* National Dairy Council, Rosemont, IL.
- *Winning Spirit Nutrition,* Nutritional Education Video Tape, University of Arizona Cooperative Extension, Tucson, AZ.
- *The Swimmers Diet,* Berning, J. R. and Gregg, S. G., Gatorade, 847 West Jackson St., Chicago, IL 60607.
- *Racing Fuel,* United States Swimming, 1750 East Boulder St., Colorado Springs, CO 80909.

REFERENCES

1. **Whitney, E. N. and Rolfes, S. R.,** *Understanding Nutrition,* West Publishing Company, MN, 1993.
2. **Calloway, D. H. and Spector, H.,** Nitrogen balance as related to caloric and protein intake in active young men, *Am. J. Clin. Nutr.,* 2, 405, 1954.
3. **Butterfield, G.,** Amino acid and high protein diets, in *Perspectives in Exercise Science and Sports Medicine, Vol. 4, Ergogenics: Enhancement of Performance in Exercise and Sport,* Lamb, D. R. and Williams, M. E., Eds., Brown and Benchmark, Indianapolis, 1991, 87.
4. **Fox, E. L.,** *Sports Physiology,* Saunders College Publishing, Philadelphia, 1979, 35.
5. **Ernst, N. D., Cleeman, M. D., Mullis, R., Sooter-Bochenek, J., and Van Horn, L.,** The national cholesterol education program: implications for dietetic practitioners from the adult treatment panel recommendations, *J. Am. Diet. Assoc.,* 88, 1401, 1988.

6. **Costill, D. L.,** Carbohydrates for exercise: dietary demands for optimal performance, *Int. J. Sports Med.,* 9, 1, 1988.
7. **Coleman, E.,** *Diet, Exercise and Fitness,* Nutrition Dimension, San Marcos, CA, 1993.
8. **Sherman, W. M.,** Carbohydrate, muscle gycogen and improved performance, *Phys. Sportsmed.,* 15, 157, Feb. 1987.
9. **Costill, D. L., Sherman, W. M., Fink, W. J., Maresh, C., Witten, M., and Miller, J. M.,** The role of dietary carbohydrate in muscle glycogen resynthesis after strenuous running, *Am. J. Clin. Nutr.,* 34, 1831, 1981.
10. **Roberts, K. M., Noble, E. G., Hayden, D. B., and Taylor, A. W.,** Simple and complex carbohydrate-rich diets and muscle glycogen content of marathon runners, *Eur. J. Appl. Physiol.,* 57, 70, 1988.
11. **Ivy, J. L., Miller, W., Dover, V., Goodyear, L. G., Sherman, W. M., Farrell, S., and Williams, H.,** Endurance improved by ingesting of a glucose polymer supplement, *Med. Sci. Sports Exerc.,* 15, 466, 1983.
12. **Ivy, J. L., Datz, A. L., Cutler, C. L., Sherman, W. M., and Coyle, E. F.,** Muscle glycogen synthesis after exercise: effect of time of carbohydrate injestion, *J. Appl. Physiol.,* 6, 1480, 1988.
13. **Coyle, E. F., Coggan, A. R., Hemmert, M. K., and Ivy, J. L.,** Muscle glycogen utilization during prolonged strenuous exercise when fed carbohydrate, *J. Appl. Physiol.,* 61, 165, 1986.

Chapter **4**

NUTRITIONAL CONCERNS OF RECREATIONAL STRENGTH ATHLETES

Jaime S. Ruud
Ira Wolinsky

CONTENTS

0-8493-7914-8/95/$0.00+$.50

I. INTRODUCTION

What are the dietary requirements of strength athletes? Are their nutritional needs different from other sport groups? These are questions frequently asked by recreational athletes who primarily use resistance exercise regardless of their level of conditioning and commitment to training.

The purpose of this chapter is to examine the nutritional considerations for recreational athletes participating in bodybuilding, weightlifting, wrestling, and self-defense. Although a variety of nutritional factors can affect strength performance, three major areas of interest to these athletes are protein requirements, dietary supplements, and "making weight".

Before discussing the nutritional considerations of these individuals, it is important to distinguish among the different types of exercise and sport. Athletes who lift weights or use progressive resistance exercise solely to improve the external configuration and appearance of the body are bodybuilders.[1] The amount of weight moved or the level of resistance is of no consequence. This differs from weightlifters who train for the purpose of increasing resistance and the amount of weight lifted or moved by specific muscle groups in clearly defined categories which are usually grouped by weight classification. Additionally, "weight training" is a system of conditioning in which athletes lift weights for increasing muscular strength, endurance, and mass; they usually focus on the muscle groups most used in their sport.

II. NUTRITIONAL PROFILE OF STRENGTH ATHLETES

A. BODYBUILDING AND WEIGHTLIFTING

1. Definition and Dietary Habits of Bodybuilders

Bodybuilding is a demanding sport that involves years of dedicated training to artistically sculpt the body's muscles to high aesthetic standards.[2] It is a subjective sport, similar to gymnastics and diving, where athletes are judged on appearance, presentation, balance, symmetry, and compulsory rounds. The goal of bodybuilding is to maximize lean tissue and minimize fat tissue so that the muscular structure underneath is prominently seen.[3] The winning physique is determined by the athlete who possesses a low percentage body fat level and a high degree of muscularity, which is well proportioned and symmetrical. However, many recreational bodybuilders do not compete but follow the same training routines as competitors in order to achieve a more desirable body configuration.

There are two distinct phases of training in bodybuilding.[4] The first is a "bulking phase" where the individual focuses on building strength and muscle mass. The second phase is an external body reduction or "cutting phase" initiated just before competition to yield maximum visibility of muscle mass which requires reducing superficial fat to a minimum.[4,5]

The eating habits of bodybuilders are truly unique to the sport. Surveys show that bodybuilders often base their dietary strategies on advice from more advanced bodybuilders, bodybuilding magazines, and "nutrition stores".[4,5] This suggests that there exists a general lack of sound nutrition knowledge.

Case studies illustrate the diet, exercise, and drug regimens of these individuals.[4-8] Steen[5] studied a male bodybuilder who was preparing for contest. The athlete had been following a rigid, monotonous diet prescribed by another bodybuilder. His average calorie intake during the "bulking phase" was 4193 calories a day and the percentage of calories from carbohydrate, protein, and fat was 72, 23, and 5%, respectively. The foods consumed most often included chicken, turkey, tuna packed in water, egg whites, brown rice, whole grain cereal, vegetarian beans, tea, and water. During the 3 months prior to competition, the athlete had lost 11 pounds in 6 weeks. During the weight reduction phase, his average calorie intake was 3020 calories and percentage of calories from carbohydrate was 65%, from protein, 29%, and from fat, 6%. As calories were restricted further, the athlete reported feeling "irritable and difficult to get along with". In an attempt to promote temporary swelling of the muscles the day of the contest, the bodybuilder carbohydrate loaded. During the off-season he consumed a multivitamin/multimineral supplement and 60 to 100 g of amino acids. Prior to competition, his use of supplements increased. Sodium and water were restricted just before competition to produce dehydration which the bodybuilder believed would "make the skin paper thin and tight over the musculature to give definition". Six different anabolic steroids were used either orally or by injection during the off-season.

2. Anabolic-Androgenic Steroids

Anabolic-androgenic steroids, derivatives of the male hormone testosterone, can increase muscle mass quickly; however, there are numerous constraints upon their success and concerns about their abuse as presented in the position stand of the American College of Sports Medicine (Appendix E). It is commonly believed that they will be successful in all individuals who use them and this may be why bodybuilders who desire more lean mass and less body fat, and weightlifters, who want to increase the maximum amount of weight they lift, use these steroids. It is estimated that approximately 90% of male professional bodybuilders and 80% of female professional bodybuilders use steroids.[9] Although the prevalence of steroid use among recreational bodybuilders is not known, it is felt that these are the most abused drugs among recreational athletes.

Anabolic steroids commonly are used in "cycles", periods lasting 6 to 12 weeks.[10] However, it is not uncommon for individuals to use these drugs on a continuous basis and increase their doses or alter different types of steroids prior to competition to achieve the desired effects.

Steroid use can result in serious physical effects in men including: decreased sperm production and shrinkage of testicles, increased blood pressure, increased blood cholesterol levels, and liver diseases.[9] In women, steroid use can cause increased facial hair, male pattern baldness, deepened voice, and decreased breast tissue. While the effects of the drugs are often reversible in men, this does not seem to be the case with women who tend to retain the secondary sexual characteristics of males after drug use is discontinued.

Anabolic steroids can also produce negative psychological effects. The habitual user often becomes irritable and aggressive to the point of being difficult to get along with. Several court cases have thus far been tried in which the "steroid defense" was used as an explanation for behavior which was violent and led to murder. Thus far, no courts have accepted this as an excuse. And, even when people stop using steroids, they show a greater prevalence of depression, excessive sleep, guilt, and impaired concentration for quite some time.[9]

3. Rapid Weight Loss

Rapid weight loss is another part of the competition preparation of many bodybuilders and weightlifters. Hickson et al.[4] studied a 27-year-old bodybuilder before competition and reported that he followed a strict, high-protein, moderate carbohydrate diet. The bodybuilder "cut" 7.1 kg (15 1/2 lb) over a 26-day period. Some weight loss was lean body tissue, indicating that the rate of weight loss was too fast.

Starvation or extremely low-calorie diets are not recommended, ever. Prolonged fasting or diets that severely restrict calories result in the loss of lean body mass, large amounts of body water, electrolytes, minerals, and glycogen. Rapid weight loss methods can adversely affect health and performance and may result in:

- Decreased strength and power
- Decreased speed and agility
- Decreased endurance
- Increased colds and infections
- Low energy levels
- Moodiness or irritability

Kleiner et al.[11] evaluated the dietary habits of 19 male and 8 female bodybuilders and found that energy, fat, and fluid restrictions were the primary changes in dietary patterns. The men reported consuming high-protein, low-fat, low-calorie diets. The female bodybuilders' diets were particularly low in dietary calcium. The authors concluded that the dietary practices of bodybuilders may place them at risk for future health problems.

Athletes of all levels and ages experiment with fad diets in an effort to improve physical appearance or performance. When individuals are unable to reach their weight and strength goals, they often turn to fad diets. The problem is that fad diets promote quick weight loss, but it is primarily water weight, not fat loss, and the weight is quickly regained. Fad diets eliminate major food groups such as dairy products or meats, are nutritionally unbalanced, and teach poor eating habits.

4. Dietary Concerns of Bodybuilders and Weightlifters

It has been written that "bodybuilders seem to believe that nothing succeeds like excess. That if something is good for you, twice as much is even better. That too much is never enough."[12] Back in the 1970s this theory held true. Bodybuilders constantly put their bodies through radical changes. During the bulking phase, they ate enormous amounts of food to gain weight, then 10 weeks into competition they would "cut" 30 to 50 lb rapidly, using starvation diets, drugs, and diuretics. All of these dietary practices pose potential risks to the athlete's health and ability to perform.

Today, more enlightened bodybuilders take a more "gradualistic" approach.[2] Athletes stay in "contest" shape year-round. Off-season calorie intakes are not so drastic. The bodybuilder loses a smaller amount of weight slowly, over a longer time period. Nevertheless, bodybuilders continue to take part in nutritional practices that have little scientific basis and can be very costly, both monetarily and health-wise; supplements and drugs are expensive and, when taken in large amounts, can be hazardous to one's health.[13]

5. Protein Requirements

Protein is the nutrient most often associated with strength performance. Do athletes participating in strength sports such as bodybuilding and weightlifting require more protein than nonathletes? Studies in this area of sports nutrition are inconclusive.

The Recommended Dietary Allowance (RDA) of protein for sedentary persons is 0.8 g/kg a day.[14] Studies show that protein needs of strength athletes are greater; between 1.0 and 1.5 g/kg body weight a day.[15,16] This level is provided by a typical American diet, as long as adequate calories are consumed. Many people, however, already eat more protein than they need, and there appears to be little benefit to consuming more than 2.5 g of protein a day.[16] Eating more protein than you need will not increase muscle mass and strength unless accompanied by exercise. Without the proper strength training program, protein is converted to carbohydrate or fat and stored in the body, thereby leading to increased body weight without increased muscle mass.

To measure changes in protein metabolism, scientists use a procedure known as nitrogen balance. Nitrogen is one of the products resulting from protein breakdown. By measuring the amount of nitrogen consumed in the diet and the amount excreted by the body, it is surmised how protein is being used. A positive nitrogen balance means that the athlete is consuming enough protein and the body is using that protein to build muscle tissue. However, when protein intake is not adequate, a negative nitrogen balance will occur. In this case, the body may be using its own protein stores for energy instead of building and repairing body tissues.

Athletes should carefully consider the quality of dietary protein. Protein is found in many foods, both animal and plant sources. Amino acids are the building blocks of protein. Twenty-two amino acids have been identified in foods. Of these 22 amino acids, 9 cannot be made by the body and must come from the foods we eat. If these nine "essential" amino acids are not eaten in the correct proportions or ratio, the body's ability to make protein is impaired, which may lead to decreases in muscle mass and strength. In order to increase muscle protein, all of the amino acids must be present in the correct ratio. If this does not occur, muscle mass does not increase regardless of the high level of any one particular amino acid.

It is important to eat foods that contain the right balance of essential amino acids. High quality protein (meat, milk, fish, and chicken) provides a mixture of amino acids in proportions similar to our own tissue proteins. Plant proteins tend to be deficient in one or more of the essential amino acids, especially tryptophan or lysine. Cereal proteins are inferior to the proteins found in soybeans, beans, and other legumes. Therefore, a varied diet is more likely to provide an adequate mixture of amino acids than a diet that limits major food groups.

Furthermore, if an athlete has too much of one amino acid, the body will not be able to utilize the other amino acids as well. This should be a concern of athletes who consume large amounts of single amino acid supplements or high-protein powders.

Although strength training can be very intense, the duration of exercise is short, and protein is not the most important energy source. Short-term, high intensity exercise such as weightlifting relies mostly on carbohydrate for energy. Therefore, if athletes want to gain muscle mass, they need to become involved in a resistive weight-training program and eat plenty of carbohydrates, then check to make sure they are consuming adequate protein.

6. Dietary Supplementation

Many strength athletes have experimented with dietary supplements in hopes of improving performance. At elite or professional levels, athletes are under great pressure to perform and success is often measured in milliseconds or millimeters. Hence, they are often motivated to try dangerous practices. However, many of these same practices are followed at the recreational level, since all athletes tend to search for the shortcuts to arduous training regimens.

The practice of supplementation is widespread among strength athletes. Studies of bodybuilders[5,11,13] and weightlifters[17] have reported a high prevalence of supplement use. Faber and Spinnler Benade[13] studied 76 male bodybuilders and reported that 63% used vitamin and mineral supplements, and 59% consumed high-protein powders. Use of these supplements was recommended by other bodybuilders, not by trained nutritionists. The bodybuilders averaged 19 pills a day, with 1 subject consuming 87 pills a day. There are many reasons why bodybuilders and weightlifters take nutritional supplements, but most often it is to compensate for less than adequate diets, or to increase muscle mass and strength. Weightlifters studied by Burke et al.[17] believed that their training loads subjected them to increased nutrient requirements that could not be met by food alone.

Bodybuilders and weightlifters are susceptible to misinformation about muscle growth and development because they want quick results and because they do not understand the dietary requirements for muscle gain or muscle hypertrophy. Instead, they consume protein powders and supplements in the belief that since muscle is made of protein, at least, in part, supplements will provide extra energy and increase muscle mass and strength. But protein, per unit of measure, actually provides far less energy than fat or carbohydrate.

Athletes need to be aware that taking large doses of protein powders and amino acid supplements may lead to metabolic imbalances and toxicity. Many athletes do not read labels and therefore have no idea what and how much they are taking. A survey of popular strength and fitness magazines reported that the doses for amino acids ranged from 350 mg for some single amino acids to 40,000 mg for unspecified amino acids.[18]

7. Dietary Recommendations: A Summary

A balanced diet that contains 1.0 to 1.5 g of protein per kg of body weight per day, 30% of the total calories as fat, and 5 g of carbohydrate per kg of body weight is recommended for recreational strength athletes of all ages. Many different dietary patterns will provide good nutrition. Most nutrition experts support the Dietary Guidelines For Americans[19] and the Food Guide Pyramid[20] (see Chapter 7) as the foundation for a healthy diet. The pyramid emphasizes each of the six food groups and the appropriate number of servings within each group. No one food group is more important than another. Good nutrition is a function of the total amount of food eaten over several days.

Paying close attention to nutrition before, during, and after competition and during training is important to any strength conditioning program. Contrary to popular belief, protein is not the most important nutrient needed for building muscle mass. Research on protein and amino acid supplements shows no beneficial effects on strength, power, hypertrophy of muscle, or physiological work capacity.

Exercise is the single most important factor for increasing the size and strength of muscles. Individuals need to eat a high-carbohydrate diet and consume adequate calories to meet energy needs. Fluids are also important. The athlete must maintain adequate fluid intake at all times to avoid dehydration. Replacing body fluids will conserve strength and power and reduce the risk of injury.

B. WRESTLING

Like bodybuilding and weightlifting, the training and nutritional practices of wrestlers are specific to the sport. The objective of wrestling is to establish physical control over the opponent which requires agility and strength, but the way this is accomplished varies among the different styles of wrestling (e.g., scholastic, collegiate, international, and olympic).

In wrestling, an athlete needs strength, speed, stamina, and skill to win a match. Therefore, training and conditioning methods often include both anaerobic and aerobic activities. Many wrestlers lift weights to increase strength and power, and run for cardiovascular fitness.

Regardless of the level of competition, there are weight classifications, and certain match and weigh-in regulations in wrestling. Wrestlers often choose a weight class below their normal weight because they believe they will gain an advantage over an opponent or they need to fill a vacant position on the team.[21] Unfortunately, the weight loss methods used to achieve weight classifications can lead to poor performance, poor eating habits, and poor health.

1. Weight Control Practices

The tradition of "making weight" is an integral part of wrestling.[22] A variety of weight loss methods are used to achieve weight classifications.[22-24] Restricting food intake rapidly and severely is one of the most common weight loss techniques, followed by increased exercise, restricting fluids, and use of a sauna. Less frequently used, but more extreme methods are laxatives, diuretics, induced vomiting, and spitting.

Weight fluctuations among wrestlers are frequent, rapid, and large. Steen and Brownell[22] reported that during season, college wrestlers cut weight an average of 15 times. Weight fluctuations of 5.0 to 9.1 kg each week of the season were reported by 41% of the college wrestlers and 35% had lost 0.5 to 4.5 kg over 100 times in their life.

Research has repeatedly shown that rapid weight loss methods can adversely affect athletic performance. According to the American College of Sports Medicine[25] (Appendix F), the short-term physiological effects of "making weight" include a decrease in performance, a loss of muscular strength and endurance, lower plasma and blood volumes, depletion of carbohydrate (glycogen) stores, and dehydration. This will, therefore, lead to strength decrements and may also impair the immune system. In young athletes, weight-cutting practices may alter normal growth and development.

The psychological effects of making weight also are important considerations. One study reported that when trying to make weight, the wrestlers experienced moderate to severe fatigue, anger, anxiety, and feelings of isolation.[22] Depression, low-self esteem, and preoccupation with food were also evident. These personality features are considered warning signs of an eating disorder.[26]

The two most common eating disorders are anorexia nervosa and bulimia nervosa. Anorexia nervosa is self-imposed starvation in an obsessive effort to lose weight. Bulimia nervosa is defined as recurring episodes of uncontrolled binge-eating, followed by purging. Vomiting, laxative abuse, and intense exercise are methods often used to relieve guilt and avoid weight gain. Oppliger et al.[27] reported that 1.7% of high school wrestlers met the criteria for bulimia nervosa, a rate higher than expected for adolescent males.

Although some wrestlers exhibit pathogenic weight control behaviors during the season, many are able to resume normal eating habits during the off-season. Still, at least some of these individuals may develop eating disorders and the warning signs are not always obvious. The physical signs of anorexia — significant weight loss and body distortion — are much easier to recognize than those of bulimia because the bulimic usually appears within normal weight range.[28] If an athlete strives for a weight that is below the ideal competitive weight set for that athlete and continues to lose weight even during the off-season, there is cause for concern and professional medical treatment is recommended.

2. Dietary Intakes of Wrestlers

Are the dietary intakes of wrestlers adequate? That may depend on the time of year (preseason, during competition, post-season). Steen and McKinney[29] found that during the season, 37% of the wrestlers did not meet the RDA for calories. Furthermore, calorie intakes fluctuated throughout the season. One wrestler reportedly consumed 334 calories the day before a match, 4214 calories the evening following the match, and 5235 calories the next day. Many of the wresters did not meet two thirds of the RDA for protein, vitamins A and C, pyridoxine, iron, zinc, and magnesium. The wrestlers preferred foods they believed were low in calories, such as salads, vegetables, fruits, and juices. In another study, Horswill et al.[30] found that adolescent wrestlers who reduced their body weight by approximately 6% had low energy intakes (54% of the RDA) which had a negative affect on protein status.

Tipton[31] recommends that wrestlers consume a slightly higher protein intake (1.5 g/kg body weight), a lower percentage of fat (25% of total calories), and a higher percentage of their calories from carbohydrate (approximately 60%). The daily minimum calorie intake should not go below 1500 calories a day for the wrestler weighing 100 pounds, and no less than 2200 calories a day for wrestlers weighing approximately 185 pounds.[31]

3. Recommended Methods of Making Weight

Athletes will find that they have more power, endurance, and speed for competition if they either stay in the weight category in which they naturally belong or reduce to their best competitive weight (when fully hydrated) early in the season and stay at that weight throughout the season. Wrestlers who are not fully mature should not consider making weight until growth is terminated. In males, this may not be until age 25 when the growth plates are completely closed.

The Wisconsin Minimum Weight Project encourages wrestlers to adopt healthy nutrition and weight-loss habits. This program prohibits wrestlers from losing more than 3 lb a week and requires them to maintain a minimum of 7% body fat. Wrestlers have to forfeit matches in which they weigh less than their established minimum body weight.[32]

The minimum weight for wrestling competition should be based on body composition, body fat, and fat-free percentages.[21] This will provide the lowest competitive weight compatible with optimal performance, good health, and normal growth. The most practical method of determining percent body fat is with skin-fold calipers. Skinfold measurements are more accurate than body weight alone and are easily obtained in a routine clinical setting or from exercise physiologists well trained in their use. Measurements generally are taken at three anatomical sites, the triceps, waist, and below the scapula. Once you know percent body fat and body weight, you can use the formula in Table 1 to calculate the best competing weight.

C. SELF-DEFENSE (MARTIAL ARTS)

Today, many recreational athletes incorporate martial arts training into strength and conditioning programs. Martial arts training mandates developmental balance in opposing muscle groups.[33] The skills required for this type of training include

Table 1 Formula To Calculate Minimum Weight for Wrestling

1. Multiply body weight by percent body fat to estimate fat weight.
2. Subtract fat weight from body weight to estimate fat-free weight.
3. Divide fat-free weight by 0.93 to estimate minimum weight with 7% body fat.[a]

[a] Use 0.95 to calculate minimum weight with a 5% body weight.

From Tipton, C. M., in *Sports Science Exchange,* Gatorade Sports Science Institute, 2, 1990.

strength, flexibility, endurance, and agility. As with most athletes, martial artists view good nutrition as one of the elements of optimal training and conditioning.

Little information exists regarding the nutritional requirements of martial arts. What has been written is often based on ancient disciplines and myths. For example, "natural foods", such as tofu, honey, garlic, nutritional yeast, herbal teas, and wheat germ, are highly promoted while refined or processed foods, sugar, and caffeine-containing beverages are discouraged.[34]

Unfortunately, many people believe if a food is "natural" it is safer for you or more healthful. This is not always the case. Some natural food products may be toxic. For example, there are aflatoxins in grains and vegetables, and poisons in mushrooms. Many herbal teas contain harmful substances which act like drugs when consumed in large amounts. Ginseng, an herbal root sold in whole or capsule form as an extract, powder, paste or tea, is promoted as an "energizer". However, at doses as low as 3 g/day, high blood pressure and symptoms such as insomnia, nervousness, confusion, depression, and edema have been reported.[35]

A person who is physically fit and eats a well-balanced diet will be able to function better defensively than one who does not.[36] A good diet is one that provides adequate calories and all other nutrients (carbohydrates, protein, fat, vitamins, minerals, and water) in the right amounts.

Calorie requirements vary from person to person and depend on body size, age, level of training, and climate. Athletes who are maintaining their weight are eating enough. Calorie intake should balance energy expended. Table 2 shows the number of calories burned per hour for 2 individuals, 1 weighing 205 lb and the other weighing 125 lb, each engaging in various types of sports, including judo and karate. This information may be used to compare activities other than those mentioned in this chapter.

The need for some vitamins and minerals may increase during strenuous exercise, but this increase is small and can be accomplished by eating a variety of foods and consuming adequate calories. Many of today's foods are "fortified" with vitamins and minerals, thus contributing to a person's total daily intake. On the other hand, if you are restricting food intake to lose weight, or omit entire food groups from your diet, a vitamin/mineral supplement may be beneficial. A single daily multivitamin that provides no more than 100% of the Recommended Dietary Allowance is recommended. While supplements can prevent inadequate intake of some nutrients, they will not make up for a poor diet. Athletic performance of all types depends on learning proper nutrition and putting these practices into daily life.

TABLE 2 Comparison of Approximate Kilocalories Used per Hour for Two Different Weight Individuals

	Weight	
Activity	**125 lb (kcal/h)**	**205 lb (kcal/h)**
Archery	268	420
Baseball — Infield or outfield	234	382
Pitching	299	488
Basketball — Moderate	352	575
Vigorous	495	807
Bicycling — On level, 5.5 mph	251	409
On level,13.0 mph	537	877
Canoeing — 4mph	352	565
Dancing — Moderate	209	341
Vigorous	284	464
Fencing — Moderate	251	409
Vigorous	513	837
Football	416	678
Golf — Twosome	271	443
Foursome	203	332
Handball or hardball — Vigorous	488	797
Horseback riding — Walk	165	270
Trot	338	551
Motorcycling	182	297
Mountain climbing	503	820
Rowing — Pleasure	251	409
Rowing machine or sculling (20 strokes/min)	684	1116
Running — 5.5 mph	537	887
7.0 mph	669	1141
9.0 mph	777	1269
9.0 mph, 2.5% grade	907	1480
9.0 mph, 4% grade	959	1564
12.0 mph	984	1606
In place, 140 counts/min	1222	1993
Skating — Moderate	285	465
Vigorous	513	837
Skiing — Downhill	483	789
Level, 5.0 mph	586	956
Soccer	447	730
Squash	520	849
Swimming — Backstroke, 20 yd/min	194	316
40 yd/min	418	682
Breaststroke, 20 yd/min	241	392
40 yd/min	482	786
Butterfly	586	956
Crawl, 20 yd/min	241	392
50 yd/min	532	869
Sidestroke	418	682
Tennis — Moderate	347	565
Vigorous	488	797

TABLE 2 Comparison of Approximate Kilocalories Used per Hour for Two Different Weight Individuals (continued)

Activity	Weight 125 lb (kcal/h)	Weight 205 lb (kcal/h)
Volleyball — Moderate	285	465
Vigorous	489	797
Walking — 2.0 mph	176	286
110–120 paces/min	260	425
4.5 mph	331	540
Downstairs	333	544
Upstairs	869	1417
Water skiing	391	638
Wrestling, judo, or karate	643	1049

Note: **1.** Calculations can be done for 1 min of activity by dividing the value found in the table by 60 (60 min/h). This number can then be multiplied by the minutes of the activity if it lasts less than 1 h (i.e., 20 min of wrestling for a 125-lb wrestler = 643 kcal per hour/60 min/h = 10.7 kcal/min. 10.7 kcal/min × 20 min = 214 kcal/20 min).
2. Calculations can also be done for different body weights by dividing either column by the total body weight to find the calories for each pound. This number can be multiplied by the weight of the individual to find kcal/h (i.e., a 100-lb wrestler: 643 kcal/125 lb/h/125 lb = 5.1 kcal/lb/h. 5.1 kcal/lb/h × 100 lb = 510 kcal/h).
3. The above data can also be completely personalized by first calculating an individual number of kcal/h for a specific body weight (2 above) dividing by 60 min/h for the specific cost per minute, and then multiplying by the number of minutes of activity.

Adapted from *Nutrition for Sport Success,* Swanson Center for Nutrition, Inc., 1984, 6. With permission.

REFERENCES

1. **Katch, V. L., Katch, F. I., Moffatt, R., and Gittleson, M.,** Muscular development and lean body weight in body builders and weightlifters, *Med. Sci. Sports Exer.,* 12, 340, 1980.
2. **Dobbins, B.,** Is bodybuilding a sport?, *Muscle Fitness,* August, 147, 1991.
3. **Potteiger, J. A. and Hopkins, D. R.,** Nutritional and body composition changes in female bodybuilders during preparation for competition, *Int. J. Sport Nutr.,* 2, 297, 1992.
4. **Hickson, J. F., Johnson, T. E., Lee, W., and Sidor, R. J.,** Nutrition and the precontest preparations of a male bodybuilder, *J. Am. Diet. Assoc.,* 90, 264, 1990.
5. **Steen, S. N.,** Precontest strategies of a male bodybuilder, *Int. J. Sport Nutr.,* 1, 69, 1991.
6. **Lama-Hildebrand, N., Saldanha, L., and Endres, J.,** Dietary and exercise practices of college-aged female bodybuilders, *J. Am. Diet. Assoc.,* 89, 1308, 1989.
7. **Sandoval, W. M. and Heyward, V. H.,** Food selection patterns of bodybuilders, *Int. J. Sport Nutr.,* 1, 61, 1991.

8. **Heyward, V. H., Sandoval, W. M., and Colville, B. C.,** Anthropometric, body composition and nutritional profiles of bodybuilders during training, *J. Appl. Sport Sci. Res.,* 3, 22, 1989.
9. **Catlin, D., Wright, J., Harrison P., and Liggett, M.,** Assessing the threat of anabolic steroids, *Phys. Sportsmed.,* 21, 37, 1993.
10. **Friedl, K. E. and Yesalis, C. E.,** Self-treatment of gynecomastia in bodybuilders who use anabolic steroids, *Phys. Sportsmed.,* 17, 67, 1989.
11. **Kleiner, S. M., Bazzarre, T. L., and Litchford, M. D.,** Metabolic profiles, diet, and health practices of championship male and female bodybuilders, *J. Am. Diet. Assoc.,* 90, 962, 1990.
12. **Demey B.,** Easy does it contest prep, *Muscle Fitness,* September, 146, 1990.
13. **Faber, M. and Spinnler Benade, A. J.,** Nutrient intake and dietary supplementation in bodybuilders, *S. Afr. Med. J.,* 72, 831, 1987.
14. National Research Council, *Recommended Dietary Allowances,* 10th ed., National Academy Press, Washington, D.C., 1989.
15. **Tarnopolsky, M. A., Atkinson, S. A., MacDougall, J. D. Chesley, A., Phillips, S., and Schwarcz, H. P.,** Evaluation of protein requirement for trained strength athletes, *J. Appl. Physiol.,* 73, 1986, 1992.
16. **Lemon, P. W. R., Tarnopolsky, M. A., MacDougall, J. D., and Atkinson, S. A.,** Protein requirements and muscle mass/strength changes during intensive training in novice bodybuilders, *J. Appl. Physiol.,* 73, 767, 1992.
17. **Burke, L. M., Gollan, R. A., and Read, R. S. D.,** Dietary intakes and food use of groups of elite Australian male athletes, *Int. J. Sport Nutr.,* 1, 378, 1991.
18. **Philen, R. M., Ortiz, D. I., Auerbach, S. B., and Falk, H.,** Survey of advertising for nutritional supplements in health and bodybuilding magazines, *J. Am. Med. Assoc.,* 268, 1008, 1992.
19. U.S. Department of Agriculture and U.S. Department of Health, Education and Welfare, *Nutrition and Your Health: Dietary Guidelines for Americans,* 3rd ed., Home and Garden Bulletin No. 232., U.S. Department of Agriculture, Washington, D.C., 1990.
20. U.S. Department of Agriculture, *The Food Pyramid,* U.S. Government Printing Office, Washington D.C., 1992.
21. **Horswill, C. A.,** When wrestlers slim to win: what's a safe minimum weight?, *Phys. Sportsmed.,* 20, 91, 1992.
22. **Steen, N. S. and Brownell, K. D,** Patterns of weight loss and regain in wrestlers: has the tradition changed?, *Med. Sci. Sports Exerc.,* 22, 762, 1990.
23. **Marquart, L. M. and Sobal, J.,** Weight loss practices among high school wrestlers, *Int. J. Sport Nutr.,* 2, 297, 1992.
24. **Nitzke, S. A., Voichick, S. J., and Olson, D.,** Weight cycling practices and long-term health conditions in a sample of former wrestlers and other collegiate athletes, *J. Athletic Training,* 27, 257, 1992.
25. American College of Sports Medicine Position Stand, Weight loss in wrestlers, *Med. Sci. Sports Exerc.,* 8, xi, 1976.
26. **Mallick, M. J., Whipple, T. W., and Huerta, E.,** Behavioral and psychological traits of weight-conscious teenagers: a comparison of eating disordered patients and high- and low-risk groups, *Adolescence,* 23, 157, 1987.
27. **Oppliger, R. A., Landry, G. L., Foster, S. W., and Lamrecht, A. C.,** Bulimic behaviors among interscholastic wrestlers: a statewide survey, *Pediatrics,* 91, 826, 1993.
28. **Wichmann, S. and Martin, D. R.,** Eating disorders in athletes: weighing the risks, *Phys. Sportsmed.,* 21, 126, 1993.
29. **Steen, S. N. and McKinney, S.,** Nutrition assessment of college wrestlers, *Phys. Sportsmed.,* 14, 100, 1986.
30. **Horswill, C. A., Park, S. H., and Roemmich, J. N.,** Changes in the protein nutritional status of adolescent wrestlers, *Med. Sci. Sports Exerc.,* 22, 599, 1990.
31. **Tipton, C. M.,** Making and maintaining weight for interscholastic wrestling, in *Sports Science Exchange*, Gatorade Sports Science Institute, Chicago, IL, 2, 1990.

32. Wrestling with weight cycling, *Phys. Sportsmed.,* 20, 24, 1992.
33. **Hemba, G.,** A contemporary application to sports strength and conditioning, *Natl. Strength Cond. Assoc. J.,* 13, 31, 1991.
34. **Parulski, G. R.,** *Black Belt Judo*, Contemporary Books, Chicago, IL, 1985, 199.
35. **Contursi, J., Kleiner, S., and Mielcarek, J,** Nutrient and quasi-nutrient supplement consumption, in *Sports Nutrition: A Guide for the Professional Working with Active People*, Vol. 2, Benardot, D., Ed., The American Dietetic Association, Chicago, IL, 1993, 238.
36. **Wyness, G. B.,** *Practical Personal Defense*, Mayfield Pub. Co., Palo Alto, CA, 1975, 99.

Chapter 5

NUTRITIONAL CONCERNS OF RECREATIONAL ATHLETES WHO CROSS-TRAIN

Ann C. Snyder
Ralph S. Welsh
Robert J. Hanisch

CONTENTS

0-8493-7914-8/95/$0.00+$.50

I. INTRODUCTION

Cross-training can be defined as using two or more different types of exercises in a training and/or fitness program. With such a broad definition, cross-training has many different interpretations and uses. The use of cross-training grew in popularity during the 1970s and 1980s as the sport of triathlon grew. Triathletes, because of the very nature of their sport, must train in three different activities: swimming, cycling, and running. Quite possibly as the single sport athletes (runners, cyclists, or swimmers) began to cross-train for triathlons, they started to perceive that their performance in their initial sport could be maintained and at the same time their training became more interesting as the different activities were performed. Thus, the number of people cross-training grew. The immense popularity of cross-training has inspired some apparel companies to attach this term to various products such as clothing and shoes; even some equipment such as bicycles have cross-training names. In addition, a new magazine has emerged entitled *Cross-Trainer: The Journal of Total-Body Fitness.*

Historically, however, cross-training did not start with the sport of triathlon. One of the first instances of an athletic event which required more than one discipline occurred at the original Olympic Games in 776 BC when the pentathalon event was performed consisting of the broad jump, javelin throw, 200-m run, discus throw, and a wrestling match.[1] Today many multisport events exist, such as triathlons and duathlons (sometimes called biathlons). Triathlons usually consist of swimming, cycling, and running, and duathlons cycling and running, but they can also include Nordic skiing, in-line skating, canoeing, and/or rowing. Other modern day multisport events include the Olympic biathlon event (Nordic skiing and shooting) and the track and field decathlon and pentathlon. To compete in any of these multisport events, one would have to train in each of the different activities. However, we must differentiate between the athletes who cross-train to become competitive for a multisport event and those who cross-train to either enhance a single sport or their health in general.

For a single sport athlete, cross-training might mean combining weight (resistance) training with a running program or it could mean Nordic skiing in the winter instead of cycling. For recreational athletes, cross-training could mean incorporating a wide variety of activities like running, swimming, cycling, and resistance training into a fitness program to enhance health. Indeed, by definition cross-training can involve any of a number of different activities, such as resistance training, cycling, running, swimming, skating, skiing, aerobic dance, rowing, or jumping rope.

Sport-specific training (single sport training) has been the dominant type of training for many decades since the first information pertaining to the specificity of training became available. That is, in general the body adapts to an exercise training overload both centrally and peripherally.

Central adaptations that occur involve the heart and the circulatory system. For example, with aerobic endurance training a greater cardiac output and an increased ability of the body to transport oxygen to the muscles would occur.[2]

Peripheral adaptations that occur are primarily in the muscles. Following an aerobic endurance training program the peripheral adaptations include: increases in the number of capillaries in the muscle (the blood vessels which allow oxygen to enter the muscle), increases in the number and activity of the oxidative enzymes (the enzymes used to provide energy for aerobic endurance activities), and greater carbohydrate stores.[2] All of the central and peripheral adaptations following aerobic endurance training would lead to a greater maximal oxygen uptake ($\dot{V}O_2max$) and increased endurance capacity.[2] (See Chapter 3 for more discussion on the adaptations following aerobic endurance training.)

With resistance training the central adaptations include an increased thickness of the left ventricle of the heart.[3] While following resistance training the peripheral adaptations that occur include: increased muscle fiber size, increased high energy phosphate stores proportional to increases in muscle mass, and enhanced muscular recruitment.[3] (See Chapter 4 for more discussion on the adaptations following resistance training.)

All of these adaptations, both central and peripheral, lead to a greater ability to perform activity, but primarily a greater ability in the activity performed, since the peripheral adaptations are going to be specific to the muscles used, thus the specificity of training.[4] Therefore, if an athlete wants to run faster, the best method of training would involve a large amount of running in the training program. "Crossover" benefits do exist from cross-training, especially if overall fitness rather than time to the finish line is the goal. However, the degree of cross-training benefits will be dependent on the person's initial fitness level.

Depending on the activities performed, one of the benefits of cross-training is that peripheral adaptations generally occur to a greater muscle mass than occurs with single sport training. That is, utilizing a greater number of muscle groups with cross-training (such as including swimming with a running training program) should maintain central adaptations, but could also cause peripheral adaptations in previously nontrained musculature. Cross-training can also reduce the risk of injury, if the time spent performing a single sport is reduced to a safe level.[5] With running, a significant relationship has been found between the distance run a given month and the number of days missed the next month due to injury.[6] With cross-training, the individual activities are usually not performed on consecutive days; thus, the body has more time to recover and the injury rate could be reduced. However, an athlete who performs more than one type of exercise activity is not immune from injury. Thus, new activities must be incorporated very carefully into a training program.[7] One other benefit of performing cross-training that needs to be mentioned is that by performing different types of exercise, variety is added to the training program, and participation and adherence can therefore be enhanced.

II. TYPES OF CROSS-TRAINING ACTIVITIES

As stated before, the specific activities involved in a cross-training program can vary greatly depending on the individual and the goals of the training program.

However, most physical activities can be classified as either aerobic endurance activities (continuous movement activities which require oxygen) or muscular strength and endurance activities (high intensity activities primarily anaerobic in nature and therefore not requiring oxygen). Activities such as running, cycling, swimming, aerobic dance, rowing, jumping rope, Nordic skiing, and bench stepping, when performed at an intensity that can be performed for greater than 20 min, are aerobic endurance in nature. Resistance training or any of the previously mentioned activities performed at a high intensity such that the exercise can last less than 2 min (intervals) would be muscular strength and endurance activities. Both types of training are important for overall fitness and the requirements of daily living.

A. AEROBIC ENDURANCE ACTIVITIES

In general, the greater the muscle mass used during an exercise bout, the greater will be the aerobic requirement and thus the greater the energy expenditure. The muscle mass utilized during an activity will vary depending on the activity performed. For example, rowing and Nordic skiing utilize many muscle groups (arms, shoulders, back, and legs), while running and cycling utilize primarily the muscles of the leg and thus use a smaller muscle mass than rowing or Nordic skiing. With other activities such as aerobic dance and swimming, the muscles used are dependent on how the activities are performed. Whatever the muscle mass, a rhythmic activity, such as those mentioned above, should be performed in order to enhance cardiovascular and thus central adaptations as well as peripheral adaptations.

For the most part, aerobic endurance-based activities utilize carbohydrates as an energy source, with some contribution from fats depending on the intensity and duration of the activity.[8] The lower the intensity and the longer the duration, the greater will be the utilization of fats during exercise.[8] For significant adaptations to occur with training, aerobic endurance activities should be performed for at least 20 min a session with a goal of expending at least 300 kcal (or calories) per exercise session at least 3 to 4 times a week.[9] Table 1 lists the time required to expend 300 kcal for various aerobic endurance activities. The degree to which the central and peripheral adaptations occur following aerobic endurance training will depend on the intensity, duration, and frequency of the exercise bouts and appropriate combinations of exercise training along with planned recovery.

B. MUSCULAR STRENGTH AND ENDURANCE ACTIVITIES

As with aerobic activities, the muscles utilized during muscular strength and endurance activities are dependent on the activities performed. With a resistance training program the exercises performed should incorporate a large muscle mass involving the arms, legs, back, and abdomen. Two distinctly different types of training can be performed with resistance training, one to enhance muscular strength and one to enhance muscular endurance. To enhance muscular strength,

TABLE 1 Time Required To Expend 300 kcal of Different Aerobic Endurance Activities for Three Body Weights[10-12]

	Body Weights		
	59 kg	68 kg	77 kg
Activities	(min for 300 kcal expenditure)		
Aerobic dancing			
Medium intensity	49	43	38
High intensity	38	33	29
Cycling			
Leisure, 5.5 mph	79	69	61
Leisure, 9.4 mph	51	44	39
Racing	30	26	23
In-line skating	32	27	24
Jumping rope			
70/min	31	27	24
125/min	29	25	22
145/min	26	22	20
Rowing	55	47	42
Running, horizontal			
11.5 min/mi	38	33	29
9.0 min/mi	26	23	20
8.0 min/mi	24	21	19
7.0 min/mi	22	19	17
6.0 min/mi	20	17	15
5.5 min/mi	18	15	13
Nordic skiing, hard snow			
Level, moderate speed	43	37	33
Level, walking speed	36	31	27
Uphill, maximum speed	19	16	14
Swimming, freestyle			
20 yd/min	73	63	55
25 yd/min	58	50	44
35 yd/min	47	41	36
50 yd/min	33	28	25
Treading, fast	30	26	23
Treading, normal	82	71	63
Walking, normal pace			
Asphalt road	63	55	49
Fields and hills	62	54	47

resistance training is performed with heavy resistance (70 to 100% of the 1 repetition maximum, 1RM) and thus a low number of repetitions (1 to 8 repetitions) with a long period of rest for recovery (2 to 6 min).[13] To enhance muscle endurance, a program such as "circuit" training can be used, in which the athlete will perform 10 to 16 different exercises at 50 to 70% 1RM, with 3 sets of 12 to 15 repetitions of each exercise performed in each set.[14]

The sets for a given exercise are separated by other exercises utilizing a different muscle mass to allow the muscles to recover in between the sets, but there is very little time in between each exercise (<30 seconds).[14] Since the rest period is short in circuit training and heart rate can be increased greatly,[15,16] some aerobic benefit can also be obtained from circuit training. However, due to the fact that the heart rate-oxygen uptake relationship is much different during resistance training than during more aerobic endurance type training (partly due to stroke volume not increasing as much during resistance training), the aerobic adaptations as measured by $\dot{V}O_2max$ are small (≈5%) compared to those following aerobic endurance training (≈20%).[14,16] While maximal aerobic ability does not change greatly following resistance training, cycling time to exhaustion has been shown to increase 33 to 47% with resistance training.[17,18]

Muscular strength and endurance can also be enhanced by performing several bouts of high intensity activity for less than 2 min interspersed with rest periods (i.e., interval training). The skill requirements of an activity (i.e., Nordic skiing, speed skating, in-line skating) might limit the ability of an individual to perform at higher intensities, and thus care should be taken initially.

The primary adaptations to muscular strength and endurance activities include an increase in muscle size, muscle strength, and ability to perform high intensity activity over a period of time as well as various adaptations to the nervous and metabolic systems. The primary energy source of this high intensity activity is carbohydrates; however, the total energy expenditure is generally less than that used during aerobic endurance exercise since the "actual" exercise duration is shorter (Figure 1). Along with meeting the demands of the exercise activity more easily following muscular strength and endurance activities, everyday living activities such as carrying groceries or luggage and lifting a child, just to mention a few, will also be enhanced because of the muscular adaptations to the muscular strength and endurance training.

C. COMBINING ACTIVITIES

The central and peripheral adaptations of both aerobic endurance and muscular strength and endurance activities are important to the overall health and fitness of a person. Therefore, cross-training if performed appropriately would appear to be beneficial. With cross-training, central adaptations which occur during single sport training should theoretically be maintained, while peripheral adaptations should also occur, usually to a greater extent than with just single sport training. However, again the adaptations are dependent on the initial fitness level, activities performed, and the intensity, duration, and frequency at which these activities are performed.

While little is available in the research literature concerning cross-training, the available information deals with the crossover effects of different types of training. As would be expected from the specificity of training concept, muscularly and metabolically similar activities seem to be the most beneficial in enhancing performance of a single activity. That is, in moderately to well trained athletes, stair-climbing and cycling training have both been shown to enhance running ability,[19,20] while swimming and arm ergometry training did not enhance running ability.[21] Likewise, training either the arms or the legs with cycling activity did not

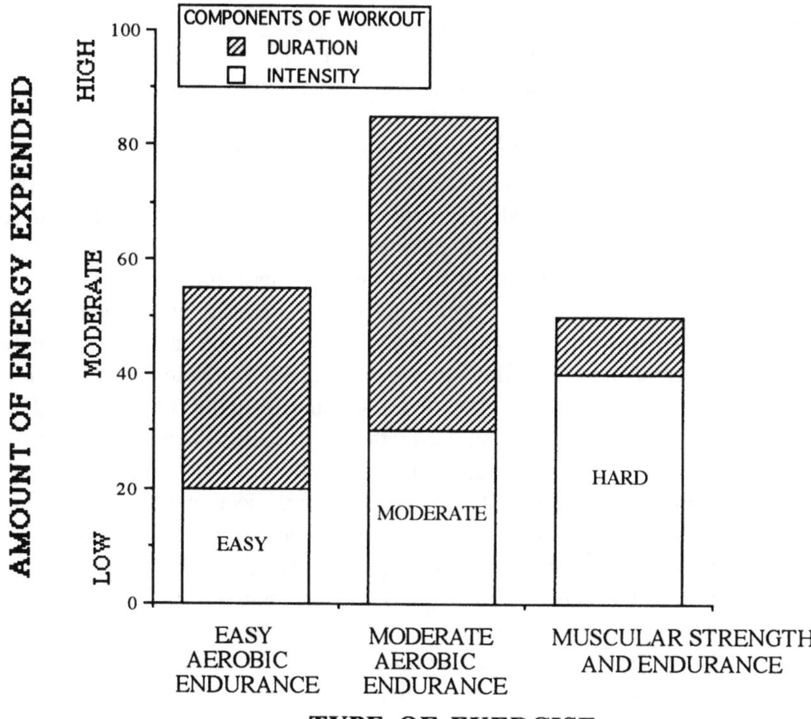

Figure 1. Example of how intensity, duration, and type of exercise affect energy expenditure.

enhance the ability of the nontrained limb (either the legs or the arms).[22] Similarly, resistance training using actions similar to those of swimming (i.e., dips, chins, lateral (lat) pull-downs, elbow extensions, and bent arm flys) did not enhance swimming performance in well-trained swimmers.[23] However, in all instances, improvements did occur in the cross-training activity (i.e., swimming, arm ergometry, resistance exercise).

A number of studies have examined the crossover effects of aerobic endurance and resistance training. When untrained subjects were trained using either aerobic endurance training (5 to 6 5-min high intensity exercises ≈90 to 100% of maximal oxygen uptake, $\dot{V}O_2max$), resistance training, or a combination of the 2 training programs for 7 to 10 weeks, aerobic ability was similarly increased in the aerobic endurance and concurrent-trained subjects, but strength gains were greater in the strength-trained only subjects (26 to 44% strength gain) than in the concurrently trained subjects (20 to 25% strength gain).[24,25] Possibly, the detrimental effect of aerobic endurance training on strength development is due to an increase in the slow twitch muscle fiber (aerobic muscle fibers) population and a decrease in the fast twitch muscle fiber (aerobic and anaerobic muscle fibers) population that occurs as a result of the endurance training.[26] Other investigations have observed similar increases in muscular strength following concurrent resistance and aerobic endurance training when compared to the gains in muscular strength which followed just resistance training.[27,28] Thus, in untrained individuals the adaptations of resistance training may be compromised when aerobic endurance training is performed concurrently; however, increases in strength do occur.

The carry-over effect of the adaptations to resistance and aerobic endurance training when performed separately has also been examined by having subjects perform either an aerobic endurance program (4 days/week, 30 min/day) or a high resistance/low repetition strength program (4 days/week, 5 sets of 4 maximal contractions) utilizing the same muscle mass for 7.5 weeks.[29] The subjects then had a 5.5-week hiatus and then performed the other training program. Resistance training followed by aerobic endurance training resulted in an initial increase in muscle fiber cross-sectional area (following the resistance training), but by the end of the aerobic endurance training, the muscle fiber cross-sectional area was less than during the control period at the beginning of the investigation. Aerobic endurance training followed by resistance training resulted in an initial increase in the muscle fiber cross-sectional area (following the aerobic endurance training program) and then a further increase in the muscle fiber cross-sectional area following the resistance training program. The results indicated that caution should be used in combining muscular endurance training with muscular strength training if muscle hypertrophy is desired since the adaptability of muscle to exercise training may be restricted by the oxygen requirements of the muscle fiber.[29] Others have shown that concurrent resistance and aerobic endurance training have resulted in a decrease in the capillary density (a typical adaptation following resistance training) and thus the oxygen delivery to the muscle fiber.[30]

Performing resistance training once an aerobic endurance training program has been initiated has shown positive benefits. Strength gains in athletes compared with those of previously sedentary individuals following 12 weeks of resistance training were comparable.[27,31] Similarly, adding a resistance training regimen (3 days/week for 10 weeks) to the training program of aerobic endurance trained athletes resulted in a 30% increase in muscular strength, no change in $\dot{V}O_2$max, but a 20% increase in endurance time of exercise performed at 80 to 85% of $\dot{V}O_2$max.[7] Possibly, the increase in endurance following resistance training is due to a greater ability to recruit muscle fibers.[7]

A number of the investigations examining the effects of concurrent resistance and aerobic endurance training have used small numbers of males and females as subjects. In all reported instances, the males and females have adapted to the training similarly.[24,28,31]

Finally, changes in muscular strength following aerobic endurance training have been examined. Initially, no changes in muscular strength were observed following the performance of high intensity (approaching $\dot{V}O_2$max) intervals (6 5-min exercises) for 6 days/week for 10 weeks.[24] More recently, however, cycling at 90% of $\dot{V}O_2$max, 5 days/week for 7 weeks or stairclimbing at 80 to 85% of maximum heart rate, 4 days/week for 12 weeks resulted in increased isokinetic strength at speeds slower than 180°/second.[32,33]

Thus, the types of physical activity to be performed in a cross-training program will be dependent on the goals of the program. If cross-training is being used to enhance a single sport performance such as running, then muscularly similar activities should be performed; however, the overall central and peripheral adaptations due to the added cross-training activity will be minimal. On the other hand, if overall fitness and health are the goal, then the training activities should involve a large muscle mass, with performance in any one activity probably less than optimally possible. Finally, if gains in muscular strength are the sole reason for training, then cross-training probably is not appropriate. As most recreational athletes are more interested in the health/fitness aspect than the performance aspect of exercise training, we will concentrate more on this area.

When designing a cross-training program week, 3 to 4 days of the program should incorporate an aerobic endurance activity, with a goal of at least a 300 kcal expenditure from exercise each day.[9] Two to three days of the program should involve muscular strength and endurance activities.[9] Finally, 1 to 2 days of the program should be recovery days with no physical activity performed. One of the foundations of beginning the program is not to perform the same activity on consecutive days, but rather allow the body to recover from the previous day's activity by performing a different one. Also, when combining resistance and aerobic endurance training, greater adaptations have been observed when the training program had aerobic endurance training on separate days from resistance training.[30] Possibly separate days of training produced greater adaptations because when both resistance and aerobic endurance training were performed on the same day, the total training effort was decreased due to the amount of activity to be performed.[30] Thus, another key to a good cross-training program is not just spending the appropriate time performing the activities, but performing the appropriate activities in the proper time sequence.

Aerobic endurance activities should be performed 3 to 4 days per week. The activity should be performed at an intensity sufficient to elicit a heart rate of approximately 60 to 90% of age-predicted maximal heart rate (220 minus age, but the prediction can vary ±10 beats/minute) and should be performed until at least 300 kcal are expended. The activity could be any of those previously listed or any other activity which is rhythmic in nature and maintains an elevated heart rate. Due to technology and safety of performance, some activities will be more aerobically challenging than others. Lower energy expenditure and lower heart rates were observed when subjects performed exercise on a stair stepping device when compared to running on a treadmill, possibly due to the work rate being less on the stair stepping device and/or that the step returns to the starting position automatically once it is depressed.[34] On the other hand, energy expenditure during in-line skating has been observed to be less than that of cycling and running, as safety became an issue when intensity (i.e., speed) increased with in-line skating.[12] Thus, with some activities, duration will have to be increased to have a comparable energy expenditure when the intensity of the activity cannot be as great.

By definition cross-training is fulfilled by the inclusion of both aerobic endurance and muscular strength and endurance activities. The aerobic endurance exercise performed could be the same type (but may be performed at different intensities) for each of the 3/4 days. However, the greater the muscle mass utilized, the greater will be the overall adaptations; thus, different aerobic endurance activities could also be performed. As training adaptations occur and as time for exercise permits, the amount of activity can be increased; however, probably no more than a 5 to 10% increase in duration **or** intensity should occur per week. Table 2 gives examples of different weekly cross-training programs which alter exercise intensity and/or activity performed.

Important components of any exercise bout are the warm-up and cool-down periods. Prior to the beginning of any aerobic endurance exercise, the body should be warmed-up with at least a 5-min low intensity activity using muscles similar to those to be used during the exercise bout. The purpose of the warm-up period is to increase body and thus muscle temperature to enhance circulation and muscle contractility. Following the warm-up period, a brief period of static stretching should occur, making sure to stretch the muscle groups to be used during the activity. After the active warm-up and stretching periods, the aerobic endurance exercise should be performed. Following the exercise bout, low intensity activity should be performed to allow the body to get back to homeostasis (i.e., near the resting state). The cool-down period helps the cardiovascular and temperature regulation systems return back to the sedentary state. The heart rate during the cool-down period should get to around 60% of the age-predicted maximal heart rate before the cool-down is completed.

Because the intensity of the aerobic endurance portion of the cross-training program is moderate to hard, the energy sources for the activity will be carbohydrates and fats. With lower intensity activities a greater percentage of fats will be utilized for energy, but the caloric cost per minute will be lower.[8] Conversely, with higher intensity activities a greater percentage of the energy will be derived from carbohydrates and the caloric cost per minute will be higher.[8] Thus, from a caloric expenditure point of view, the greater the intensity and the longer the duration the greater will be the caloric cost. However, different goals of the training program will dictate the amount and degree which intensity and duration contribute to each exercise session. An advantage of cross-training is that different muscle groups are trained throughout a program using different activities, and thus overtraining and also injury may not be as predominant as with single sport training. However, injury can occur if new activities are started too aggressively, or if total training time is increased at a rate greater than that suggested.[5-7]

The muscular strength and endurance portion of the cross-training program should be performed 2 to 3 days per week. If resistant training is to be performed, probably a more circuit-type program is appropriate. The cross-trainer performing resistance training for general muscle adaptations should perform 3 sets of anywhere from 10 to 18 different types of activities, with 12 to 15 repetitions in each set. Of course, the number of exercises, sets, and repetitions will vary depending on the desired benefits. Consecutive sets of the same activity should be interspersed with a set of a different activity, preferably using a different muscle mass, and activities utilizing a large muscle mass should be performed before those

TABLE 2 Examples of Different Weekly Cross-Training Programs

	MON.	TUES.	WED.	THURS.	FRI.	SAT.	SUN.
Example #1 Early Phase							
Aerobic endurance	Easy		Mod		Hard		
Resistance training		C.T.		C.T.		C.T.	
Recovery							Rec
Example #1 Later Phase							
Aerobic endurance		Easy	Mod		Hard		Easy long
Resistance training		C.T.		C.T.		C.T.	
Recovery	Rec						
Example #2 Early Phase							
Aerobic endurance (old)	Easy		Mod		Hard		
Aerobic endurance (new)		Easy		Easy		Easy	
Resistance training	C.T.			C.T.			
Recovery							Rec
Example #2 Later Phase							
Aerobic endurance (old)	Easy		Mod		Hard		
Aerobic endurance (new)		Hard		Mod		Easy	
Resistance training	C.T.		C.T.		C.T.		
Recovery							Rec
Example #3 Early Phase							
Aerobic endurance (old)	Easy		Mod		Hard		
Aerobic endurance (new #1)		Mod		Easy		Easy	
Aerobic endurance (new #2)	Mod		Easy		Easy		
Recovery							Rec
Example #3 Later Phase							
Aerobic endurance (old)	Easy		Mod		Hard		
Aerobic endurance (new #1)		Mod		Easy		Hard	
Aerobic endurance (new #2)	Mod		Hard		Easy		
Recovery							Rec

Note: Easy = 40–60% maximal heart rate; Mod = 60–80% maximal heart rate; Hard = 80–100% maximal heart rate; C.T. = circuit training; Rec = recovery day; Easy long = easy intensity of long duration.

utilizing a small muscle mass. Thus, sets utilizing the legs could be performed in combination with sets utilizing the shoulders or the back and abdomen, such as legs (squats, leg extensions, leg curls, toe raises), back and abdomen (abdominal crunches, extensions), and shoulders and arms (bench press, military press, push ups, dips, lat pulls, rowing). As with the aerobic endurance activities, prior to performing any resistance training exercises a warm-up period should be performed which incorporates at least 5 min of a low intensity aerobic activity followed by low intensity resistance training exercises similar to those to be performed during the exercise session.

High-intensity short duration (interval training) activities can also be performed to enhance muscular strength and endurance. If interval training is to be used, 4 to 10 repetitions of a high intensity activity lasting less than 2 min should be performed with sufficient active recovery in between repetitions to allow the heart rate to drop to around 70% of maximum. Due to the high intensity of the activity, 15 to 20 min of active warm-up, using an activity similar to that to be performed during the exercise bout, should be performed prior to any interval training. Following both resistance training and interval training, a cool-down should be performed until the heart rate gets to about 60% of the age-predicted maximum.

III. NUTRITIONAL NEEDS OF CROSS-TRAINING

Even though cross-training for the recreational athlete can and does mean a number of different things depending on the initial fitness level, goals, and number of activities performed, the nutritional needs of the cross-training athlete are clear. As previously described, by definition cross-training is the inclusion of more than one type of physical activity into a training program; however, for the purposes of the nutritional needs, we will presume that the cross-trainer is performing 3 to 4 days of aerobic endurance activity and 2 to 3 days of resistance or interval training every 7 days as described above.

A. PROPER NUTRITION DURING TRAINING

Since more time is spent during the training phase than in competition, even for the most competitive of athletes, proper nutrition during the training phase is very important. As demonstrated by the food guide pyramid (Chapter 7), carbohydrates (from breads, cereal, rice, and pasta group; vegetable group; and fruit group) should make up the largest percentage of food consumed per day. For active people the consumption of carbohydrates is as or more important than is that for sedentary people. The reason is that carbohydrates are the primary source of energy during most of the activities outlined for cross-training, with the relative contribution of carbohydrates increasing as the intensity of the activity increases. Typically, people consume 40 to 45% of their diet as carbohydrates, well below the 55 to 60% recommended for sedentary people (RDA) and the 60 to 70% recommended for athletes.[35] Table 3 contains examples of 500 kcal high carbohdyrate meals.

1. Carbohydrate Utilization and Intake

The sources of carbohydrates within the body are very limited; glycogen is stored in the muscle (1600 kcal for 70-kg or 150-lb person) and liver (280 kcal for 70-kg person) while glucose circulates in the blood (80 kcal for 70-kg person).[36] For practical purposes, however, the available carbohydrate is less than the total amount stored, as glycogen stored in the muscle can only be used for energy in that specific muscle. That is, exercising only the leg muscles results in carbohy-

TABLE 3 Examples of High Carbohydrate Meals of Approximately 500 kcals

Breakfast

85 g (3 oz) bagel, toasted with
 28 g (1 oz) light cream cheese
335 ml (1$^1/_2$ cup) skim milk
(18% protein, 68% carbohydrate, 14% fat)

28 g (1 cup) corn flakes with
 237 ml (1 cup) skim milk
2 slices whole-wheat toast with
 9 g (2 tsp) margarine
320 g (2 cup) canteloupe cubes
(14% protein, 67% carbohydrates, 19% fat)

4 12-cm (5-in) pancakes with
 145 g (1 cup) blueberries, fresh or frozen unsweetened
237 ml (1 cup) skim milk
(12% protein, 83% carbohydrates, 5% fat)

Lunch

1 vegetarian sandwich
 2 slices Italian bread
 28 g (2 oz) part-skim mozzarella cheese
 slices of zucchini, tomato, onion, and green pepper
 14 g (1 tbsp) reduced-calorie margarine
 Garlic powder, basil, pepper
1 small banana
(18% protein, 55% carbohydrates, 27% fat)

1 cup vegetable soup
1 peanut butter sandwich
 2 slices wheat bread
 32 g (2 tbsp) peanut butter
3 medium prunes
(12% protein, 55% carbohydrates, 33% fat)

1 medium baked potato topped with
 28 g (1 oz) American cheese and
 2 g (0.25 cup) chopped broccoli
1 nectarine
(12% protein, 68% carbohydrates, 20% fat) **(continued)**

drates utilized from the leg muscles, the liver, and the blood. Glycogen stored in the arm muscles is not available for utilization by the leg muscles.

Due to the limited stores, and usage of carbohydrates during physical activity, body carbohydrates must be replaced with dietary carbohydrates. For physical activities lasting less than 60 to 90 min at a moderate intensity (70% maximal oxygen uptake, approximately 80% maximal heart rate), muscle glycogen should not be depleted if normal muscle glycogen stores were available prior to the

Table 3 (continued)

Dinner

1 serving vegetarian lasagna
1 small dinner roll with
 5 g (1 tsp) margarine
1 serving tossed salad with
 32 g (2 tbsp) part-skim mozzarella cheese
1 small pear
(18% protein, 40% carbohydrates, 42% fat)

1 serving vegetable stir fry and rice
(11% protein, 64% carbohydrates, 25% fat)

1 serving vegetable chili
28 g (1 oz) part-skim mozzarella cheese
1 serving tossed salad with
 30 ml (2 tbsp) reduced-calorie salad dressing
85 g (0.5 cup) peaches, sliced
(27% protein, 57% carbohydrates, 16% fat)

exercise bout; however, they will be utilized.[35] Activities lasting longer can deplete carbohydrate stores if the intensity remains elevated.[36]

Carbohydrates can be classified as simple or complex depending on how many carbon atoms the carbohydrate has (simple carbohydrates have 6 to 12 carbon atoms; complex carbohydrates have many more carbon atoms, upwards to 180.) Simple carbohydrates are commonly known as sugars. While breads, cereals, rice, and pasta are high in complex carbohydrates, fruits and some vegetables generally have a mix of complex and simple carbohydrates. In trained athletes both complex and simple carbohydrates have been shown to replenish muscle and liver glycogen comparably for the first 24 h following activity; however, complex carbohydrates resulted in more muscle glycogen stored 48 h after the activity.[37] Thus, complex carbohydrates should make up the greatest percentage of food in the diet. Examples of foods high and low in carbohydrates can be found in Table 4.

2. Fat Utilization and Intake

Depending on the intensity of the exercise bout, fats (in the form of fatty acids) are also utilized for energy, but to a much lesser extent. That is, the lower the intensity the greater the contribution from fats. However, unlike carbohydrates, most people have an abundant supply of fats, with the typical 70-kg person having approximately 110,000 kcal just from fat stores (in contrast to the approximately 2000 kcal of carbohydrate already discussed).[37] As most people have a large supply of stored fats and since consuming a high fat diet will probably reduce endurance ability, dietary fat intake should be reduced as much as possible. While many people consume a diet which contains upwards to 40 to 45% of fat,[38] the recommended intake of fat is less than 30% of the daily food intake.[39] As a rule of thumb, if a food item has 3 g of fat or less per 100 kcal the item will be

TABLE 4 Examples of Foods High and Low in Carbohydrates (CHO) Composed of Simple and Complex Carbohydrates

	% CHO	Simple	Complex
High Carbohydrate Foods			
♦ Bananas	91	X	X
♦ Apple juice	100	X	X
♦ Bagels	76		X
♦ Baked potato	91		X
♦ Spaghetti with marinara sauce	75		X
♦ Cherrios	71		X
♦ Nondiet soda	100	X	
♦ Jelly beans	100	X	
♦ Honey	100	X	
♦ Vegetable stir fry	64	X	
♦ Vegetarian baked beans	78		X
♦ Fruit cocktail	96	X	
♦ Oatmeal	69		X
♦ Pancakes (buttermilk)	79		X
♦ Plain popcorn (air popped)	83		X
Low Carbohydrate Foods			
♦ Cheddar cheese	1		
♦ Sliced turkey	3		
♦ Spaghetti with Alfredo sauce	44		
♦ Scrambled eggs	9		
♦ Croissant	44		
♦ Sausage pizza	40		
♦ Quiche Lorraine	30		
♦ Baked beans with beef	54		
♦ Cheese manicotti	40		
♦ Cream of broccoli soup	39		
♦ Guacamole dip	23		
♦ Tofu	12		

less than 30% fat. Of this fat intake, most should be from unsaturated fats (typically from vegetable sources) with as small an amount as possible from saturated fat (typically from animal sources), as intake of saturated fat has been associated with cardiovascular disease. Table 5 lists high and low fat foods and their percentage of saturated and unsaturated fats. Additional information can be found in Chapter 7.

While caffeine has been ingested to increase the fatty acid concentration in the blood, and thus stimulate the utilization of fats during exercise, much conflict and controversy exist over the use of this procedure as an ergogenic aid to exercise, especially since people have different tolerances to caffeine ingestion.[40] Finally, as adaptations occur to aerobic endurance training, greater utilization of fats for energy will occur; however, as shown above, for most people there is no need to replenish the fat that is utilized during activity.[8]

TABLE 5 Examples of Foods High and Low in Fat with Saturated and Unsaturated Percentages

	Fat %	Saturated (%)	Unsaturated (%)
High Fat Foods			
⊗ French fries	50	21	79
⊗ Cheese danish	62	20	80
⊗ Butter	100	62	38
⊗ Hamburger	52	45	55
⊗ Corn oil	100	13	87
Low Fat Foods			
♥ Cod	7	13	87
♥ Corn flakes	0	0	0
♥ Pita bread	5	9	81
♥ Apple	5	16	84
♥ Green beans	6	22	88

3. Protein Utilization and Intake

Protein is used very minimally as an energy source (up to 6%) during exercise when the exerciser is in a normal nutritional state.[41] Therefore, the need to replenish protein as an energy source is minimal. A small amount of protein is necessary for normal physiological functioning of the body and, therefore, the recommended intake of protein is 0.8 g protein · kg body weight^{-1} · day^{-1} or approximately 12 to 15% of the nutrient intake.[42] For active people, the recommendation for protein intake is increased to 1.0 to 1.5 g protein · kg body weight^{-1} · day^{-1}, but the percentage remains at 12 to 15% as active people will have an increased caloric intake.

Protein can be complete and incomplete, and can be obtained from animal and vegetable sources. Incomplete proteins, usually from vegetable sources, lack one or more of the essential amino acids (the building blocks of protein). Thus, combining of vegetable sources of protein is important to ensure adequate intake of all of the essential amino acids. Complete proteins, usually from animal sources, contain all of the essential amino acids, but can also be high in saturated fat. Table 6 lists both complete and incomplete sources of protein.

4. Fluid Ingestion

Because exercise increases body temperature which results in an increase in sweating and thus the loss of fluids from the body, proper hydration is very important throughout the nonexercise part of the day. If an athlete begins the exercise bout with an already reduced hydration level, body temperature can increase more than would be expected due to a decrease in the sweat response, which can be detrimental not only to the performance of the exercise but also to life. Dehydration, or loss of body fluids, can occur with as little as a 1% loss in body weight during physical activity, while performance and temperature regulation are affected by as little as a 2% loss in body weight.[43] Thus, throughout the day fluids should be consumed, not only to replenish the fluid lost from the last

TABLE 6 Examples of Food Sources of Complete and Incomplete Protein

Complete Protein Foods	Incomplete Protein Foods
♦ Chicken	♦ Nuts
♦ Fish	♦ Soybeans
♦ Turkey	♦ Rice
♦ Beef	♦ Kidney beans
♦ Eggs	♦ Corn
♦ Dairy products	
♦ Rice and beans	
♦ Tofu	

exercise bout, but also to ensure that the body is euhydrated (in a normal hydration state) before the next bout of exercise occurs. Recommended fluid consumption during the day would be at least 240 ml (8 oz) of fluid with each meal and at least 240 ml of fluid in between each meal.[40] Thus, 5 to 6 240-ml servings of fluid should be consumed each day. Alcoholic and caffeinated fluids should be avoided when rehydration is the purpose of the consumption as both of these types of drinks can act as a diuretic and thus increase the loss of fluids.[40] In the sedentary condition, thirst appears to counterbalance the need for fluid; however, during exercise the need for fluid is generally greater than the thirst.[43] Therefore, the need to enter an exercise bout in a euhydrated state is even greater. For most exercise activities lasting less than 60 min and performed in a normal environment (i.e., not hot and humid), water is the main ingredient lost in sweat and should be replenished as such.[44] For activities lasting longer than 60 minutes and those performed in a hot and humid environment, electrolyte (sodium, potassium, chloride, and magnesium) loss could also be significant.[44] In the conditions where a large electrolyte loss occurs, carbohydrate/electrolyte solutions should be consumed.[44] During exercise 120 to 240 ml (4 to 8 oz) of fluid should be consumed every 15 to 20 min, with 240 to 480 ml (8 to 16 oz) consumed after the exercise is completed.[40] Additional information about fluids and hydration can be found in Chapter 8.

5. Mineral and Vitamin Needs

The consumption of a diet which contains about 60% carbohydrates, 25% fats, and 15% proteins will usually provide all of the recommended vitamins and minerals in at least the minimal levels. Two minerals, however, may need special attention, calcium and iron. Calcium is used by the body primarily for bone formation but is also used in the transmission of nerve impulses and in the contraction of muscle. Calcium is found primarily in dairy products (i.e., milk, cheese, yogurt), but can also be found in certain vegetables (i.e., broccoli) and also in some fish (i.e., oysters, salmon, and sardines). Many people, both sedentary and athletic, do not consume the recommended daily amount of calcium.[45] In elite male runners, stress fractures have not been associated with low calcium intake,[46] but low calcium intake theoretically can cause a retardation in bone growth.[40] Reduced bone growth can be a significant problem for females who have low estrogen levels, whether they are postmenopausal or secondary amenorrheic, which will be compounded by a low intake of calcium.[40] Two to three servings of dairy products (i.e., milk, cheese, or yogurt) are recommended daily to ensure proper calcium intake.

Iron is another mineral that depending on a person's nutrient intake could be deficient in the diet. Iron intake is associated with caloric intake; that is, there are roughly 6 mg of iron for every 1000 kcal consumed in a balanced diet. As many females consume only 2000 to 2500 kcal (roughly 12 to 15 mg iron), iron intake is quite frequently less than the RDA (iron RDA for females = 15 mg).[45,47] Males on the other hand generally consume around 3000 kcal (or roughly 18 mg of iron) and therefore generally exceed the RDA (iron RDA for males = 10 mg).[48] The type of iron consumed also affects the amount of iron that the body absorbs. Heme iron is found in meats, poultry, and fish and is readily absorbed (≈23%) by the body, whereas nonheme iron found in plants and vegetables is not as readily absorbed (≈5%).[49] Consuming heme iron with nonheme iron will enhance the absorption of the nonheme iron; likewise, ascorbic acid (vitamin C) is known to increase the absorption of iron.[49] Conversely, tannic acid (found in tea) inhibits the absorption of iron.[49] Many athletes, both recreational[47] and elite,[45,46,50] are known to consume diets that contain little heme iron which may result in mild cases of iron deficiency (as depicted by lower serum ferritin levels).[47] Recently we showed that subjects who were mildly iron deficient utilized carbohydrates to a greater extent than noniron deficient subjects, which could decrease performance if activities lasting longer than 60 min are performed.[51] With activities lasting less than 60 min, there will probably not be a decrement in performance if the athlete started the activity with normal muscle glycogen levels and was only mildly iron deficient.

B. NUTRIENT INTAKE AND EXERCISE

With the consumption of a balanced and well-rounded food intake, as described above, exercise performed during a cross-training program should not be limited by diet; however, a few tips about nutrient intake and the exercise bout are warranted.

1. Pre-Exercise and Exercise Food Intake

People exercise and perform competitively at all times of the day; thus, their nutritional needs could be different throughout the day. After an overnight fast (as would occur after one night of sleeping), decreases occur in the levels of liver glycogen; therefore, food should be consumed prior to the performance of an exercise bout on a given day. If exercise is to be performed in the early morning, a high carbohydrate dinner and bedtime snack should be consumed the night before. A high carbohydrate snack (i.e., bagel and juice) or liquid meal (i.e., Instant Breakfast®, GatorPro®) should then be consumed in the morning prior to the exercise to relieve the hunger feelings and replenish the liver glycogen. If exercise is to be performed at noontime, a large high carbohydrate breakfast (i.e., cereal, waffles, bread, juices) should be consumed. If exercise is to be performed in the evening, a high carbohydrate breakfast, lunch (i.e., baked potato, thick crust pizza), and afternoon snack should be consumed. Remember, as stated before, fluids should be consumed at all meals and at least once in between meals to maintain proper hydration of the body.

Unless the activity to be performed is longer than 60 min, there will probably be no benefit to consuming carbohydrate either immediately before or during the exercise bout (unless muscle glycogen levels are low to start with). With trained athletes, the literature is mixed as to whether carbohydrate consumption 30 to 45 min prior to long duration exercise is beneficial or not.[35] Therefore, if carbohydrate consumption is necessary, due to the length of the exercise bout or due to low muscle glycogen levels, a carbohydrate snack should be consumed in a time frame 1 to 2 h prior to the exercise in sugar-sensitive people.

In long duration activities (greater than 90 min), carbohydrate consumption immediately prior to[52,53] and during[54,55] exercise has been shown to increase blood glucose levels and prolong low intensity exercise.[54] Sports drinks which are generally between 5 to 8% carbohydrate are good sources of carbohydrate during an exercise bout with a low enough carbohydrate content so that gastric emptying is not impaired, but sufficient carbohydrate content to provide some for the body.[35] Soft drinks (approximately 11% carbohydrate) and juices (approximately 13%) have a little more carbohydrate in them and thus should probably be diluted before consumed during an exercise bout, as absorption by the body may be delayed otherwise.[44] As cold fluids are absorbed faster than warm fluids, drinks consumed during an exercise bout should also be chilled.[44] Solid foods can also be consumed during an exercise and are generally well tolerated at low intensity levels of exercise. Each performer should experiment with pre-exercise meals and supplemental nutrition during exercise, as unexpected performance impairing problems (i.e., stomach aches) could occur.[56]

2. Post-Exercise Food Intake

In well-trained athletes, muscle glycogen resynthesis has been found to be greatest when carbohydrate is consumed within 2 h post-exercise.[57] Thus, following each exercise bout approximately 300 kcal of carbohydrate should be consumed within the first 2 h to begin the resynthesis of muscle glycogen and prepare the muscles for the next exercise bout. Even though with cross-training we have advised that the same activity not be performed on consecutive days, the same muscles will probably be used to some extent on consecutive days; therefore, the resynthesis of muscle glycogen is very important. Table 7 lists high carbohydrate food sources which contain approximately 300 kcal that could be consumed within 2 h post-exercise. In addition to carbohydrate consumption following exercise, fluid consumption as discussed earlier must also occur.

TABLE 7 Examples of High Carbohydrate (CHO) Foods of Approximately 300 kcals

Food	CHO %
♦ 109 g (0.75 cup) raisins (310 kcal)	95
♦ 350 ml (12 oz) nondiet soda (150 kcal)	94
28 g (1 oz) pretzels (100 kcal)	
10 jelly beans (60 kcal)	
♦ 1 bagel (175 kcal)	86
20 g (1 tbsp) jelly (50 kcal)	
1 banana (100 kcal)	
♦ 28 g (8 oz) low fat yogurt (230 kcal)	80
1 apple (70 kcal)	
♦ 66 g (2 cups) Cheerios (160 kcal)	75
175 ml (0.75 cup) skim milk (60 kcal)	
175 ml (0.75 cup) apple juice (80 kcal)	
♦ 140 g (1 cup) cooked spaghetti (150 kcal)	74
175 ml (0.75 cup) marinara spaghetti sauce (40 kcal)	
2 slices of white bread (120 kcal)	

IV. SUMMARY

Cross-training is a type of exercise training which involves more than one activity, preferably aerobic endurance and resistance or interval exercise, performed alternately. The health and fitness benefits from cross-training probably exceed those from single sport training as similar central adaptations, but greater overall peripheral adaptations should occur. Cross-training can also lead to less injury and boredom if performed correctly. Nutritional requirements of people who cross-train are similar to those of the general population; however, a greater emphasis should be placed on carbohydrate consumption and the timing of the meals. Special attention should also be made to the intake of fluids throughout the day and to the intake of the minerals calcium and iron, especially in women. While consumption of carbohydrates and fluids prior to and during an exercise bout might enhance the performance depending on the duration, they will not completely make up for inadequate nutritional practices prior to the exercise. Thus, proper nutrition throughout the training and exercise periods is required to ensure maximal benefits from cross-training.

REFERENCES

1. **Poole, L. and Poole, G.,** *History of Ancient Olympic Games*, Ivan Obolensky Inc., New York, 1963, 54.
2. **Holloszy, J. O.,** Biochemical adaptations to exercise: aerobic metabolism, in *Exercise and Sport Sciences Reviews, Vol.1,* Wilmore, J. H., Ed., Academic Press, New York, 1973, 45.
3. **Kraemer, W. J., Deschenes, M. R., and Fleck, S. J.,** Physiological adaptations to resistance exercise implication for athletic conditioning, *Sports Med.,* 6, 246, 1988.

4. **Astrand, P-O. and Rodahl, K.,** *Textbook of Work Physiology,* 3rd ed., McGraw-Hill, New York, 1986, 463.
5. **Murphy, P.,** Cross-training may not reduce injury rate, *Phys. Sportsmed.,* 15, 49, 1987.
6. **Lysholm, J. and Wiklander, J.,** Injuries in runners, *Am. J. Sports Med.,* 15, 168, 1987.
7. **Hickson, R. C., Dvorak, B. A., Gorostiaga, E. M., Kurowski, T. T., and Foster, C.,** Potential for strength and endurance training to amplify endurance performance, *J. Appl. Physiol.,* 65, 2285, 1988.
8. **Gollnick, P. D.,** Energy metabolism and prolonged exercise, in *Perspectives in Exercise Science and Sports Medicine, Volume 1: Prolonged Exercise,* Lamb, D. R. and Murray, R., Eds., Benchmark Press, Indianapolis, IN, 1988, 1.
9. American College of Sports Medicine, *Guidelines for Exercise Testing and Prescription,* 4th ed., Lea & Febiger, Philadelphia, 1991, 1.
10. **McArdle, W. W., Katch, F. I., and Katch, V. L.,** *Exercise Physiology: Energy, Nutrition and Human Performance,* 3rd ed., Lea & Febiger, Philadelphia, 1991, 804.
11. **Richard, D. and Birrer, R.,** Exercise stress testing, *J. Family Practice,* 26, 433, 1988.
12. **Snyder, A. C., O'Hagan, K., Clifford, P., Hoffman, M., and Foster, C.,** Exercise responses to in-line skating, cycling, and running, *Int. J. Sports Med.,* 14, 29, 1993.
13. **Kraemer, W. and Koziris, L. P.,** Olympic weightlifting and power lifting, in *Perspectives in Exercise Science and Sports Medicine, Volume 7: Physiology and Nutrition of Competitive Sport,* Lamb, D. R. and Knuttgen, H, Eds., Benchmark Press, Indianapolis, IN, 1994, 1.
14. **Gettman, L. R. and Pollock, M. L.,** Circuit weight training: a critical review of its physiological benefits, *Phys. Sportsmed.,* 9, 44, 1981.
15. **Fleck, S. J.,** Cardiovascular adaptations to resistance training, *Med. Sci. Sports Exerc.,* 20, S146, 1988.
16. **Hurley, B. F., Seals, D. R., Ehsani, A. A., Cartier, L.-J., Dalsky, G. P., Hagberg, J. M., and Holloszy, J. O.,** Effects of high-intensity strength training on cardiovascular function, *Med. Sci. Sports Exerc.,* 16, 483, 1984.
17. **Hickson, R. C., Rosenkoetter, M. A., and Brown, M. M.,** Strength training effects on aerobic power and short-term endurance, *Med. Sci. Sports Exerc.,* 12, 336, 1980.
18. **Marcinik, E. J., Potts, J., Schlabach, G., Will, S., Dawson, P., and Hurley, B. F.,** Effects of strength training on lactate threshold and endurance performance, *Med. Sci. Sports Exerc.,* 23, 739, 1991.
19. **Loy, S. F., Holland, G. J., Mutton, D. L., Snow, J., Vincent, W. J., Hoffmann, J. J., and Shaw, S.,** Effects of stairclimbing versus run training on treadmill and track running performance, *Med. Sci. Sports Exerc.,* 25, 1275, 1993.
20. **Mutton, D. L., Loy, S. F., Rogers, D. M., Holland, G. J., Vincent W. J., and Heng, M.,** Effect of run versus combined cycle/run training on $\dot{V}O_2max$ and running performance, *Med. Sci. Sports Exerc.,* in press.
21. **Hector, L., Green, M. A., Schrager, M., Snyder, A. C., Welsh, R., and Foster, C.,** Longitudinal evaluation of the cross-training hypothesis, *Med. Sci. Sports Exerc.,* 25, S169, 1993.
22. **Bhambhani, Y. N., Eriksson, P., and Gomes, P. S.,** Transfer effects of endurance training with the arms and legs, *Med. Sci. Sports Exerc.,* 23, 1035, 1991.
23. **Tanaka, H., Costill, D. L., Thomas, R., Fink, W. J., and Widrick, J. J.,** Dry-land resistance training for competitive swimming, *Med. Sci. Sports Exerc.,* 25, 952, 1993.
24. **Hickson, R. C.,** Interference of strength development by simultaneously training for strength and endurance, *Eur. J. Appl. Physiol.,* 45, 225, 1980.
25. **Dudley, G. A. and Djamil, R.,** Incompatibility of endurance- and strength-training modes of exercise, *J. Appl. Physiol.,* 59, 1446, 1985.
26. **Dudley, G. A. and Fleck, S. J.,** Strength and endurance training, are they mutually exclusive, *Sports Med.,* 4, 79, 1987.
27. **Bell, G. J., Peterson, S. R., Wessel, J., Bagnall, K., and Quinney, H. A.,** Physiological adaptations to concurrent endurance training and low velocity resistance training, *Int. J. Sports Med.,* 12, 384, 1991.

28. **Sale, D. G., MacDougall, J. D., Jacobs, I., and Garner, S.,** Interaction between concurrent strength and endurance training, *J. Appl. Physiol.*, 68, 260, 1990.
29. **Jackson, C. G. R., Dickinson, A. L., and Ringel, S. P.,** Skeletal muscle fiber area alterations in two opposing modes of resistance-exercise training in the same individual, *Eur. J. Appl. Physiol.,* 61, 37, 1990.
30. **Sale, D. G., Jacobs, I., MacDougall, J. D., and Garner, S.,** Comparison of two regimens of concurrent strength and endurance training, *Med. Sci. Sports Exerc.,* 22, 348, 1990.
31. **Hunter, G., Demment, R., and Miller, D.,** Development of strength and maximum oxygen uptake during simultaneous training for strength and endurance, *J. Sports Med. Phys. Fitness,* 27, 269, 1987.
32. **Tabata, I., Atomi, Y., Kanehisa, H., and Miyashita, M.,** Effect of high-intensity endurance training on isokinetic muscle power, *Eur. J. Appl. Physiol.,* 60, 254, 1990.
33. **Loy, S. F., Conley, L. M., Sacco, E. R., Vincent, W. J., Holland, G. J., Sletten, E. G., and Trueblood, P. R.,** Effects of stairclimbing on $\dot{V}O_2$max and quadriceps strength in middle aged females, *Med. Sci. Sports Exerc.,* 26, 241, 1994.
34. **Luketic, R., Hunter, G. R., and Feinstein, C.,** Comparison of stairmaster and treadmill heart rates and oxygen uptakes, *J. Strength Conditioning Res.,* 7, 34, 1993.
35. **Sherman, W. M. and Lamb, D. R.,** Nutrition and prolonged exercise, in *Perspectives in Exercise Science and Sports Medicine, Volume 1: Prolonged Exercise*, Lamb, D. R. and Murray, R., Eds., Benchmark Press, Indianapolis, IN, 1988, 213.
36. **Cahill, G. F., Aoki, T. T., and Rossini, A. A.,** Metabolism in obesity and anorexia nervosa, *Nutr. Brain,* 3, 1, 1979.
37. **Costill, D. L., Sherman, W. M., Fink, W. J., Maresh, C., Witten, M., and Miller, J. M.,** The role of dietary carbohydrates in muscle glycogen resynthesis after strenuous running, *Am. J. Clin. Nutr.,* 34, 1831, 1981.
38. Food and nutrient intakes of individuals in one day in the United States, Spring 1977, *Nationwide Food Consumption Survey 1977–78 USDA*, Preliminary Report No. 2, Washington, D.C., Sept. 1980.
39. Committee on Nutrition, American Heart Association, *Circulation*, 58, 762A, 1978.
40. **Benardot, D.,** *Sports Nutrition*, The American Dietetic Association, Chicago, 1993,1.
41. **Lemon, P. W. R. and Mullin, J. P.,** Effect of initial muscle glycogen levels on protein catabolism during exercise, *J. Appl. Physiol.,* 48, 624, 1980.
42. Food and Nutrition Board, National Academy of Sciences, *Recommended Dietary Allowances,* 10th rev. ed., National Academy Press, Washington, D.C., 1989.
43. **Greenleaf, J. E.,** Problem: thirst, drinking behavior, and involuntary dehydration, *Med. Sci. Sports Exerc.,* 24, 645, 1992.
44. **Gisolfi, C. V. and Duchman, S. M.,** Guidelines for optimal replacement beverages for different athletic events, *Med. Sci. Sports Exerc.,* 24, 679, 1992.
45. **Kaiserauer, A., Snyder, A. C., Sleeper, M., and Zierath, J.,** Nutritional and physiological influences on menstrual function of distance runners, *Med. Sci. Sports Exerc.,* 21, 120, 1989.
46. **Snyder, A. C. and Clark, N.,** Stress fractures of male distance runners: lack of association with nutritional practices, *Nutr. Res.,* 13, 995, 1993.
47. **Snyder, A. C., Dvorak, L. L., and Roepke, J. B.,** Influence of dietary iron source on measures of iron status among female runners, *Med. Sci. Sports Exerc.,* 21, 7, 1989.
48. **Snyder, A. C., Schulz, L. O., and Foster, C.,** Voluntary consumption of a carbohydrate supplement by elite speed skaters, *J. Am. Diet. Assoc.,* 89, 1125, 1989.
49. **Monsen, E. R., Hallberg, L., Layrisse, M., Hegsted, D. M., Cook, J. D., Mertz, W., and Finch, C. A.,** Estimation of available dietary iron, *Am. J. Clin. Nutr.,* 31, 134, 1978.
50. **Brooks, S. M., Sanborn, C. F., Albrecht, B. H., and Wagner, W. W.,** Diet in athletic amenorrhea, *Lancet,* 1, 559, 1984.
51. **Welsh, R., Snyder, A. C., and Kastello, G.,** Muscle glycogen utilization during exercise in iron deficient rats, *Med. Sci. Sports Exerc.,* 25, S193, 1993.

52. **Snyder, A. C., Lamb, D. R., Baur, T., Connors, D., and Brodowicz, G.,** Maltodextrin feedings immediately before prolonged cycling at 62% $\dot{V}O_2$max increases time to exhaustion, *Med. Sci. Sports Exerc.,* 13, 126, 1983.
53. **Snyder, A. C., Moorhead, K., Luedtke, J., and Small, M.,** Carbohydrate consumption prior to repeated bouts of high intensity exercise, *Eur. J. Appl. Physiol.,* 66, 141, 1993.
54. **Coyle, E. F., Coggan, A. R., Hemmert, M. K., and Ivy, J. L.,** Muscle glycogen utilization during prolonged strenuous exercise when fed carbohydrates, *J. Appl. Physiol.,* 61, 165, 1986.
55. **Coggan, A. R. and Coyle, E. F.,** Reversal of fatigue during prolonged exercise by carbohydrate infusion or ingestion, *J. Appl. Physiol.,* 63, 2388, 1987.
56. **Worme, J. D., Doubt, T. J., Singh, A., Ryan, C. J., Moses, F. M., and Deuster, P. A.,** Dietary patterns, gastrointestinal complaints, and nutrition knowledge of recreational triathletes, *Am. J. Clin. Nutr.,* 51, 690, 1990.
57. **Ivy, J. L., Katz, A. L., Cutler, C. L., Sherman, W. M., and Coyle, E. F.,** Muscle glycogen synthesis after exercise: effect of time of carbohydrate ingestion, *J. Appl. Physiol.,* 64, 1480, 1988.

Chapter 6

NUTRITIONAL CONCERNS FOR THE VEGETARIAN RECREATIONAL ATHLETE

Rosemary A. Ratzin

CONTENTS

0-8493-7914-8/95/$0.00+$.50

I. INTRODUCTION

Fueling the body becomes an important issue and critical component of a lifetime training regimen for the recreational athlete, one whose goal is exercise for health and wellness and not necessarily competition. Questions consistently arise with respect to diet; particularly, what nutritional practices will improve performance and perhaps enhance competition but, most importantly, what practices will support a comprehensive wellness program. The recreational athlete's dilemma regarding diet, then, is unique and complex.

One such unique and healthful approach to a diet is vegetarianism. This chapter will explore vegetarianism — a meatless dietary regimen — which has become increasingly more popular in the American population. Areas that will be covered are (l) a brief history of meatless eating; (2) what is and what is not a vegetarian; (3) nutritional status of vegetarians; (4) a brief history of the vegetarian athlete; (5) how to go about eating a healthy meatless diet; (6) dietary considerations for the vegetarian recreational athlete; and (7) vegetarian periodicals.

II. HISTORY

The nutritional needs of individuals have been met by various forms of vegetarianism for longer than is often recognized. Majumder[1] stated that vegetarianism was perceived as a fad diet in the 1960s and its advocates were identified as followers of various cults. Interestingly, the fad diet so identified has a history of nearly 2000 years; vegetarian historians usually agree that the founder of the philosophical vegetarian movement was Pythagoras, the Greek mathematician.[2] In fact, up until 1847 vegetarians referred to themselves as "Pythagoreans".[3]

Vegetarianism has faded in and out of history since the time of ancient Greece. However, in the U.S., vegetarian practices are usually traced back to an English minister, William Metcalfe, who emigrated to Philadelphia, PA in 1817 with a number of his followers. A Presbyterian minister, Sylvester Graham, was converted to vegetarianism by a member of Metcalfe's church.[4] The Reverend Graham went on to become a well-known health reform lecturer advocating vegetarianism and is most remembered for inventing the graham cracker. In 1850 the American Vegetarian Society was established, and vegetarianism experienced a decline in the 1860s. It has been suggested by Roe[5] that this decline in enthusiasm was due to involvement in the American Civil War.

An individual influenced by Graham was John Harvey Kellogg, M.D., a Seventh-Day Adventist and a vegetarian. In 1876, Dr. Kellogg became the first administrator of a type of health spa known as the Battle Creek Sanitarium, Battle Creek, MI. It was here that the breakfast cereal industry emerged as an outgrowth of Dr. Kellogg's experimentation to provide a healthful and palatable vegetarian dietary program for the sanitarium patrons and workers.[6]

Since the Civil War, vegetarianism largely faded out and had not been widely publicized until the Woodstock generation. The attraction for this regimen did not subside after Woodstock but rather continues to increase. A position paper of the American Dietetic Association that addressed vegetarianism stated:

> The attention focused today on personal health habits is unprecedented, as more and more Americans adopt health-promoting life-styles that include alterations in diet and exercise patterns. Simultaneously, there has been an increased interest in vegetarian diets.[7]

As meatless eating gains popularity, the question arises: what exactly is a vegetarian? It appears that there are as many different kinds of vegetarians as there are types of individuals. In order to avoid confusion, the term "vegetarian" warrants definition.

III. WHAT IS AND WHAT IS NOT A VEGETARIAN

Every individual is on a diet, as "diet" is loosely defined as food and drink consumed each day. Vegetarianism is a dietary practice of abstaining from the ingestion of animal flesh which includes red meat, poultry, fish, and seafood. This dietary regimen is usually divided into three to five types of adherents, and the definitions that follow are those that are usually accepted among vegetarians. The following three types are the most common:

1. Lacto-ovo vegetarian - A vegetarian who combines milk products and eggs with a diet of vegetables, fruits, nuts, seeds, legumes, and grains.
2. Lacto vegetarian — A vegetarian who consumes milk products but no eggs with a diet of vegetables, fruits, nuts, seeds, legumes, and grains.
3. Vegan — This type of vegetarian excludes both milk products and eggs and consumes a diet derived exclusively from plant protein.

The latter or vegan diet is based on a philosophy of life that promotes the desire to minimize exploitation and suffering of nonhuman animals. The vegan avoids foods of animal origin, which includes honey, and products from animals such as leather, wool, fur, down, silk, ivory, and pearl. Additionally, cosmetics and household items that contain animal ingredients or that are tested on animals are avoided.

The two less common types of vegetarians are

1. Ovo vegetarian — A vegetarian who consumes eggs but no milk products with a diet of vegetables, fruits, nuts, seeds, legumes, and grains.
2. Fruitarian — A vegetarian who extends the philosophy of nonexploitation to plants as well as animals.

The fruitarian diet usually consists of consuming those parts of the plant that are cast off or dropped from the plant and that do not involve the destruction of the plant itself.[8]

Mention should be made of the diet known as macrobiotics, formerly known as "Zen" Macrobiotics. It is a philosophy that includes and revolves around a nutritional system which claims to prevent and cure many diseases. The diets prescribed, of which there are ten, are largely vegetarian, with heavy emphasis on whole-grain cereals and avoidance of sugar and fluids. Fish and fowl are included in the lower five levels of this diet. The highest diet, which is diet seven, is composed of 100% cereal. This diet is based on the teachings of the movement's founder, George Ohsawa (1893–1966), who combined Zen Buddhism and Chinese philosophies to create the macrobiotic movement.[9]

Following Woodstock, macrobiotics became very popular. Because of problems resulting from the restrictive nature of macrobiotics when practiced at the higher levels, the American Medical Association strongly opposed this diet:

> . . . when a diet has been shown to cause irreversible damage to health and ultimately lead to death, it should be roundly condemned as a threat to human health.[10]

The followers of macrobiotics have revised and updated the diet since the seventies. They have also dropped the term "Zen" from the name of this regimen. Depending on how it is followed, macrobiotics may or may not be a vegetarian diet.

Dwyer[11] investigated individuals following various forms of vegetarianism, and these individuals were referred to as "new" vegetarians. Also, the term "alternate life-style diet" describing vegetarianism surfaced in the literature around the same time. Additionally, the terms "semi-vegetarian" or "near vegetarian" (usually meaning one who ingests fish and fowl but no red meat, but can also refer to infrequent meat intake) and "pesco-vegetarian" (ingests fish but no chicken or red meat) emerged. All these terms refer to type or quantity and frequency of flesh foods consumed. Perhaps a better descriptor for some of these regimens would have been "low-meat diet" and not vegetarian.

Vegetarianism appears to be on a continuum of a diet consisting solely of plant foods to a diet restricting certain kinds of flesh foods or limiting the frequency of flesh foods. Unfortunately, it is not a singly defined diet. However, when perplexed as to what is and what is not a vegetarian, Dr. Harvey Kellogg's definition can be used: when patrons of the Battle Creek Sanitarium put the question, he would reply that if what you want to eat can get away from you, don't eat it — that's a vegetarian.[12]

IV. NUTRITIONAL STATUS OF VEGETARIANS

There are many reasons for adopting a vegetarian diet, and some include: focus on health, budgetary constraints, religious affiliation, ecological concerns, and other moral and ethical issues revolving around treatment of nonhuman animals. Whatever the reason for adopting and adhering to a vegetarian diet, certainly the most critical topic which needs to be addressed is whether an individual following this regimen can maintain adequate growth and ultimate health. The American Dietetic Association,[7,13,14] the American Academy of

Pediatrics, Committee on Nutrition,[15] and the National Academy of Sciences, Committee on Nutritional Misinformation[16] all acknowledged that a vegetarian diet can adequately meet nutritional needs.

Jaffa[17] followed a California fruitarian family for approximately 2 years (2 females, 30 and 33 years; and 3 children, 6, 9, and 13 years) and reported that all appeared to be in good health other than the children being below average in height and weight. A fruitarian diet was maintained by this family for a period of 5 to 7 years. This study demonstrated that it was possible to exist on the most restricted plant-based diet.

The research that has been conducted on the less restrictive lacto-ovo form of vegetarianism[18-22] and on the more restrictive vegans[23-27] indicated that vegetarians presented with normal blood findings, lower body weights, and lower skinfold measurements. Caloric intake was reported as adequate to low. Macronutrient intake was usually sufficient, and the protein content of vegetarian diets was successful in meeting nutritional needs. The scientific literature showed that inadequate protein intake was not a concern in this type of diet.

Vitamin intake was usually adequate in vegetarians. However, the B vitamins and in particular vitamin B_{12} have been reported as being low.[18] Vitamin B_{12} generally causes concern among vegetarians because the information that is popular in the press indicates that vitamin B_{12} can only be derived from animal sources. Immerman[28] disagreed with this popular notion and reported that this vitamin might be found in root vegetables or in the soil of poorly washed root vegetables, mung beans and mung bean sprouts, comfrey leaves, peas and whole wheat, ground nuts, lettuce, alfalfa, some batches of turnip greens, and fermented soybean products. Immerman stated that although a vegetarian diet is generally thought to be low in vitamin B_{12} intake, a review of the literature indicated that most studies that have found vitamin B_{12} deficiency have been unconvincing. He further stated that vegans who have been evaluated usually have had a normal vitamin B_{12} status. In studies where deficiency was discovered, the vegetarians also presented with other complications such as tropical sprue, hookworms, and partial gastrectomy — conditions which would affect vitamin B_{12} status. Therefore, it was concluded that vitamin B_{12} intake should not be a problem among the majority of healthy, adult vegetarians.

The area of mineral intake should, however, present concern among vegetarians. The literature reveals those minerals that are generally indicated as being low are calcium, iron, and zinc.[29,30] Because vegetarians were so consistently low in certain mineral intake, complementing a meatless diet with a mineral supplement might be a consideration to ensure adequate mineral intake.

In the area of disease, a vegetarian lifestyle is associated with risk reduction for a number of chronic, degenerative diseases such as obesity, coronary artery disease, hypertension, diabetes, certain cancers[7] and possibly osteoporosis, kidney stones, and diverticular disease.[31] Other researchers[32-39] have demonstrated lower rates of cancer, hypertension, and coronary heart disease among the vegetarian population. It is not surprising, then, that serum cholesterol levels were repeatedly reported as being low in vegetarians as compared to controls.[40-45]

In summary, the research did support as healthy those adult individuals who were practicing a meatless dietary regimen. The potential problem areas most frequently reported were low caloric intake along with low levels of certain minerals and vitamins. Mineral intake represented the most serious potential hindrance for following vegetarian diets. The low weights and low skinfolds described in vegetarians are not a major concern, as this would tend to be a more desirable state of health than obesity. Low blood pressures and low levels of serum cholesterol were reported, and again, this would generally be considered a desirable state of health. Low incidence of certain diseases would be advantageous as well. The research on the various forms of vegetarianism generally indicated that these individuals were healthy, and vegetarianism may be beneficial in certain health states where lower weight, blood cholesterol, and blood pressure levels are sought.

V. VEGETARIAN ATHLETE

Heavy meat eating for enhanced performance became a training diet with the ancient Greek athletes. Consider the following:

> Ever since the ancient Greek Olympic hero Milo of Croton won fame on a reputed training diet of twenty pounds of meat and eighteen pints of wine a day (as well as twenty pounds of bread), it had been popularly assumed that athletes required flesh for victory.[46]

The early history of diet and performance is summarized by Whorton.[47] The standard diet for collegiate teams in the late 1800s consisted of two kinds of meat served at all three meals. Also, most training guides recommended that beef be served rare. This resulted in meat being so rare that at some training tables it was referred to as “red rags”. These primitive thoughts regarding training diets appear at times to continue to permeate certain sports even today.

Still, early vegetarian athletes followed a stricter dietary and training regimen than did their meat-eating contemporaries in spite of jokes being made about them. Also at this time alcoholic beverages were considered ergogenic aids and their consumption around competition was considered appropriate behavior. In the 1908 Olympics, for example, some marathoners drank cognac to enhance performance while a walker in a 100-km race in Germany in the same year reportedly consumed 22 glasses of beer and a half bottle of wine.[48] Again, vegetarian athletes exhibited a different standard of practice, and because they were exposed to the health practices of the day and reportedly did not imbibe, their performance most likely was exemplary.

Fisher[49] conducted experiments that were designed to investigate the effects of thorough mastication of food upon endurance while allowing his subjects, nine male Yale University students, choice in their diets during the length of the experiment. All types of food were available, and the subjects were encouraged to eat meat. Some of the subjects gravitated towards a meatless diet. In 1 of the 7 endurance tests, Fisher noted that a vegetarian was able to perform 1000 deep knee bends, whereas none consuming meat were able to meet or exceed that record.

In 1934 Wishart[50] reported the results of a dietary study on a 48-year-old male vegetarian Olympic cyclist, who was tested on a bicycle ergometer. Four experimental meatless diets with different levels of protein were used in this study; however, none represented a typical mixed diet. The subject was reported to have excelled on a high protein intake provided mainly by eggs and milk. This high protein diet was not initially a part of the experiment but was a diet of the subject's choice.

Not many studies have surfaced since 1934. Meyer et al.[51] investigated the effect of a predominantly fruit diet on the athletic performance of 9 university and high school students (6 males and 3 females, 17 to 24 years old). The subjects exercised for 1 h daily in addition to running at least 20 km per day. This training program lasted for 1 year prior to the experiment. The subjects were then asked to run 8 km as fast as possible, their times were recorded, and different diets then followed. After 14 days on a predominantly fruit diet, the best times were recorded and compared for all subjects; however, the results were not statistically significant.

Hanne, Dlin, and Rostein[52] investigated physical fitness, anthropometric, and metabolic parameters in 29 male vegetarian athletes and 29 controls (17 to 60 years). These athletes trained from 5 to 8 h/week and participated in a variety of activities. No significant difference in heart rate, blood pressure, aerobic capacity, predicted $\dot{V}O_2$ max or in anaerobic capacity was found between vegetarians and age-matched nonvegetarian controls.

Few modern studies have compared athletic ability of vegetarian vs. meat-eating subjects. Nieman[53] stated that the fact that vegetarianism is not a single-defined diet, coupled with the impact that training and lifestyle may have on the individual, makes definition of specific influences of the diet on performance unclear. Although this is apparently true, many individuals who exercise regularly are adopting heart healthy diets and, in particular, meatless diets because of the apparent health benefits. Therefore, the next topic emerges: how should one eat when following a vegetarian diet?

VI. HOW TO GO ABOUT EATING A HEALTHY MEATLESS DIET

Before proceeding to recommendations regarding existing vegetarian diets or for those desiring to change their diets to that of a vegetarian, two areas with respect to impressions of vegetarians and the dietary regimens that they follow will be briefly discussed: (1) how do vegetarians fare regarding nutrition knowledge, and (2) are vegetarians accepted and supported by professionals in the field of nutrition? Two studies will be mentioned that address these topics.

Freeland-Graves et al.[54] conducted a study in which 106 vegetarians and 106 nonvegetarians, who were matched for age, gender, residence, and nutrition training, were tested in relation to general principles of nutrition and concepts related to vegetarianism. The results indicated that the vegetarians scored significantly higher in the total test as well as the general and vegetarian nutrition subtests than did the nonvegetarians.

Another study of interest was conducted by Strobl and Groll[55] in which a questionnaire was mailed to a random sample of 312 members chosen from the current membership list of the California Dietetic Association. The goal of the questionnaire was to assess present knowledge of vegetarianism, to reveal prevailing attitudes towards vegetarians, and to identify present counseling practices with vegetarians. It was found that knowledge was below the predicted mean score and attitudes were slightly above neutral in support of vegetarianism. Although respondents recognized that there were economic and health benefits to vegetarianism, they did not support the client's choice to eliminate meat from their diet.

While both studies were conducted in the early 1980s, they are significant in that these data showed that individuals following vegetarian diets were generally nutritionally aware; however, they were unsupported by professionals in the nutrition community. The American Dietetic Association has since responded to the needs of the vegetarian population by the formation of the Vegetarian Nutrition Dietetic Practice Group within its organization[56] and the publication of a daily food guide for vegetarians.[57] However, having been given a brief history of vegetarianism, is it not time for recognition that this is not a fad diet? Additionally, it is time for acknowledgment that the majority of those who choose to follow various patterns of meatless dietary regimens are healthy individuals cognizant of healthy eating patterns. With this in mind, the following are guidelines to eating a healthy meatless diet.

For the transition to a vegetarian diet, simply continuing the same eating pattern except for eliminating meat and/or increasing consumption of high-fat dairy products in place of meat would seem to be misguided and an unhealthy approach to change. If an individual is going to make lifestyle changes in their diet, it would seem that improving their present diet to a healthier eating pattern would be a first step. Once this is accomplished, alterations to an existing healthy diet can usually occur without compromising nutritional status. The manner in which an individual makes the movement to vegetarianism is very individual; some stop eating red meat, then fowl, and finally fish and seafood. Others proceed less gradually and exclude flesh foods all at once. However one chooses to change to a meatless diet, in the process one should follow guidelines for healthy eating based on current recommendations from reputable sources. Therefore, three sets of guidelines are recommended to follow; they are as follows:

1. Dietary Guidelines for Americans[58] (general dietary recommendations)
2. Food Guide Pyramid[59] (general daily food guide)
3. Eating Well — The Vegetarian Way[57] (specific daily food guide for vegetarians)

TABLE 1 Comparison of Food Guide Pyramid[59] to Food Guide for Vegetarians[57]

Food Guide Pyramid	Food Guide for Vegetarians
6–11 servings bread, cereal, rice, pasta	6 or more servings
3–5 servings vegetable group	4 or more servings
2–4 servings fruit group	3 or more servings
2–3 servings milk, yogurt, and cheese	up to 3 servings, optional
2–3 servings meat, poultry, fish, dry beans, eggs, and nuts	2–3 servings legumes and meat substitutes

Note: Both guides recommend limited calories from fats and sweets. Serving sizes are the same for both guides except the meat/legume group; 1 serving counts as the following:

Bread Group	1 slice bread, 1/2 cup cooked rice, pasta, cereal or 1 oz dry cereal
Vegetable Group	1/2 cup cooked or 1 cup raw
Fruit Group	1 piece fruit, 1/2 cup juice, 1/2 cup canned fruit
Dairy Group	1 cup milk or yogurt, 1-1/2 oz natural cheese or 2 oz process cheese
Meat/Legume Group	
Pyramid	2-1/2 to 3 oz cooked lean meat, poultry, or fish, and 1/2 cup cooked beans, 1 egg, 1/3 cup nuts, or 2 tbsp peanut butter counts as 1 oz lean meat ($1^1/_2$ cup cooked beans count as 3 oz meat or 1 serving.)
Vegetarian	1/2 cup cooked beans, 4 oz tofu, 8 oz soy milk, 2 tbsp nuts or seeds (eggs are optional — 1 egg or 2 egg whites equal 1 serving, 3–4 limit of yolks per week)

Both the Dietary Guidelines and Food Guide Pyramid are discussed elsewhere; refer to Chapter 7 for a detailed explanation of these guidelines and recommendations. What is presented here is a comparison between the Food Guide Pyramid and the daily food guide for vegetarians. Both sets of recommendations are similar, and Table 1 contrasts and compares them for healthy adults.

In making the transition to a vegetarian diet, follow the Food Guide Pyramid and eat a healthy, regular, mixed diet. Once a healthy eating pattern is established, one can then make changes to a meatless regimen following the food guide for vegetarians, eating at least the minimum number of servings. Additionally, one can also follow the new Vegetarian Food Pyramid (Figure 1).

Listed in Table 2 are three selected days from an economical 4-week lacto-ovo vegetarian meal plan that was developed by the Vegetarian Resource Group.[60] These menus were designed as follows: week 1 uses ordinary foods that can be prepared quickly and easily; week 2 introduces common recipes; week 3 uses new foods requiring longer preparation; and week 4 eliminates animal products.

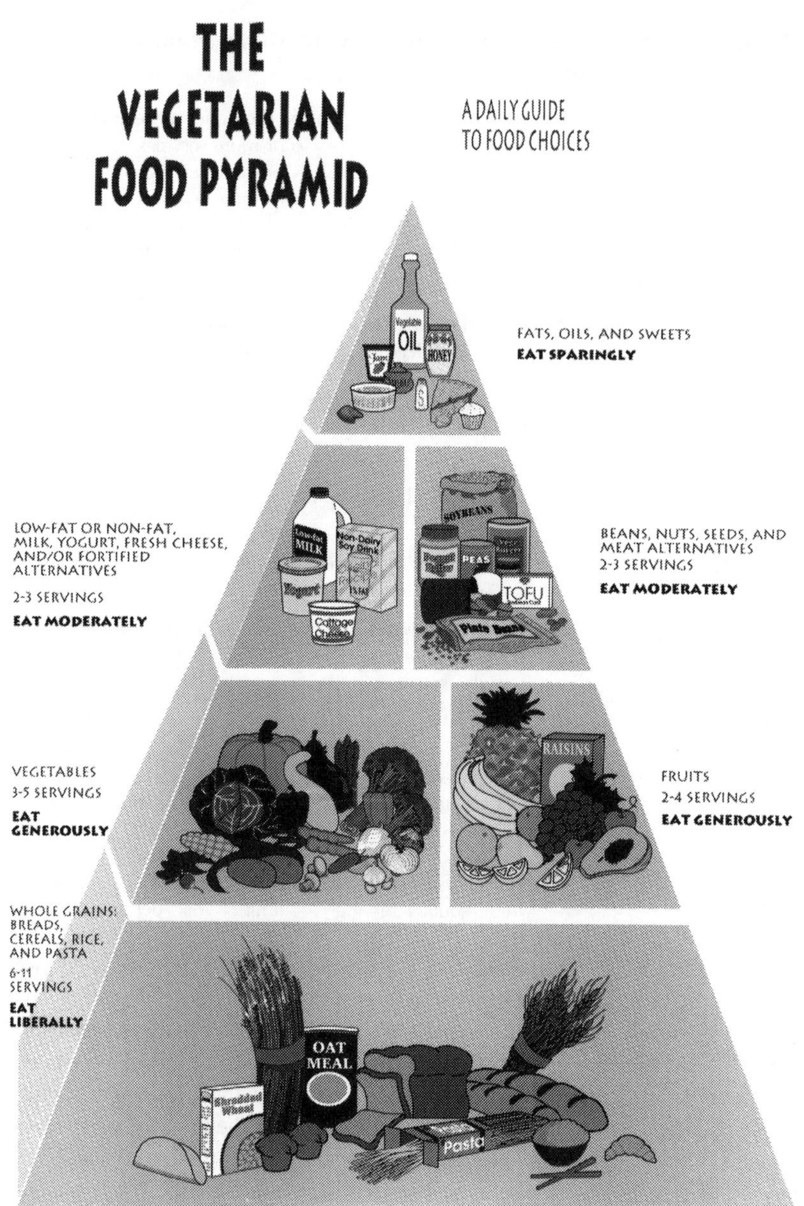

Figure 1. The vegetarian food pyramid. (From The General Conference Nutrition Council, Stoy Proctor, chairman and Merle Porter, designer, © The Health Connection, 1-800-548-8700 or 301-790-9735. With permission.)

TABLE 2 Menu Suggestions for Transition to a Vegetarian Diet

	Day 1 (Week 1)
Breakfast	Sliced cheese, toast, orange juice
Lunch	Peanut butter and jelly on whole wheat bread, celery/carrot sticks, apple
Dinner	Spaghetti with mushrooms or other vegetable, parmesan cheese, spinach, fruit salad
Snacks	Popcorn
	Day 2 (Week 2)
Breakfast	Oatmeal, raisins, milk
Lunch	Broiled cheese toast, potato salad, tomato slices, watermelon
Dinner	Pasta with frozen vegetables, green salad, garlic bread
Snack	Ice cream
	Day 3 (Week 4)
Breakfast	Potato pancakes, applesauce
Lunch	Pasta salad, pita bread, vegetable juice, watermelon
Dinner	Baked beans, Spanish rice, carrots, fresh pear
Snacks	Nut/seed/raisin mix

Note: A heart-healthy suggestion is to use low-fat or nonfat dairy products.

From *Vegetarian J.*, IV, 3, 1985.

In addition to the suggestions in Table 2, other nutrition information pertaining to vegetarian diets should be mentioned. There are two basic nutrition concepts which are necessary to emphasize at this point. They apply equally to healthy eating in general and vegetarianism in particular:

1. Caloric (energy) intake must be adequate to meet activity requirements
2. Consume a wide variety of foods[14]

Based on the findings in the scientific literature, the vegetarian needs to be aware of the importance of adequate caloric intake. On a vegetarian diet, where meat intake is eliminated, a decrease in fat kilocalories generally occurs. Therefore, meeting energy needs can be problematic. Most adults require between 2000 and 3000 kcal/day, with women needing around 2000 and men requiring closer to 3000.[61] Again, the vegetarian must be mindful of adequate caloric intake, and the foods consumed should constitute a wide variety of nutrients. If vegetarians follow these two recommendations, then the possibility of nutrient deficiencies decreases.

Perhaps the most concern on meatless regimens centers around adequate protein intake and the notion that proteins need to be complemented at every meal. The research has shown that vegetarian diets are adequate in protein intake, and it is no longer necessary to complement proteins at the same meal.[14] As long as a wide variety of foods is consumed, all essential amino acids should be provided in the diet. As a matter of course, most individuals complement proteins without paying attention to them, i.e., peanut butter and jelly sandwiches, bean-based soups with a slice of bread, combining beans and rice, or eating a bean burrito. Complementary proteins were discussed previously; refer to Chapter 3. However, the vegetarian should be aware of good sources of plant protein, and they include: grains, legumes (beans, lentils, peas, and peanuts), nuts, seeds, low-fat dairy products, and foods such as tofu.

The intake of mineral elements should be of concern to vegetarians, especially calcium, iron, and zinc. Good sources of calcium are broccoli, greens (kale, collard, mustard, and turnip), low-fat dairy products, and fortified soy milk. Sources of iron include dried fruit, prune juice, spinach, and dried beans. Including a good source of vitamin C such as orange or tomato juice, citrus fruit, or broccoli at meal time will enhance iron absorption. Sources of zinc include peas, lentils, and wheat germ.

Vitamin B_{12} intake will be adequate if low-fat dairy products and/or eggs are included in a vegetarian diet. However, if one follows the vegan regimen, then fortified foods such as breakfast cereals or soy milk should be consumed. Also, on the vegan regimen, attention should be paid to riboflavin (vitamin B_2) and vitamin D. Vegetarian sources of riboflavin include broccoli, asparagus, and almonds. Where exposure to sunlight is adequate, vitamin D status should be adequate as well.[30]

To make vegetarian meal planning healthful and nutritionally sound, it is important to take in adequate calories and eat a wide variety of foods. Also, limiting the amount of sweets and fatty foods will help enhance the quality of the diet. To make the transition to vegetarianism, follow the guidelines and recommendations as mentioned to ensure a healthy diet. However, when activity level increases, what modifications to a vegetarian diet should a recreational athlete make?

VII. DIETARY CONSIDERATIONS FOR THE VEGETARIAN RECREATIONAL ATHLETE

Since vegetarian diets are usually higher in carbohydrate intake, many endurance athletes choose to follow this dietary regimen. It is well known that when glycogen stores are depleted, activity stops and that the higher carbohydrate intake of a vegetarian diet enhances glycogen stores. Endurance athletes such as runners, bicyclists, and distance swimmers who train at a high level for approximately an hour or more a day might find that a vegetarian regimen is of greater benefit to them than a regular, mixed diet.[62] They must also pay close attention to their protein intake as they utilize more protein to produce energy during the activity. It has also been suggested that strength athletes would benefit from a slightly higher intake of protein above the RDA. However, the research is conflicting as to recommendation for protein intake for athletes.[62] In general, Americans tend to exceed the recommendations of the RDA of 0.8 to 1.0 g of protein per kilogram body weight.

Few recent investigations relating vegetarian diet to performance have been published. One recent study investigated sedentary vegetarian and nonvegetarian males who were placed on an aerobic conditioning program. Prior to and after 6 weeks of exercising, there was no significant difference in aerobic power between both groups of subjects.[8] In another study, male endurance athletes were placed on a lacto-ovo vegetarian diet for 6 weeks and then on a mixed, meat-rich diet for 6 weeks. No significant changes in performance were reported at the end of the study.[63] These data suggest that there is no effect of vegetarian diet on performance.

There is a question as to whether or not the recommendations for the vegetarian recreational athlete should be similar to those of the meat-eating recreational athlete. One of the issues in meatless diets is the known low caloric intake of vegetarians. Low energy increases the possibility of nutrient deficiencies. It was previously mentioned that the energy requirement for adult women is about 2000 kcal/day and for adult men is about 3000 kcal/day. Age, body size, and activity level will affect the actual number of kilocalories needed in a day. An athlete will most certainly require more energy and the vegetarian recreational athlete needs to account for the additional amount. Active individuals usually consume between 2000 and 5000 kcal/day. To estimate energy intake for individuals who participate in low to moderate exercise activities use Table 3, based on the 1989 Recommended Dietary Allowances.[61] If the activity level increases, then the calculations for additional energy expenditure can be found in Table 2 of Chapter 4.

Consuming adequate calories to support activity can be challenging to the vegetarian recreational athlete. These individuals tend to develop an eating pattern called "grazing" in which they eat small quantities of food at frequent intervals throughout the day in order to consume enough calories. Some practical suggestions that might help are the following:

1. Instead of three meals per day, try eating five or six smaller meals
2. Increase the number of snacks
3. Eat higher calorie foods

Clark[64] offers vegetarian athletes suggestions to meet the need for increasing caloric intake such as eating two peanut butter sandwiches at lunch time. Also included in her book are many meatless recipes, which are fast to prepare as well as nutritious.

There are sources of information that will allow the recreational athlete to more accurately calculate energy intake,[62] but one can follow several simpler practices to monitor the conditioning response. Weight can be monitored, and there should not be great fluctuations in weight gain and weight loss over the longer term. To determine hydration needs (Chapter 8), weight can be taken

TABLE 3 How To Estimate Daily Energy Intake for Light To Moderate Activity

Age Category by Gender	kcal/kg	kcal/lb
	Males	
11–14	55	25
15–18	45	20.5
19–24	40	18.2
25–50	37	16.8
51+	30	13.6
	Females	
11–14	47	21.4
15–18	40	18.2
19–24	38	17.3
25–50	36	16.4
51+	30	13.6

Note: (1) Calculation: First determine your weight in either kg or lb. Then find your age category by gender and estimated kcal equivalent. Multiply this number times your weight to determine approximate daily energy intake. (2) Example: A 100-lb female who is 22 would multiply 100 lb × 17.3 kcal/lb = 1730 kcal/day. With higher than moderate levels of activity, see Table 2 in Chapter 4 and add this to the daily estimate.

From *Recommended Dietary Allowance,* 10th ed., National Academy Press, Washington, D.C., 1989.

before and after a workout. The level of fatigue during a workout is a good indicator of glycogen stores; undue tiredness usually indicates that glycogen levels are low. Performance should also be monitored and, particularly if no improvements are seen or there are decrements, steps can be taken to enhance carbohydrate intake in the diet. By following these simple practices and observing the body's response to exercise, the recreational vegetarian athlete is better able to determine if any dietary modifications should be made.

VIII. SUMMARY

In summary, general recommendations for the vegetarian recreational athlete are challenging to make because:

1. The term vegetarian recreational athlete is a new concept
2. There are various types of vegetarians
3. There are other forms of flesh-restricted diets that are labeled vegetarian

Therefore, the general recommendations for the vegetarian recreational athlete include those of the meat-eating recreational athlete. However, where an individual is a true vegetarian, then it is recommended that they follow the daily food guide given for nonexercising vegetarians. In addition to these guidelines, vegetarian recreational athletes must pay close attention to the importance of adequate caloric intake to support the additional energy expenditure of increased exercise. The athlete must also be aware of the need for adequate intake of the minerals calcium, iron, and zinc and a mineral supplement may be considered if exercise levels increase to the point of weight loss during a workout. When planned correctly following the suggestions given, the diet of the vegetarian recreational athlete should be nutritionally adequate.

IX. FURTHER INFORMATION — VEGETARIAN PERIODICALS

The following are periodicals that give current information on vegetarianism and meatless recipes.

- *Vegetarian Gourmet*
  2 Public Ave.
  Montrose, PA 18801
  (Published quarterly — primarily recipes; gives 3-day seasonal menus)
- *Vegetarian Journal*
  P. O. Box 1463
  Baltimore, MD 21203
  (410) 366-VEGE
  (Published bimonthly by The Vegetarian Resource Group, a nonprofit educational organization; can order cookbooks and educational materials)
- *Vegetarian Times*
  P. O. Box 446
  Mount Morris, IL 61054
  Subscription Information: 1-800-435-9610
  (Published monthly — can order cookbooks recommended by VT)
- *Veggie Life*
  Box 57159
  Boulder, CO 80322
  (Published bimonthly)

REFERENCES

1. **Majumder, S. K.,** Vegetarianism: Fad, faith, or fact?, *Am. Sci.,* 60, 175, 1972.
2. **Dombrowski, D. A.,** *The Philosophy of Vegetarianism,* The University of Massachusetts Press, Amherst, 1984, 35.
3. **Ireland, C.,** Vegetarian timeline, *Vegetarian Times,* February, 56, 1992.
4. **Giehl, D.,** *Vegetarianism, A Way of Life,* Harper & Row, New York, 1979, 208.
5. **Roe, D. A.,** History of promotion of vegetable cereal diets, *J. Nutr.,* 116, 1355, 1986.
6. **Hardinge, M. G. and Crooks, H.,** Non-flesh dietaries. I. Historical background, *J. Am. Diet. Assoc.,* 43, 545, 1963.
7. American Dietetic Association, A.D.A. reports, position of the American Dietetic Association: Vegetarian diets — technical support paper, *J. Am. Diet. Assoc.,* 88, 351, 1988.
8. **Ratzin, R. A.,** Effect of aerobic conditioning on resting serum testosterone levels and muscle fiber types in vegetarian and nonvegetarian sedentary males, Doctoral dissertation, University of Northern Colorado, Greeley, CO, 1990.
9. **Erhard, D.,** The new vegetarians, part two — the Zen macrobiotic movement and other cults based on vegetarianism, *Nutr. Today,* 20, 1974.
10. American Medical Association, Council on Foods and Nutrition, Zen macrobiotic diet, *J. Am. Med. Assoc.,* 218, 397, 1971.
11. **Dwyer, J. T., Mayer, L. D. V. H., Kandel, R. F., and Mayer, J.,** The new vegetarians, Who are they?, *J. Am. Diet. Assoc.,* 62, 503, 1973.
12. **Sussman, V. S.,** *The Vegetarian Alternative,* Rodale Press, Emmanus, PA, 1978, 10.
13. American Dietetic Association, Position paper on the vegetarian approach to eating, *J. Am. Diet. Assoc.,* 77, 61, 1980.
14. American Dietetic Association, Position of The American Dietetic Association: Vegetarian diets, *J. Am. Diet. Assoc.,* 93, 1317, 1993.
15. American Academy of Pediatrics, Committee on Nutrition, Nutritional aspects of vegetarianism, health foods and fad diets, *Pediatrics,* 59, 460, 1977.
16. National Academy of Sciences, Committee on Nutritional Misinformation, *Vegetarian Diets, A Statement of the Food and Nutrition Board, Division of Biological Sciences, Assembly of Life Sciences, National Research Council,* U.S. Government Printing Office, Washington, D.C., May, 1974.
17. **Jaffa, M. E.,** Nutrition investigations among fruitarians and Chinese, USDA Agric. Bull., 107, 1901.
18. **Hardinge, M. and Stare, F. J.,** Nutritional studies of vegetarians. I. Nutritional, physical, and laboratory studies, *J. Clin. Nutr.,* 2, 73, 1954.
19. **Harland, B.F. and Peterson, M.,** Nutritional studies of lacto-ove vegetarian Trappist monks, *J. Am. Diet. Assoc.,* 72, 259, 1978.
20. **Simons, L. A., Gibson, C., Paino, C., Hosking, M., Bullock, J., and Trim, J.,** The influence of a wide range of absorbed cholesterol on plasma cholesterol levels in man, *Am. J. Clin. Nutr.,* 31, 1334, 1978.
21. **Armstrong, B., Clarke, H., Martin, C., Ward, W., Norman, N., and Masarei, J.,** Urinary sodium and blood pressure in vegetarians, *Am. J. Clin. Nutr.,* 32, 2472, 1979.
22. **Taber, L. A. L. and Cook, R. A.,** Dietary and anthropometric assessment of adult omnivores, fish-eaters, and lacto-ovo vegetarians, *J. Am. Diet. Assoc.,* 76, 21, 1980.
23. **Ellis, F. R. and Montegriffo, V. M. E.,** Veganism, clinical findings and investigations, *Am. J. Clin. Nutr.,* 23, 249, 1970.
24. **Abdulla, M., Andersson, I., Asp, N., Berthelsen, K., Birkhed, D., Decker, I., Johansson, C., Jagerstad, M., Kolar, K., Nair, B., Nilsson-Ehle, P., Norden, A., Rassner, S., Akesson, B., and Ockerman, P.,** Nutrient intake and health status of vegans. Chemical analysis of diets using the duplicate portion sampling technique, *Am. J. Clin. Nutr.,* 34, 2464, 1981.
25. **Burslem, J., Schonfeld, G., Howald, M. A., Weidman, S. W., and Miller, J. P.,** Plasma apoprotein and lipoprotein lipid levels in vegetarians, *Metabolism,* 27, 711, 1978.

26. **Sanders, T. A. B., Ellis, F. R., and Dickerson, J. W. T.,** Studies of vegans: the fatty acid composition of plasma choline phosphoglycerides, erythrocytes, adipose tissue, and breast milk, and some indicators of susceptibility to ishcemic heart disease in vegans and omnivore controls, *Am. J. Clin. Nutr.,* 31, 805, 1978.
27. **Freeland-Graves, J. H., Bodzy, P. W., and Eppright, M.A.,** Zinc status of vegetarians, *J. Am. Diet. Assoc.,* 77, 655, 1980.
28. **Immerman, A. M.,** Vitamin B_{12} status on a vegetarian diet, a critical review, *World Rev. Nutr. Diet,* 37, 38, 1981.
29. **Ratzin, R. A.,** Vegetarianism: a review and critique of the scientific literature, Unpublished master's research project, University of Colorado, Boulder, CO, 1982.
30. University of California at Berkeley Wellness Letter, *The New Vegetarianism,* 9, March 1993.
31. **Guthrie, H. A.,** *Introductory Nutrition,* 7th ed., Times Mirror/Mosby College Publishing, St. Louis, 1989, chap. 20.
32. **Lemon, F. R., Walden, R., and Woods, R. W.,** Cancer of the lung and mouth in Seventh Day Adventists, *Cancer,* 17, 486, 1964.
33. **Phillips, R. L.,** Role of life-style and dietary habits in risk of cancer among Seventh-Day Adventists, *Cancer Res.,* 35, 3513, 1975.
34. **Phillips, R. L., Lemon, F. R., Beeson, L., and Kuzma, J. W.,** Coronary heart disease mortality among Seventh-Day Adventists with differing dietary habits: a preliminary report, *Am. J. Clin. Nutr.,* 31, S191, 1978.
35. **Haines, A. P., Chakrabarti, R., Fisher, D., Meade, T. W., North, W. R. S., and Stirling, Y.,** Haemostatic variables in vegetarians and non-vegetarians, *Thrombosis Res.,* 19, 139, 1980.
36. **Armstrong, B., van Merwyk, A. J., and Coates, H.,** Blood pressure in Seventh-Day Adventist vegetarians, *Am. J. Epidemiol.,* 105, 444, 1977.
37. **Armstrong, B., Clarke, H., Martin, C., Ward, W., Norman, N., and Masarei, J.,** Urinary sodium and blood pressure in vegetarians, *Am. J. Clin. Nutr.,* 32, 2472, 1979.
38. **Beilin, L. J., Rouse, I. L., Armstrong, B. K., Margetts, B. M., and Vandongen, R.,** Vegetarian diet and blood presdure levels: incidental or causal association?, *Am. J. Clin. Nutr.,* 48, 806, 1988.
39. **Fraser, G. E.,** Determinants of ischemic heart disease in Seventh-Day Adventists: a review, *Am. J. Clin. Nutr.,* 48, 833, 1988.
40. **Walden, R. T., Schaefer, L. E., Lemon, F. R., Sunshine, A., and Wynder, E. L.,** Effect of environment on the serum cholesterol-triglyceride distribution among Seventh-Day Adventists, *Am. J. Med.,* 36, 269, 1964.
41. **West, R. O. and Hayes, O. B.,** A comparison between vegetarians and non-vegetarians in a Seventh-Day Adventist group, *Am. J. Clin. Nutr.,* 21, 853, 1968.
42. **Burslem, J., Schonfeld, G., Howald, M. A., Weidman, S. W., and Miller, J. P.,** Plasma apoprotein and lipoprotein lipid levels in vegetarians, *Metabolism,* 27, 711, 1978.
43. **Sanders, T. A. B., Ellis, F. R., and Dickerson, J. W. T.,** Studies of vegans: the fatty acid composition of plasma choline phosphoglycerides, erythrocytes, adipose tissue, and breast milk, and some indicators of susceptibility to ishcemic heart disease in vegans and omnivore controls, *Am. J. Clin. Nutr.,* 31, 805, 1978.
44. **Simons, L. A., Gibson, C., Paino, C., Hosking, M., Bullock, J., and Trim, J.,** The influence of a wide range of absorbed cholesterol on plasma cholesterol levels in man, *Am. J. Clin. Nutr.,* 31, 1334, 1978.
45. **Ornish, D., Brown, S., Scherwitz, L., Billings, J., Armstrong, W., Ports, T., McLanahan, S., Kirkeeide, R., Brand, R., and Gould, K. L.,** Can lifestyle changes reverse coronary heart disease?, *Lancet,* 336, 129, 1990.
46. **Whorton, J. C.,** *Crusaders for Fitness, the History of American Health Reforms,* Princeton University Press, New Jersey, 1982, 227.
47. **Whorton, J. C.,** Muscular vegetarianism: the debate over diet and athletic performance in the progressive era, *J. Sport History,* 8, 58, 1981.

48. **Whorton, J. C.,** *Crusaders for Fitness, the History of American Health Reforms,* Princeton University Press, New Jersey, 1982, 233.
49. **Fisher, I.,** The effect of diet on endurance, based on an experiment with nine healthy students at Yale University, *Conn. Acad. Arts Sci.,* 13, 1, 1906.
50. **Wishart, G. M.,** The efficiency and performance of a vegetarian racing cyclist under different dietary conditions, *J. Physiol.,* 82, 189, 1934.
51. **Meyer, B. J., de Bruin, E. J. P., Brown, J. M. M., Bieler, E. U., Meyer, A. C., and Grey, P. R.,** The effect of a predominantly fruit diet on athletic performance, *Plant Foods for Man,* 1, 239, 1975.
52. **Hanne, N., Dlin, R., and Rostein, A.,** Physical fitness, anthropometric and metabolic parameters in athletes, *J. Sports Med.,* 26, 180–185, 1986.
53. **Nieman, D. C.,** Vegetarian dietary practices and endurance performance, *Am. J. Clin. Nutr.,* 48, 754, 1988.
54. **Freeland-Graves, J. H., Greninger, S. A., Vickers, J., Bradley, C. L., and Young, R. K.,** Nutrition knowledge of vegetarians and non-vegetarians, *J. Nutr. Educ.,* 14, 21, 1982.
55. **Strobl, C. M. and Groll, L,** Professional knowledge and attitudes on vegetarianism: implications for practice, *J. Am. Diet. Assoc.,* 79, 568, 1981.
56. VEGEDINE, Association of Vegetarian Dietitians and Nutrition Educators, *Issues in Vegetarian Dietetics,* IV, 1, 1990.
57. American Dietetic Association, *Eating Well — The Vegetarian Way,* Chicago, 1992.
58. U. S. Department of Agriculture and U. S. Department of Health and Human Services, *Nutrition and Your Health: Dietary Guidelines for Americans,* 3rd ed., Washington, D.C., 1990.
59. U. S. Department of Agriculture and U. S. Department of Health and Human Services, *Food Guide Pyramid, A Guide to Daily Food Choices,* Washington, D.C., 1991.
60. Four weeks of menus, *Vegetarian J.,* IV, 3, 1985.
61. Food and Nutrition Board, *Recommended Dietary Allowance,* 10th ed., National Academy Press, Washington, D.C., 1989.
62. **Williams, M. H.,** *Nutrition for Fitness and Sport,* 3rd ed., Wm. C. Brown Pub., Dubuque, IA, 1992, chap. 12.
63. **Raben, A., Kiens, B., Richter, E. A., Rasmussen, L. B., Svenstrup, B., Micic, S., and Bennett, P.,** Serum sex hormones and endurance performance after a lacto-ovo vegetarian and a mixed diet, *Med. Sci. Sports Exerc.,* 24, 1290, 1992.
64. **Clark, N.,** *Nancy Clark's Sports Nutrition Guidebook,* Leisure Press, Champaign, IL, 1990.

Chapter 7

SPECIAL CONSIDERATIONS FOR THE POST-HEART ATTACK RECREATIONAL ATHLETE TO REDUCE DIETARY RISKS OF HEART DISEASE

Jennifer Anderson

CONTENTS

0-8493-7914-8/95/$0.00+$.50

I. INTRODUCTION

Experiencing a heart attack or myocardial infarction is a warning to the affected individual. The survivor is given a new lease on life and a golden opportunity to make simple changes in lifestyle that will improve the odds it will not happen again.

Heart disease is known as a lifestyle disease. We develop it, in part, because of certain habits or a way of living that we have. These habits are under our control and we can change them. Many individuals can reduce the level of the cholesterol in the blood to a safe level by making a food change in what and how they eat. Combined with increased activity and terminated smoking the contribution of these lifestyle risk factors to heart disease can be diminished. Diabetes and hypertension (high blood pressure) are also risk factors for heart disease, but they are not habits, rather diseases that we can control with diet and perhaps medication. Exercise is also used to help control hypertension and the position statement of the American College of Sports Medicine can be found in Appendix D.

Most postinfarct patients participate in a supervised cardiac rehabilitation program where they have followed a carefully constructed exercise plan. They often then become recreational athletes of many types with aerobic exercise most often being the activity of choice. Aerobic exercise is known to diminish the risk

TABLE 1 Types of Foods To Increase and Decrease in the Diet To Reduce Cardiovascular Disease Risk Factors

	Category of Food	Examples of Foods
Increase	↑ Nutrient-dense food	Lean meats, low-fat dairy, vegetables, legumes
	↑ Fiber-rich food	Dried peas, beans, whole-grain breads, whole-grain cereals, fruits, vegetables
	↑ A variety of foods	
Decrease	↓ Fatty foods	Animal fat, butter, margarine, oil, shortening, peanut butter, nuts
	↓ High cholesterol foods	Egg yolk, whole milk, cream, cheese, shrimp
	↓ Sugary foods	Doughnuts, pastries, cookies, cakes
	↓ Salty foods	Chips, cheese, processed meats, pickled foods
	↓ Too much food	

factors for cardiovascular disease if done properly. The current recommendations suggested by the American College of Sports Medicine can be found in Appendix G. The question then often becomes what to eat and how to follow the advice of the hospital or rehabilitation registered dietitian. Making changes in shopping, cooking, and eating will be the key to success in reducing dietary contributions to risk factors for cardiovascular disease. This chapter will review current recommendations and make suggestions for positive dietary lifestyle changes.

II. FOOD RISK FACTORS

Just a few changes in what and how much you eat can usually decrease your blood cholesterol levels. Positive changes can occur if certain types of foods are either increased or decreased in the diet as illustrated in Table 1.[1]

Fats (Triglycerides, Saturated, Monounsaturated, and Polyunsaturated Fats) — Too much fat in the food you eat can end up as fatty deposits in veins, arteries, and the heart, which lessen the flow of blood or close it off altogether. Too much fatty food may also make you overweight. There is no evidence that the body needs as much fat as Americans eat.

Cholesterol — A high level of cholesterol in the blood (serum cholesterol) has long been associated with heart disease. Most people with atherosclerosis have an increased serum cholesterol level. Research indicates that one of the factors that contributes to high serum cholesterol is diet — eating either food with high cholesterol levels or food containing too much fat, especially saturated fat.

Sugar, Salt — Americans tend to eat too much sugar and salt. The U.S. Dietary Guidelines recommend that consumption of salt and sugar be decreased.[2] Sugary foods provide mainly calories without vitamins or other essential nutrients and may contribute to obesity. The connection between salt consumption and hypertension has not been firmly established but is important for those persons sensitive to sodium (salt) or who have hypertension to decrease intake.

Overweight —Weight adds to the effect of all of the other risk factors, making them doubly serious. Excess body weight in the form of subcutaneous fat increases the work of the heart, as it must push more blood through more territory. People who are overweight often have high blood pressure and higher levels of cholesterol and triglycerides in their blood. Reducing weight often diminishes the level of fats in the blood, lowers blood pressure, and improves glucose intolerance. Extra pounds carried around the middle and upper body now appears to be of greater risk where heart disease is of concern than that excess carried on the thighs. A person with a "pear shape" or triangular silhouette is at lower risk of heart disease than a person with an "apple shape" or inverted triangle silhouette.

A. HEART HEALTH FACTORS

There is a tendency to think only about the things that are hazardous to our health and not about the positive things a person can do to improve his/her well-being. Food can have a very positive effect; the results are unlikely to be sudden or dramatic, but they are sure.

1. Basic Balance

One of the best defenses against disease is a good, balanced diet. A balanced diet is one of wide variety to supply protein, vitamins, and minerals, as well as fats and carbohydrates, so that the body is maintained in top working condition. When the body is in such excellent shape, it is more able to handle stress and to fight off disease.

2. Nutrient-Dense Foods

Getting enough nutrients each day without consuming too many calories at the same time is of concern in our sedentary society. A major benefit of exercise is simply the fact that there is a need for more calories. Foods that are high in protein, vitamins, and minerals for the amount of calories they have are often referred to as nutrient-dense foods and, when added to exercise, can lead to a stable weight and a reduction of cardiovascular risk factors.

3. Fiber

Dietary fiber is composed of the tough cell walls of plant foods; it is not usually broken down by the digestion process for use in the body but, instead, passes on through and is excreted. It is also capable of absorbing water and other substances as it traverses the intestines. Major sources of dietary fiber are fruits, vegetables, nuts, and whole grain products. Fiber has recently received considerable attention because of its possible benefit in lowering blood cholesterol and preventing certain diseases of the digestive system such as constipation, colon-rectal cancer, and diverticulosis. Research shows that soluble fiber reduces the cholesterol level in the blood, and insoluble fiber helps maintain a healthy digestive system. Oat bran, legumes, and pectin are high in soluble fiber and show the most promise in lowering blood cholesterol levels.

4. Antioxidants

Beta carotene, the precursor of Vitamin A, Vitamin C, and Vitamin E are the three major nutrients whose properties are related to a decreased risk of heart disease and cancer. Vitamin E research is especially exciting for heart disease and shows that there is a greater effect of this nutrient on cardiovascular disease than has previously been recognized. More research is needed to truly document safe and effective levels of intake, but it is recommended that everyone consumes at least five servings of fruit and vegetables a day. Fruits and vegetables are rich in all antioxidants while whole grains are also rich in Vitamin E. All of the above concepts will be reviewed in greater detail and will be put into the context of a simple eating plan.

III. NUTRITION RECOMMENDATIONS

A. DIETARY GUIDELINES

First let us review the following recommendations that are drawn from the American Heart Association, the National Heart, Lung and Blood Institute (NHLBI) National Cholesterol Education Program, and the U.S. Dietary Guidelines.[2-4] Table 2 is a compilation of all of the current recommendations.

The National Heart, Lung and Blood Institute (NHLBI) of the National Institutes of Health (NIH) has a recommended intake of fat, carbohydrate, protein, and dietary cholesterol.[4] The high intake of saturated fat, dietary cholesterol, and calories are noted as the three dietary habits that typically contribute significantly to elevated blood cholesterol. Table 3 depicts these recommendations from the National Cholesterol Education Program of NHLBI, NIH.

A postinfarct or heart attack patient can benefit from following the Step II diet shown in Table 3 where saturated fat is less than 7% of total calories and dietary cholesterol is less than 200 mg/day. Cutting fat to less than 30% of total calories is a goal everyone should attempt to achieve whether the person has had a heart attack or not. If one has already had a heart attack, reducing fat to 20 to 25% of total calories is a goal to set. Table 4 gives guidelines for how to achieve these levels of fat.

As fat is so important and it is its control that will yield the most positive results, an explanation of the types of fat will aid understanding. "Saturated" and "unsaturated" are chemical terms that describe the fats in our foods. They refer to how much hydrogen is attached to the fat molecule. Table 5 illustrates the differences among fats, their characteristics, and their effects on health.

1. Cholesterol

Cholesterol is a waxy substance that is manufactured in the body and is present in certain foods we eat. In food, it is known as dietary cholesterol; when it is being transported in the blood, it is called serum cholesterol. It aids in several important body functions: forming Vitamin D (with the help of sunshine); aiding

TABLE 2 Combined Dietary Guidelines for Reduction of Cardiovascular Risk Factors from the American Heart Association, the National Heart, Lung And Blood Institute, and the U.S. Dietary Guidelines

What You Eat

1. Eat only as many calories as you need to keep your ideal body weight.
2. Reduce total fat.
3. Reduce cholesterol-rich foods.
4. Meet your carbohydrate needs with complex carbohydrates rather than with sugars.
5. Increase nutrient-dense and fiber-packed foods.

How You Eat

1. Avoid fat "binges" or frequent high-fat meals; instead, spread your fat calories throughout each day and week.
2. Eat breakfast.
3. Have regular meals at set times (3 or more).
4. Take time to fix and serve heart healthy food in attractive, tasty ways, so that meals are pleasurable.

Specific Recommendations from the American Heart Association:

1. Saturated fat intake should be less than 10% of calories.
2. Total fat intake should be less than 30% of calories.
3. Cholesterol intake should be less than 100 mg/1000 cal, not to exceed 300 mg/day.
4. Protein intake should be approximately 15% of calories.
5. Carbohydrate intake should constitute 50 to 55% or more of calories, with emphasis on increased complex carbohydrates.
6. Sodium intake should be reduced to approximately 1 g/1000 cal, not to exceed 3 g/day.
7. If alcoholic beverages are consumed, the caloric intake from this source should be limited to 15% of total calories but should not exceed 50 ml of ethanol per day.

TABLE 3 Step I and Step II Dietary Recommendation from the NHLBI of NIH To Reduce Blood Cholesterol

	Recommended Intake (% of total calories)	
Nutrient	**Step I Diet**	**Step II Diet**
Total Fat	<30	<30
Saturated	8–10	<7
Polyunsaturated	Up to 10	Up to 10
Monounsaturated	10–15	10–15
Carbohydrates	50–60	50–60
Protein	10–20	10–20
Dietary cholesterol	<300 mg/d	<200 mg/d
Total calories	Amount to achieve and maintain desirable wt.	

digestion by forming bile acids in the liver; making steroid hormones, such as estrogen; and building brain, nerve, and other tissues. Although some serum cholesterol is necessary, too much of it can accumulate and clog the arteries, causing atherosclerosis.

TABLE 4 How To Plan a Diet To Include 30 Percent of Calories from Fat Daily

Participants	Total Calories	Calories from Fat	Grams of Fat	Teaspoons of Fat[a]
Male athlete	3000–4000	900–1200	100–133	20–27
Active adult male	2500–3000	750–900	83–100	17–20
Adult male or active female	2000–2500	600–750	67–83	13–17
Adult female or elderly male	1500–2000	450–600	50–67	10–13
"Dieting" adult or elderly female	1000–1500	300–450	33–50	6–10

[a] Fats do not always come in teaspoons, but all fat must be counted in what you eat each day. For example, the fat in a hot dog cannot be measured with a teaspoon, but may be a large source of fat contributing 3 tsp/2 oz hot dog. A teaspoon of fat contains about 45 cal and 5 g. The number of teaspoons of fat that are prudent depends on how many calories you eat.

TABLE 5 Definitions of Polyunsaturated, Monounsaturated, and Saturated Fats and Their Characteristics

	Polyunsaturated	Monunsaturated	Saturated
Different fats have different amounts of hydrogen atoms	Polyunsaturated fats (oils) are missing many atoms.	Monounsaturated fats (oils) are missing only two atoms.	Saturated fats are filled with hydrogen.
How they affect our health	In most people, monounsaturated and polyunsaturated fats tend to lower blood cholesterol.		In most people, saturates tend to raise cholesterol.
At room temperature	Polyunsaturated and monounsaturated fats are liquid (so we call them oils)		Saturated fats are usually solid or firm.
Where they come from	Mostly from plants	Mostly from plants	Mostly from animals, some from plants
Examples	Safflower oil, corn oil, sunflower oil, soybean oil, cotton-seed oil, sesame oil	Olive oil, canola oil	Fat in meat, butter, lard, cheese, whole milk (cream)
Hydrogenating oils add hydrogen atoms that make oil firm like margarine			Also some from plants, coconut oil, palm oil, cocoa butter (in chocolate) Hydrogenated vegetable oil

Cholesterol levels are often high in the individual who has just had a heart attack. Levels below 200 mg/dl are classified as "desirable blood cholesterol", those 200 to 239 mg/dl as "borderline-high blood cholesterol", and those 240 mg/dl and above "high blood cholesterol".[4] These are total cholesterol values. A component of total cholesterol, LDL (Low Density Lipoprotein)-cholesterol, is a definite risk factor for heart disease. Levels of LDL-cholesterol of 160 mg/dl or greater are classified as "high-risk LDL-cholesterol", and those 130–159 mg/dl are "borderline-high-risk".

TABLE 6 Cholesterol Content in Foods

High Cholesterol	No Cholesterol
⊗ Liver, heart, tongue	♥ Plant and vegetable oils
⊗ Egg yolk	♥ Margarine
⊗ Sweetbreads	♥ Peanut butter
⊗ Ice cream	♥ Any vegetable
⊗ 4% Milkfat cottage cheese	♥ Any fruit
⊗ Whole milk	
⊗ Hard cheese	
⊗ Butter	
⊗ Mayonnaise	

A low level of HDL (High Density Lipoprotein)-cholesterol (below 35 mg/dl) is considered another risk factor for heart disease. Regular exercise will help increase HDL-cholesterol levels, one of the reasons for making a permanent lifestyle change with the addition of exercise.

B. FATS AND CHOLESTEROL

1. How are Fats Related to Blood Cholesterol?

Scientific evidence indicates that the amount and type of dietary fat can affect blood cholesterol.[3] Eating less fat, especially saturated fats, has been found to lower blood cholesterol levels. Replacing some saturated fats with polyunsaturated and monounsaturated also can be helpful in lowering blood cholesterol levels. Dietary cholesterol also can raise blood cholesterol but generally is not as important as saturated fat and total fat in the diet. Remember, high blood cholesterol levels increase risk of heart disease while lower blood cholesterol reduces risk.

2. In What Foods are Fats and Cholesterol Found?

In some foods fats are obvious, such as noticeably greasy, fried, or oily foods. In other foods, they are more invisible. Cholesterol in foods comes from animal products, but has no tell-tale signs. It is not found in food products made from plants. A food can be high in fat and cholesterol (fried egg), high in fat but low in cholesterol (peanut butter), low in fat and high in cholesterol (shrimp), or low in both (fruit). Table 6 shows foods with and without cholesterol and Tables 7 and 8 illustrate the difficulty in finding cholesterol in flesh and nonflesh foods.

3. What about Fish and Fish Oil Supplements?

Diets containing high amounts of fish have been linked with reduced risk of heart disease. The effectiveness and safety of fish oils has yet to be proven. Therefore, eating fish is encouraged, but the use of fish oil supplements is not currently recommended by the American Heart Association.

C. REDUCING FAT AND CHOLESTEROL

There are several simple actions you can take to reduce the amount of fat and cholesterol you eat. Change your eating habits by:

TABLE 7 Identifying Hard To Find Fats and Cholesterol in Nonflesh Foods

Category, Food, Serving Size	Gram Fat per Serving	Cholesterol per mg
Dairy		
Ice cream, 1 c	14	59
Egg, cooked	6	274
Cheddar cheese, 1 oz	9	30
Swiss cheese, 1 oz	8	26
Cream cheese, 1 tbsp	6	31
Sour cream, 1 tbsp	2	5
Nuts and seeds		
Peanut butter, 1 tbsp	8	0
Peanuts, 10 nuts	5	0
Sunflower seeds, 1 tbsp	4	0
Nuts (walnuts, almonds, etc.) 1/8 c av	10	0
Baked goods		
Doughnut, 1 glazed	10	11
Apple pie, 1 slice	13	13
Brownies, 1 square	5	13
Macaroon cookies, 2	2	42
Candy		
Chocolate, 1 oz	10	0
Other		
Mayonnaise, 1 tbsp	11	8
Olives, 5 giant size	5	0

- Eating more vegetables, lean meats, fish, poultry, vegetable protein sources such as: peas, lentils, beans; grains, breads, and cereals, fruit for dessert, and snacks.
- Eating less fried foods, fatty and processed meats: lunch meats, bacon, hot dogs, sausage; desserts high in fat such as: ice cream, pastries, pies, and cheesecake.

D. EVALUATE YOUR PRESENT EATING PATTERN

A diet is more effectively planned if the current pattern of eating is known. Table 9 has been provided to help determine current eating patterns.[5]

To reduce fat and cholesterol in your diet make a few simple changes. These are not difficult to do if one considers the diet as a whole. Table 10 has been provided to identify simple practices to follow to make the diet more healthy.[1]

Fats in processed foods are good examples of hidden fats. While most vegetable fats are naturally unsaturated, those in processed foods often are saturated — particularly palm oil, coconut oil, and liquid oils that have been "hardened" or "hydrogenated". Read labels to avoid hidden saturated fats. Ingredients are listed in order of weight in a product. Avoid products whose labels list oil ("hardened" or "hydrogenated") and those made with coconut or palm oil as the first ingredient. (Hint: choose products that list a liquid oil first, such as canola, soy, corn, or sunflower. Enjoy fat-free salad dressings.) Moderation is the key.

TABLE 8 Identifying Hard To See Fats and Cholesterol in Foods — Meats/Fish/Poultry

Category, Food, Serving Size	Gram Fat per Serving	Cholesterol per mg
Meat		
Regular ground beef	20	90
1 patty, cooked (3.5 oz)		
Extra lean ground beef		
1 patty, cooked (3.5 oz)	16	100
Luncheon meats, 1 slice bologna	7	13
Hot dogs, 1 (8 per lb package)	16	35
Red Meats (lean) (3 oz)		
Beef	8.7	77
Lamb	8.8	78
Pork	11.1	79
Veal	4.7	128
Organ Meats (3 oz)		
Liver	4.0	270
Pancreas (sweetbreads)	2.8	400
Kidney	2.9	329
Brains	10.7	1746
Heart	4.8	164
Poultry (3 oz)		
Chicken (without skin)		
Light	3.8	72
Dark	8.2	79
Turkey (without skin)		
Light	1.3	59
Dark	6.1	72
Fish (3 oz)		
Salmon	9.3	74
Tuna, light canned in water	0.7	55
Shellfish (3 oz)		
Abalone	0.8	90
Clams	1.7	57
Crab meat		
Alaskan king	1.3	45
Blue crab	1.5	85
Lobster	0.5	61
Oysters	4.2	93
Scallops	0.8	35
Shrimp	0.9	166

Make a change in your approach to food selection, a change which will reduce your risk factors for heart disease.

E. USING FOOD LABELS

The new food labels began appearing on packages in 1993.[6] Reading the label tells more about the food and what you are buying. This will help you evaluate

TABLE 9 Rate Your Present Eating Pattern

Check the Most Appropriate Column

	Most Days	Every 2 or 3 Days	Seldom
How often do you eat fatty meats (hot dogs, luncheon meats)?			
How often do you eat or drink high-fat dairy products (whole milk, butter)?			
How often do you eat egg yolks? Include those you use in cooking (cakes, custards)			
Do you eat snacks and processed foods without reading the ingredients and nutrition labels?			

Note: The checks in the Most Days column show you where you need to reduce fat and cholesterol in your diet. The questions above illustrate that fats and cholesterol are found in a variety of foods and often are hidden, especially in snacks and desserts. For healthy people, moderation in fat intake should become the rule of thumb! Fats, irrespective of their source, are high in calories. The first and most basic step to heart health is to eat in moderation.

TABLE 10 General Guidelines To Follow for a Healthy Diet

- ♥ Buy lean cuts of beef, pork and lamb. (Hint: sirloin, tenderloin, round, eye of round, top round, and top loin are very lean. These are termed the "Skinny Six" cuts of meat. Wild game is low in fat but has similar cholesterol content to other meat, fish, and chicken. Fish has almost no saturated fat.) White poultry meat has less fat than dark.
- ♥ Trim off visible fat before cooking. Bake, broil, simmer, grill, or poach meat, chicken, and fish. Do not add extra fat to brown meat. Remove skin from chicken and turkey before cooking, if possible, but especially before eating.
- ♥ Trimming the fat helps, but watch out for the fat you CANNOT SEE: the fat in foods such as hot dogs, mayonnaise, and deep-fried chicken and fish products.
- ♥ Use smaller portions. (Hint: A 3-oz portion is adequate and is about the size of a deck of cards.)
- ♥ Cut down on luncheon meats, bacon, and sausage. (Hint: use sliced beef or turkey in place of cold cuts.)
- ♥ Limit egg yolks to four a week. Include those you use in cooking. (Hint: egg whites contain no cholesterol. Try two whites and one yolk to replace two whole eggs.)
- ♥ All dairy fats are highly saturated and can raise the levels of cholesterol in your blood stream. It's easy to buy dairy products in a low-fat form, or find substitutes. No-fat dairy products are now appearing in your supermarket. Give them a try.
- ♥ Switch from whole milk to low-fat milk (1 percent or 2 percent). (Hint: take two or three weeks for each small change. Start by mixing whole milk with low-fat; then drink low-fat.) If you drink low-fat already, how about skim milk?
- ♥ Cut down on high-fat cheeses. Most cheese is high in fat. (Hint: low-fat cottage cheese and part-skim mozzarella cheese are low in fat. Read the label for other low-fat choices.)
- ♥ Cut down on cream, ice cream, sour cream. Frozen low-fat yogurt, sherbet, sorbet, and ice milk are all much lower in fat than ice cream. (Hint: plain low-fat yogurt is an excellent substitute for sour cream. Whip chilled evaporated skim milk and use as a topping in place of cream.) With low-fat dairy products you get fewer calories, less saturated fat, and less cholesterol, without losing the nutrients. Look for new low-fat products in your grocery store.

TABLE 11 Recommended Dietary Percentages of Total Fat, Saturated Fat, Total Carbohydrate, Dietary Fiber, and Protein

Food Component	% Calculated As[a]
Total fat	30% of total calorie intake
Saturated fat	10% of total calorie intake
Total carbohydrate	60% of total calorie intake
Dietary fiber	11.5 g per 1000 cal
Protein	10% of total calorie intake

[a] Some numbers may be rounded for nutrition labeling.

TABLE 12 Personalized Nutrition Reference Amounts for Different Calorie Levels[a]

	Calories					
Food Component	**1600**	**2000[b]**	**2200**	**2500**	**2800**	**3200**
Total fat (g)	53	65	73	80	93	107
Saturated fat (g)	18	20	24	25	31	36
Total carbohydrate (g)	240	300	330	375	420	480
Dietary fiber (g)	20[c]	25	25	30	32	37
Protein (g)	46[d]	50	55	65	70	80

Note: These calorie levels may not apply to children and adolescents, who have varying calorie requirements. For specific advice concerning calorie levels, please consult a registered dietitian or qualified health professional.

[a] Numbers may be rounded. [b] % Daily value on the label for total fat, saturated fat, carbohydrate, dietary fiber, and protein (if listed) is based on a 2000 calorie reference diet. [c] 20 g is the minimum amount of fiber recommended for all calorie levels below 2000. (Source: National Cancer Institute.) [d] 46 g is the minimum amount of protein recommended for all calorie levels below 1800. (Source: *Recommended Daily Allowances,* 1989.)

food choices in a more informed way. The new label format will allow you to buy food and plan menus that will meet your dietary goal. The format of the new labels is illustrated in Appendix H.

Daily values are the new label reference standard. These values are set by the government and use the recommendations described. Some labels use a diet of 2000 and 2500 calories. The percent of the Daily Value (% Daily Value) gives a general idea of the food's nutrient content and how it contributes to the 2000 calorie diet. Your own calorie needs may be less than or more than this daily value. But use it to quickly compare foods and see how they fit into the diet based on the 2000 calorie reference. Table 11 shows the recommended dietary percentages of total fat, saturated fat, total carbohydrate, dietary fiber, and protein. Once these percentages were established, the number of grams of each nutrient can be recommended as shown in Table 12 for each of the different calorie level diets.

TABLE 13 Nutrition Panel for Current Labeling Guidelines

Food Component	Daily Value[a]
Total fat	**65 g[b]**
Saturated fat	**20 g[b]**
Cholesterol	**300 mg**
Sodium	**2400 mg**
Potassium	3500 mg
Total carbohydrate	**300 g[b]**
Dietary fiber	**25 g[c]**
Protein	**50 g[b]**
Vitamin A	**5000 IU**
Vitamin C	**60 mg**
Calcium	**1 g**
Iron	**18 mg**
Vitamin D	400 IU
Vitamin E	30 IU
Thiamin	1.5 mg
Riboflavin	1.7 mg
Niacin	20 mg
Vitamin B_6	2.0 mg
Folate	0.4 mg
Vitamin B_{12}	6.0 mcg
Biotin	0.3 mg
Pantothenic acid	10 mg
Phosphorus	1 g
Iodine	150 mcg
Magnesium	400 mg
Zinc	15 mg
Copper	2.0 mg

Note: Items in bold are required; others are optional.

[a] Daily value for adults and children aged 4 and older. [b] Daily value based on a 2000 calorie reference diet. [c] Daily value based on 11.5 grams per 1000 calories.

The grams recommended for each nutrient increase as the total calories increase, but the proportion of each remains the same as determined from the values in Table 11. The daily values listed in Table 11 are also the basis for the nutrition label shown in Table 13 which uses the 2000 calorie diet when listing items. The nutrition label illustrated in the table shows required items on the label which are in boldface and optional items are identified in plain print. For example, total fat and saturated fat must be listed in grams while potassium amounts are optional.

F. CARBOHYDRATES

Since 1910 there has been a 50% increase in the amount of sugars and sweeteners in the American diet. Along with this we have seen a 30% increase in dietary fats. Does this mean that we are just eating more of everything? No, by and large, sugar and fat have taken the place of "complex carbohydrates", the vegetables, breads, and grains that supply many other valuable nutrients in addition to complex carbohydrates and were a greater portion of the American diet in the past.

Sugar is called a "simple carbohydrate", which means that it can be broken down easily by the body for rapid use in energy delivery to the cell. Simple carbohydrates are made up of only one or two sugar units. Complex carbohydrates (e.g., grains, cereals, breads, pasta) are made up of many sugar units linked together. Complex carbohydrates, on the other hand, take much longer to be absorbed and provide energy for a longer period of time. Sugar has another disadvantage which is considered the major one: it contains "empty" calories. It has no nutrients, no food value, and no use other than production of energy which, if it is not used for that purpose, becomes fat on your body. Fats in your diet (both the saturated and the unsaturated ones) *and* the sugar in your diet can end up as body fat if you do not use them immediately for energy.

Should we reverse the clock and go back to the complex carbohydrates? The answer is . . . Yes! If we decide to reduce the *fats* in our diet, most of us fill the void with either simple or complex carbohydrates, that is, with either sugar or grains. If we decide to reduce the *calories*, too, then we must cut down on foods that do not give us any nutrients such as sugar, as well as fats, and fill up our calorie needs with complex carbohydrates . . . the grains and cereals and vegetables. But why not eat more protein foods? Complex carbohydrates are probably preferable because most Americans consume more than sufficient amounts of protein for their needs. Eating more fruits and vegetables also increases our intake of antioxidants.

Is it not a fact that grains and cereals can also contribute to fat stores in the body? Drastic weight loss programs under physician care lead individuals to consume less than normal of all foods that could increase weight. The word "normal" is the key, however, in a modified eating plan such as the one proposed in this chapter; you would not abruptly or drastically cut down on *any* food group but slowly change the proportion of certain foods so that one is increased while another is decreased. It is the displacement of fat and sugar in your diet by foods that contain complex carbohydrates (grains, cereals, fruits, and vegetables) that is the main way these foods aid in reducing heart disease risk factors. Complex carbohydrate foods have the added advantage of being the foods where fiber and the antioxidant nutrients are found. They are also digested more slowly, stay in the system longer, and give a sensation of being "full" so that you are not hungry quickly.

G. SUGAR

1. What Is It?

It has several forms: glucose, found in fruits and vegetables; fructose, found in honey and also in fruits and some vegetables; galactose and lactose, found in milk; maltose, found in grains; and sucrose, made by refining sugar beets and cane. All of these are labeled "simple carbohydrates".

2. What Does It Do?

Sugar provides the body with substrates used for energy production and, therefore, is a source of calories. Complex carbohydrates, fats, protein, and alcohol also furnish the body with calories. Protein, fat, and complex carbohydrate foods provide other essential nutrients. Simple carbohydrates (sugar) and alcohol provide only energy (calories).

3. What If It Is Too High?

Too much sugar in your diet is stored as fat and ultimately causes obesity — a risk factor in heart disease. Also, there is an indication that in some people too much sugar increases blood triglycerides — another risk factor in heart disease. Sucrose, especially, is also linked to dental problems and is a factor to consider for diabetic persons. Eating too much sugar does not cause diabetes, but may be a factor in body weight and can be cut, especially if you wish to shed a few pounds.

4. What Is "High"?

This depends on how fast your body uses it for energy, although, in general, American diets are too high in sugar. The U.S. Dietary Guidelines state everyone should "use sugar only in moderation."

5. What Can I Do?

There are general recommendations to reduce sugar in the diet. They are

1. Decrease simple carbohydrates and, instead, get your needed calories and satisfy your appetite by increasing complex carbohydrates (remember carbohydrates should make up to 60% of your total calories).
2. Reduce the added sugar in your foods. You cannot or should not avoid all sugar because most of the foods we eat contain sugar in one form or another. But keep the amount of sugars and sweet foods you eat moderate.
3. Read labels, since many prepared and canned foods contain considerable amounts of sugar. Other terms used by manufacturers but synonymous with sugar are
   - Brown sugar
   - Cane syrup
   - Corn sugar
   - Corn syrup solids
   - Dextrose
   - Fructose
   - Glucose
   - Honey
   - Invert sugar
   - Lactose
   - Molasses
   - Natural sweeteners

H. REDUCING CALORIES BY REDUCING SUGAR

Simple carbohydrates (sugar and honey) have little nutritional value and only provide sweetness and calories — no minerals, vitamins, or fiber — just empty calories. Remember that extra sugar in your diet is stored as fat and may lead to obesity, a risk factor for heart disease. Complex carbohydrates are found in cereals, breads, pasta, grains, dried beans and peas, fruits, and vegetables. These

TABLE 14 Guidelines To Increase Complex Carbohydrates in the Diet

- ♥ Eat unsweetened cereal for breakfast or some other grain foods (whole-wheat bread, bagels, or muffins).
- ♥ Buy bread or grain products that list "whole wheat" first on the list of ingredients not just "wheat flour".
- ♥ Increase the amount of vegetables you eat. Eat at least 3 servings of vegetables each day in addition to potatoes or other starchy foods.
- ♥ Serve fruit: fresh, frozen, dried, or canned in light or unsweetened syrup for dessert. Eat at least 2 servings each day.
- ♥ Replace cookies and chips with bread sticks, unbuttered popcorn, and raw vegetables for snacks.

foods are high in vitamins and minerals, are satisfying (without containing high amounts of calories), and are a good source of fiber. Table 14 gives guidelines for increasing complex carbohydrates in the diet. As you decrease the amount of prepared foods high in sugar and eat more fruit and vegetables, you will concomitantly increase your antioxidant and fiber intake.

I. FIBER

Dietary fiber was called roughage years ago. It is found in fruits, vegetables, cereals, and grains. It is the skeletal part of plant materials and includes cellulose, hemicellulose, pectin, gum, and lignin. Fiber is not broken down by the body's digestive tract. It is usually removed when food is refined.

1. What Does It Do?

Fiber adds bulk to the diet. Unabsorbed vegetable fiber holds water and promotes more frequent bowel movements.

2. What Is Soluble Fiber?

Pectin and gum are water soluble fibers found inside plant cells. They slow the passage of food through the intestines but do nothing to increase fecal bulk. Beans (such as kidney or pinto), oat bran, barley, and some fruits and vegetables contain soluble fiber.

3. What Is Insoluble Fiber?

Fibers found inside the cell walls are water insoluble. These include cellulose, hemicellulose, and lignin. Such fibers increase fecal bulk and speed up the transit time through the digestive tract. Wheat bran and whole grains contain the most insoluble fiber, but fruits, vegetables, and beans also are good sources.

4. How Does This Affect Heart Disease?

Cholesterol is eliminated from the body through bile acids; insoluble fiber binds water, making stools softer and bulkier. Water soluble fiber binds bile acids, suggesting that a high fiber diet may result in an increased excretion of cholesterol.

TABLE 15 Examples of High and Low Fiber Foods

High-Fiber Foods	Low-Fiber Foods
♥ Whole-wheat breads	⊗ White breads
♥ Bran	⊗ Sugar
♥ Cereals, whole-grain, high-fiber breakfast cereals	⊗ Meat, fish, poultry
♥ Peanuts	⊗ Dairy products
♥ Fruit, fresh, frozen, canned in juice	
♥ Vegetables, raw and cooked	

5. What Is "High" (Or Too Low)?

A high-fiber diet supplies about 35 to 45 g of dietary fiber daily. The daily value used on the food label uses 25 g of fiber for a 2000 calorie diet. After a heart attack an individual should try to eat more fiber, and if blood cholesterol is high, the emphasis should be on soluble fiber.

The general recommendation is that people should increase the amount of fiber they consume since the American diet tends to be very low in fiber and because fiber seems to inhibit certain intestinal diseases, including cancer of the colon, hemorrhoids, and constipation. Many unsubstantiated claims are made about fiber, however, and one should be leery of specific claims or promises that dietary fiber can cure specific diseases.

The best advice is to combine dietary practices with exercise in moderation. A variety of whole-grain products, fruits, and vegetables ensures a good mixture of the different types of fiber and makes a positive contribution to the overall nutritional value of any diet. Table 15 illustrates examples of high and low fiber foods.

J. SALT

Salt, which is chemically composed of sodium and chloride, is present naturally in most foods. Some sodium is required to maintain water balance and cell pressure. It helps muscles contract and is required by the nervous system. However, too much salt can cause water retention that may lead to high blood pressure — one of the risk factors associated with heart disease.

Most adults consume about 6 to 18 g (as much as 4 tsp) of salt daily. The daily requirement for sodium is only 500 mg (1/4 tsp of salt). Most postinfarct individuals are advised to reduce salt and sodium. Table 16 has suggestions for doing this along with lists of high and low salt foods. Suggestions are provided in Table 17 for vegetables and entrees where salt is usually the seasoning choice. When additional salt is diminished or eliminated, the natural taste of food will become more pronounced and the individual will no longer enjoy high salt meals and dishes.

K. PUTTING THE PLAN TOGETHER

The Food Guide Pyramid is an outline of what to eat each day based on the most recent Dietary Guidelines published for the American population.[1] These

TABLE 16 Guidelines for Reducing Salt In the Diet and High and Low Salt Foods

- Avoid the salt habit. Do not automatically salt food before tasting or eating food.
- Cook with less salt.
- Eat less salted snacks and other high salt foods.
- Read labels for salt content.
- Try seasoning with herbs and spices

High-Salt Foods

⊗ Soups, canned and instant (bouillon cubes)
⊗ Processed foods (certain cheeses, instant and ready-to-eat cereals)
⊗ Sauerkraut
⊗ Ham, bacon, sausage
⊗ Pickles, olives
⊗ salted or smoked fish (sardines, anchovies)
⊗ Salted snack foods (potato chips, fries, pretzels, salted popcorn, nuts, crackers)
⊗ Soy sauce
⊗ Processed meats (bologna, corned or chipped beef, franks, lunch meat, smoked tongue)
⊗ Ketchup, mustard
⊗ Worcestershire sauce
⊗ Barbecue sauce
⊗ Shellfish
⊗ Dairy products
⊗ Picante sauce and other ready-made sauces

Low-Salt Foods

♥ Fresh fruits
♥ Fresh vegetables
♥ Fresh meats and poultry
♥ Fresh fish
♥ Fruit juices
♥ Dried beans/legumes

TABLE 17 Seasoning Without Your Salt Shaker

Food	Seasoning Vegetables
Asparagus	Lemon peel, thyme
Broccoli	Lemon juice, onion
Brussel sprouts	Lemon juice, mustard
Cabbage	Dill weed, caraway seeds, oregano, lemon juice, vinegar, onion, mustard, marjoram
Carrots	Marjoram, ginger, mint, mace, parsley, nutmeg, sage, unsalted butter, lemon peel, orange peel, thyme, cinnamon
Cauliflower	Rosemary, nutmeg, tarragon, mace
Celery	Dill weed, tarragon
Cucumbers	Rosemary, onion
Green beans	Basil, dill weed, thyme, curry powder, lemon juice, vinegar
Peas	Mint, onion, parsley, basil, chervil, marjoram, sage, rosemary
Potatoes	Bay leaves, chervil, dill weed, mint, parsley, rosemary, paprika, tarragon, mace, nutmeg, unsalted butter, chives
Spinach	Chervil, marjoram, mint, rosemary, mace, nutmeg, lemon, tarragon
Squash	Basil, saffron, ginger, mace, nutmeg, orange peel
Tomatoes	Basil, bay leaves, chervil, tarragon, curry powder, oregano, parsley, sage, cloves
Zucchini	Marjoram, mint, saffron, thyme

Table 17 (continued)

	Entrees
Eggs & cheese	Curry powder, marjoram, mace, parsley flakes, tumeric, basil, oregano, rosemary, garlic, mustard, mace, ginger, curry powder, allspice, lemon juice, pepper
Fish & shellfish	Basil, bay leaves, chervil, marjoram, oregano, parsley, rosemary, sage, tarragon, thyme, lemon peel, celery seed, cumin, saffron, savory, dry mustard
Poultry	Basil, saffron, bay leaves, sage, dill weed, savory, marjoram, tarragon, oregano, thyme, rosemary, paprika, curry powder, orange peel, cranberries, mushrooms
Pork	Cloves, garlic, ginger, mustard, nutmeg, paprika, sage, rosemary, savory, thyme, curry powder, oregano, apples

guidelines (Table 18) from the U.S. Department of Agriculture and Health and Human Services have been visualized in the Food Guide Pyramid (Figure 1).

The Food Guide Pyramid is the basic tool everyone should use as it addresses the total diet.[7] This should replace all former food guides, especially the Basic Four Food Groups that was designed years ago to teach nutrient adequacy. Concerns today focus on our top health problems such as heart disease and obesity. The key message in the Food Guide Pyramid is to illustrate the following key dietary recommendations:

- Eat a variety of foods
- Choose a diet low in fat, saturated fat, and cholesterol
- Use sugars only in moderation
- Choose a diet with plenty of vegetables, fruits, and grain products

These are all the facts discussed in this chapter!

The pyramid gives the image of *variety, moderation,* and *proportionality.*

- *Variety* means eating different foods from among and within all the groups.
- *Moderation* means eating fats and added sugars sparingly and limiting the foods high in fat and added sugars. This allows you to eat all foods you enjoy in limited amounts, remembering your own dietary goals.
- *Proportionality* means eating different amounts of foods from each group. All food groups are important, but we should eat more food from some groups.

Note that the icons (the dots and triangles) in the top of the Pyramid are mostly in the form of added fats or sugar. This can easily be top heavy if you choose

TABLE 18 Dietary Guidelines for Americans

- Eat a variety of foods
- Maintain healthy weight
- Choose a diet low in fat, saturated fat, and cholesterol
- Choose a diet with plenty of vegetables, fruits, and grain products
- Use sugar only in moderation
- Use salt and sodium only in moderation
- If you drink alcoholic beverages, do so in moderation and do not drive

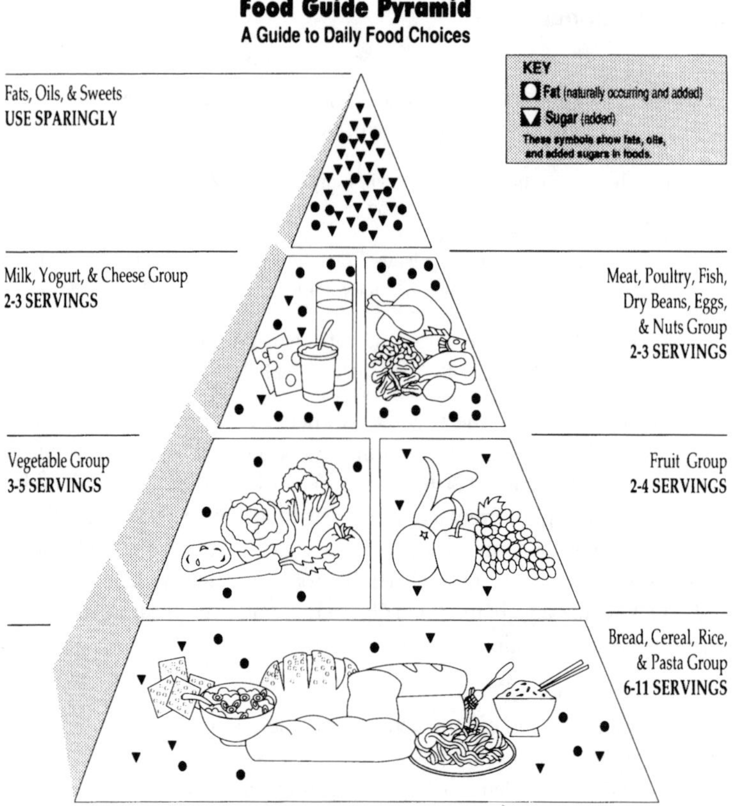

Figure 1. Food Guide Pyramid.

foods so high in fat and sugar that they spill over as a volcano, loading all the sections below in the Pyramid!

It is all a question of balance and that means proportion and moderation. If you do eat a food with a high amount of fat and sugar, decrease other foods you eat that day and make lower fat choices. No one food is good or bad. No one food or meal will cause another heart attack. It is what is eaten over the week, month, and year that ultimately counts.

Using the Pyramid as a guide, one can build a lifelong eating plan with which one can live. There is no perfect food, just a sensible eating plan built on variation, moderation, and proportionality. Appendix I describes in detail the definition of servings as related to the pyramid.

L. MODIFYING RECIPES AND COOKING TECHNIQUES

Shopping is one part of the changes needed to follow a healthier eating plan. The next is making changes in cooking. Changing to low-fat cooking techniques such as broiling, grilling, steaming, baking, braising, poaching, or stir-frying instead of frying is recommended. Low-fat toppings should be used for baked

TABLE 19 Suggestions To Reduce Fat in Cooking

- ♥ Take the skin off poultry.
- ♥ Grate cheese instead of slicing it. A little will go a long way. Look for the low- or no-fat cheese.
- ♥ Try the no-fat frozen desserts and baked products.
- ♥ Do not smear large amounts of butter on bread or slosh great dollops of salad dressing on salads. Use jams or jellies on bread without any butter and find a low-fat salad dressing or simply keep the dressing on the side and dip your fork in to get the taste of less fat.
- ♥ Do not assume that if you are a vegetarian, you are eating low-fat healthy foods; cheese and tofu are high in fat.

Additional suggestions include:

When using mayonnaise or salad dressing for salads, try substituting plain yogurt for part of the mayonnaise; fold gently or use "lite" or no-fat mayonnaise as this can cut fats by 2/3.

Substitute tomato juice for all or part of the oil when preparing commercial salad dressing mixes. Use water or vinegar for part of the oil.

Use evaporated skim milk or buttermilk to dip foods in before breading for baking.

Use aerosol vegetable sprays for frying, preparing waffle irons, and to prevent sticking in casseroles.

Use herbs to season vegetables.

For dips requiring cream cheese, select the no-fat or low-fat variety or substitute yogurt or blended cottage cheese.

potatoes in place of sour cream and butter. Plain yogurt with parsley, blended low-fat cottage cheese, grated low-fat cheese, or salsa are some suggestions for toppings. Table 19 lists suggestions for reducing fat in cooking.

M. HOW TO ADAPT YOUR OWN RECIPES AND MODIFY YOUR EATING HABITS

Determine how to change the ingredient(s) to achieve the dietary goal. Ingredient(s) can be eliminated completely, reduced in amount, or substituted with a more nutritionally acceptable ingredient. To choose the best approach, it is helpful to have a general idea of the function of the ingredient and what will happen if it is modified (Table 20). The next step is to reduce the fat and cholesterol content of recipes (Table 21) while concentrating on reducing the amount of sugar (Table 22), salt, and dietary cholesterol and saturated fat (Table 23) while increasing complex carbohydrates in the diet overall.

For more information and materials on modifying recipes, contact your County Cooperative Extension Agent or Department of Food Science and Human Nutrition, Cooperative Extension Office, Colorado State University, Fort Collins, CO 80523.

TABLE 20 Function of Fat, Eggs, Sugar, and Sodium in Recipes

Fat

Provides flavor and richness

Improves texture and tenderness in baked goods

Promotes flakiness and lightness

Promotes smoothness and creaminess

TABLE 20 Function of Fat, Eggs, Sugar, and Sodium in Recipes (continued)

Eggs
- Provide structure, elasticity, and richness
- Act as a thickener and emulsifier
- Act as leavening agents when beaten

Sugar
- Provides flavor, volume, and texture
- Increases tenderness and browning in baked goods
- Acts as a preservative in jams, jellies, and pickles
- Acts as food for yeast

Sodium
- Provides flavor
- Acts as a preservative in cured meats and brined vegetables
- Controls action of yeast

TABLE 21 Substitutions To Reduce the Amount of Fat and Cholesterol in Cooking

When the Recipe Calls For	Substitution
Sour cream	Mock sour cream: low-fat cottage cheese blended until smooth; low-fat cottage cheese plus yogurt; skim milk, low-fat ricotta cheese thinned with yogurt; plain low-fat yogurt
Whipped cream	Chilled evaporated skim milk, whipped
Chocolate	Cocoa blended with oil or margarine: 1-oz square chocolate = 3 tbsp cocoa = 1 tbsp oil or margarine.
Butter	Margarine or oil; 1 tbsp butter = 1 tbsp margarine = 3/4 tbsp oil; 1 1/4 tbsp margarine = 1 tbsp oil
Whole milk	Skim or diluted evaporated skim milk
Sugar	Use 1/4 cup powdered milk for 1/4 cup of the sugar in baked recipes; up to 1/3 cup works well
Oil	Applesauce or prune puree;[a] use to replace 1/2 to all of the oil (3/4 is ideal)

[a] Prune Puree: combine 1 1/3 cups (8 oz) pitted prunes and 6 tbsp water in container of food processor. Pulse on and off until prunes are finely chopped. Makes 1 cup. Or use prune butter. Look for this fat-free butter in the jam and jelly or baking section of your supermarket. Use as for prune puree.

TABLE 22 Suggestions for Reducing Sugar in the Diet

1. Try not adding sugar to cereals. Avoid frosted or sugar-coated cereals.
2. Add raisins, fresh fruits (such as bananas or peaches), or canned fruits packed in their own juices rather than sugar to ready-to-eat cereals for sweetening.
3. Add dried fruits the last few minutes when cooking cereals. They add flavor as well as sweetness.
4. Purchase fruits canned in their own juices or unsweetened liquid, or look for fruits canned in light syrup.
5. Top ice cream and pancakes with pureed fruits, such as apricots or peaches or applesauce, instead of syrup.
6. Use canned or frozen fruit juices singly or in favorable combinations instead of sweet, bottled drinks.

TABLE 22 (continued)

7. When freezing fruits, reduce the amount of sugar per quart or pint of fruit. When preparing fruits, toss lightly with a small amount of sugar to evenly distribute the sweetness. Fully ripe fruits are naturally sweet and require little or no added sugar.
8. Buy or make applesauce without sugar. If it's not sweet enough, add a few raisins.
9. Eat dried fruits as a snack. They are naturally sweet.
10. Eat fresh fruits in season.
11. Serve cakes without frosting. If added sweetness is desired, sift a little powdered sugar over the top of the cake. Applesauce cake, sponge cake, and other heavy, moist cakes are often served unfrosted.
12. Use less sugar in cobblers and crisps. If a recipe gives a range in the amount of sugar to use, such as in fruit pies, use the lesser amount.
13. Use very light syrup or pack in water when canning fruits.
14. Substitute 1/4 cup of nonfat dry milk for 1/4 cup of sugar in recipes.

N. DEVELOPING YOUR EATING PLAN

Try to maintain a fairly constant diet. Do not starve one day and feast the next. Enjoy eating and meal times should be pleasurable. Using the food guide pyramid as your eating plan, you will have high amounts of carbohydrate foods, moderate amounts of fat, and adequate amounts of protein. Use the pyramid to plan the amounts to eat.

Think of each day as if you are given a calorie salary, then spend it wisely. Look at the pyramid and budget your day. Over half your calories should be spent on carbohydrates to the goal of 60%. As you know by now, only 30% should come from your fat budget and 10% from protein. For growing youngsters and adolescents, 15% of their calories should come from protein, but that is enough for good growth and development and is even sufficient for the athlete. Carbohydrates would then be 55% of their salary.

You make deposits in the form of calories and your body adds them to your savings. When you need to do some work, you make a withdrawal of those calories. The savings that are not withdrawn to be spent on energy are stored as body fat. Some of us have some hefty balances! Even worse, the body, like a bank, pays us interest on those growing balances — that is as risk factors for health problems. Therefore, take a careful check of all you have learned and enjoy your exercise and eating plan.

O. PLANNING YOUR DIET

When you plan ahead of time what and how you will eat, then you have a chance to really be sure that you are

- Meeting your goals (e.g., lowering fats or calories)
- Replacing the foods you are concentrating on changing with foods that will benefit your body more . . . not ones that just happen to be on hand
- Filling *all* of your nutritional requirements

One means of achieving this is by taking into account the "nutrient density" of your food. Nutrient density is a concept that nutritionists have devised to

TABLE 23 Suggestions for Lowering Dietary Cholesterol and Saturated Fat

1. If you use margarine, select one high in polyunsaturated fats (P), in lieu of butter (or "lite" margarine). Tub soft margarines are higher in P. Check the label, amount saturated fat will be given, the first ingredient should be liquid vegetable oil.
2. Grill, rather than fry meat to remove the saturated fat. Broil or roast meat on a rack so it will remain above the drippings.
3. Use baked or boiled potatoes, rather than fried, hash browns, potato rolls or convenience precooked potatoes.
4. Use skim milk for white sauces, puddings, and all cooking.
5. Drink skim milk, if possible, or 2% if you really do not like skim milk. Try mixing 1/2 skim milk and 1/2 2% milk, gradually increasing proportion of skim milk. Check your grocery store to see if 1% or 1/2% milk is available.
6. Eat lean meat and remove skin from poultry before cooking.
7. Trim visible fat from meat before cooking. Do not add extra fat to browned meat.
8. Read food labels before you buy. White shortenings are not necessarily vegetable shortenings. They could be animal fat or a combination. Some brands use coconut oil, which is highly saturated. Items listing "vegetable oil" often mean coconut, palm kernel, or palm oil.
9. When cooking or browning hamburger, drain off the fat in a colander lined with paper towel after browning the meat; remember to use extra lean ground beef.
10. Skim fats from soups and gravies.
11. Remember that choice grade beef has the most "marbling" or fat which increases the tenderness but adds to the fat content. Lower grades of meat contain less fat, as there is much less marbling. Compare grades before you buy.
12. Substitute yogurt for sour cream and chilled, evaporated milk for whipping cream. This will greatly reduce the saturated fat and cholesterol content.
13. Replace high fat cheeses with part-skim cheeses; substitute low-fat (1%) cottage cheese for 4% butterfat cottage cheese.
14. Use egg substitutes in place of eggs in cooking, baking, and for a scrambled egg breakfast.
15. Fatless cakes and cakes using only egg whites make good low-fat and low-cholesterol desserts.
16. Use oatmeal instead of bread crumbs as an extender in meatloaf; bread crumbs soak up fat, whereas oatmeal allows it to drain off.
17. Use "no oil" salad dressings. Use "lite" mayonnaise in place of regular mayonnaise.

express a relationship between the caloric intake and nutrient intake. This is not a complex relationship and requires common sense for understanding. Nutrient density, in its simplest terms, means wisely spending your daily allotment of calories. It is found in foods whose vitamins, minerals, protein, and other components make them a good investment for the calories you spend from your account. For example, if you to were to spend one half of all the money you have in your savings account on one item, you would want that item to give you a good return on satisfaction. Comparably, your daily allowance has only so many calories with which to "buy" the nutrients that will enable you to maintain a healthy body. And, just like your hard-earned money, these calories should not be thrown away on "just anything". They should be spent wisely on those foods that will provide you with the vital nutrients for your body's "satisfaction". And, a "satisfied" body shows its appreciation by providing you with a longer and healthier life.

P. SUMMARY

This chapter was meant to give explanations and current recommendations to help reduce dietary risks for cardiovascular disease and to offer help to the individual recovering from a heart attack. However, it is also a wise and prudent diet for all Americans to follow, as heart disease is still the main cause of death in the country with the tragedy being that these diseases are often preventable and curable. Identified as related to lifestyle, the changes suggested will promote the reduction of risk for this category of diseases. Since great numbers of individuals who recover from a heart attack become recreational athletes, it is prudent for them to support their exercise habits with sound nutritional advice.

Food alone cannot make one healthy and there are no single magical nutrients. Good eating habits based on moderation and variety can, however, promote and even improve health. Enjoy eating and enjoy regular exercise; while there are no guarantees for the quantity, the quality of life will thus be enhanced.

REFERENCES

1. **Anderson, J. and Gunn, S.,** Healthy Heart Program, latest Rev., Colorado State University, Fort Collins, 1990.
2. Nutrition and Your Health: Dietary Guidelines for Americans, Third Edition, 1990, Home and Garden Bulletin, No. 232, U.S. Department of Agriculture and U.S. Health and Human Services, Washington D.C., 1990.
3. **Chait, A., Brunzell, J. D., Denke, M. A., Eisenberg, D., Ernst, N. D., Franklin, F. A., Ginsberg, H., Kotchen, T. A., Kuller, L., Mullis, R. M., Nichaman, M. Z., Nicolosi, R. J., Schaefer, E. J., Stone, N. J., and Weidman, W. H.,** Rationale of the Diet-Heart Statement of the American Heart Association, *Circulation* 88(6), 3008, 1993.
4. Second Report of the Expert Panel on Detection Evaluation and Treatment of High Blood Cholesterol in Adults *(Adult Treatment Panel II),* U.S. Department of Health and Human Services, PHS, Washington, D.C., NIH Pub. No. 93-3095, Sept. 1993.
5. **Anderson, J. and Johnson, J.,** Self-Care for a Healthy Heart., Dept. Food Science and Human Nutrition, Colorado State University, Fort Collins, Coop. Ext. Bulletin XCM-152, 1994.
6. **Boyd Browme, M.,** National Food Processors Association in Cooperation with Food and Drug Administration, U.S. Department Health and Human Services, and the Food Safety Inspection Service, USDA, Label Facts for Health Eating. Educator's Resource Guide, Mazer Corporation, Dayton, OH, 1993.
7. Food Guide Pyramid, Human Nutrition Info. Service, Home and Garden Bulletin, No. 249, U.S. Department of Agriculture, Washington, D.C., 1992. (For a copy of the Food Guide Pyramid booklet, send a check or money order for $1.00, payable to the Superintendent of Documents — Consumer Information Center, Department 159-Y Pueblo, Colorado 81009.)

Chapter 8

FLUIDS, HYDRATION, AND PERFORMANCE CONCERNS OF ALL RECREATIONAL ATHLETES

Sherrie L. Frye

CONTENTS

0-8493-7914-8/95/$0.00+$.50

I. INTRODUCTION

Water is the most abundant constituent of the human body and the single most important nutrient to life. Although water provides no food energy, it is the medium in which food and oxygen are supplied to the cells and waste products removed. One can live for several weeks without food, depending upon how much fat has been stored, but death will occur in a matter of days following a deprivation of water.

Body water performs many essential functions, but of most importance, as related to athletic performance, is the role that it plays in regulating body temperature. Increased muscular activity leads to an increase in heat production which is normally removed from the body by the evaporation of sweat. Some individuals may lose as much as 2 to 4 L sweat (6 to 8 lb body weight) per hour during strenuous activity.[1] To maintain proper water balance, fluid intake must be adequate before, during, and after exercise to minimize body weight loss and prevent the onset of heat related illness. Greater than 2% dehydration can have serious deleterious effects on physical performance and endurance.[2]

Optimal hydration is important to the health and performance of the elite, amateur, and recreational athlete. The focus of this chapter, however, will be on the recreational athlete and on the role that water plays in the achievement of performance goals and health maintenance. Topics to be presented include: the functions, requirements, distribution, and balance of water in the body; the effects of dehydration on performance; and recommendations for fluid replacement.

II. IMPORTANCE OF WATER IN THE BODY

A. BODY WATER

1. Functions

Water serves a variety of important functions in the body:

1. It provides structure and form to cells
2. It serves as a carrier of materials in solution, including other nutrients, waste products, and gases

3. It provides the medium in which physicochemical changes and reactions occur
4. It acts as a lubricant, as in saliva, the mucous secretions of the respiratory, gastrointestinal, and genitourinary tracts, and the fluid surrounding the joints
5. It provides protection to body tissue due to its resistance to compression
6. It is essential to cardiovascular function by maintaining blood volume
7. It plays an important role in regulating body temperature

2. Requirements

The adult recommendation for daily water intake under normal conditions of energy expenditure and environmental exposure is 1 ml/kcal of energy expenditure, or 2200 ml for women and 2900 ml for men. This may be increased to 1.5 ml/kcal to cover variations in activity level, sweating, and solute load, as often experienced by athletes.[3] The primary consideration in determining water requirement is the amount needed to maintain balance between water intake and water loss.

3. Distribution

Water is found in every cell in the body, with each gram of body protein holding 4 g water and each gram of fat associated with approximately 0.2 g water.[4] It follows that obese individuals would have a lower percentage of total body water than leaner individuals as they have more body fat. Since the average female has a larger percentage of body fat, as compared to her male counterpart, she also has less total body water. The typical adult female is approximately 55% water by weight as compared to 60% for the young adult male. Newborn infants are 70 to 75% water by weight, an amount that decreases progressively to 45 to 55% in the older adult.[5]

Although present in all body tissues, the amount of water present is specific to tissue type. Blood plasma is 90% water by weight, muscle tissue is approximately 72% water, fat tissue varies from 20 to 35% water, bones 25%, and teeth 15% (Figure 1).

a. *Fluid Compartments*

Body water is located in two main fluid compartments: the intracellular compartment and the extracellular compartment, as shown in Figure 2. The intracellular fluid (ICF) is the fluid contained within the cells and amounts to approximately 65% of total body water. Extracellular fluid (ECF) is the fluid outside the cells and includes: interstitial fluid (lymph); intravascular fluid (plasma); and transcellular fluid (fluid secreted by epithelial cells, such as cerebrospinal, pericardial, pleural, synovial, and intraocular fluids, as well as digestive secretions). Approximately 35% of total body water is extracellular.

It is crucial that adequate water volume be maintained in both fluid compartments. When extracellular fluid is decreased, blood volume drops, resulting in less

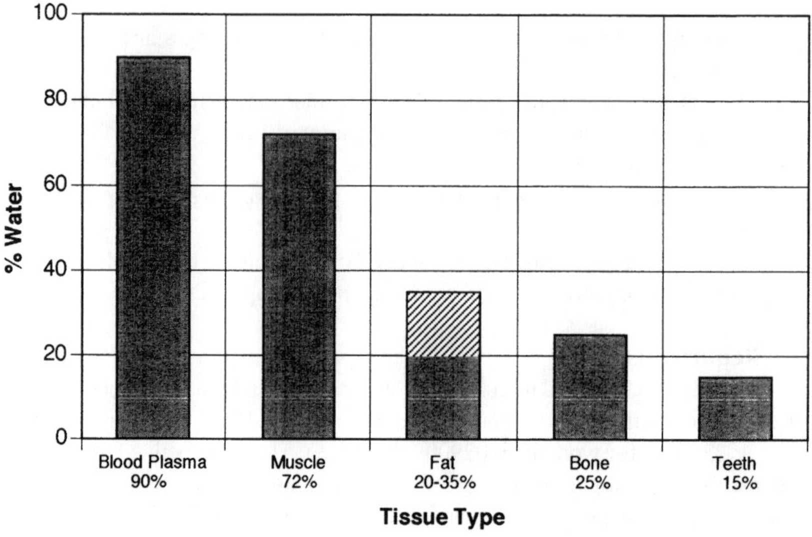

Figure 1. Water content of selected body tissues.

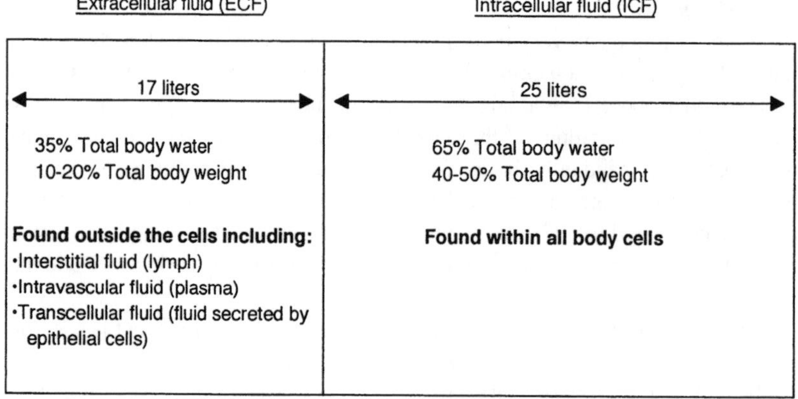

Figure 2. Fluid compartments.

oxygen supplied to cells. A decrease in intracellular fluid impairs the efficiency of cellular metabolism, including energy production. Body core temperature also rises because the heat produced by metabolic processes is being absorbed by a smaller volume of fluid.

b. Electrolytes

Electrolytes are small inorganic substances that dissociate in solution forming *ions* that carry an electrical charge, positive or negative. Cations are ions that develop a positive charge in solution and anions are ions that develop a negative charge. Sodium represents over 90% of the cations in extracellular fluid with potassium, magnesium, and calcium also present in smaller amounts. Potassium is the primary cation in intracellular fluid along with magnesium, sodium, and calcium. The primary extracellular anion is chloride, while phosphate is the primary intracellular anion.

The electrolyte concentration in the intracellular and extracellular fluid determines the movement of water within the body, and must be maintained within a narrow range.

4. Balance

When water intake is equal to water output, water balance has been achieved. Adults metabolize between 2.2 and 2.9 L of water each day in an attempt to maintain this balance. Figure 3 illustrates the concept of water balance and the sources of water input and output.

a. Water Input

Water input is provided by: (1) water consumption from various drinks, representing approximately 1500 ml/day and 60% of total water input; (2) water content of foods, contributing 750 ml/day and 30% of total water input (fruits and vegetables are particularly high in water content); and (3) the water that is produced from the oxidation of food, or metabolic water, amounting to 250 ml/day and 10% of total body water input. The amount of water produced from the oxidation of 100 g of fat, carbohydrate, and protein is 107, 55, and 41 ml, respectively.

b. Water Output

Water is lost from the body as: (1) urine, which contributes approximately 1500 ml/day or 60% or total water output; (2) insensible water loss through the skin and lungs, amounting to 700 ml/day or 28% of total body output; (3) sweat, which represents approximately 200 ml/day or 8% total water output under average conditions; and (4) the remaining 4% of total water output or 100 ml is lost in the feces each day.

B. WATER AND PHYSICAL PERFORMANCE

1. Thermoregulation

Normal adult body temperature is approximately 98.6°F (37°C). Death will occur when temperature falls below 80°F (27°C) or rises above 108°F (42°C). These values are for oral temperature, as core temperature is approximately 1°F (0.6°C) higher. Among the many factors that contribute to heat production in the body are resting or basal heat production provided through normal oxidative processes of food; disease; a higher basal rate; the specific dynamic action of food; shivering; unconscious muscular contraction; and exercise.[6] The means by which heat loss is accomplished includes conduction, convection, radiation, and evaporation.

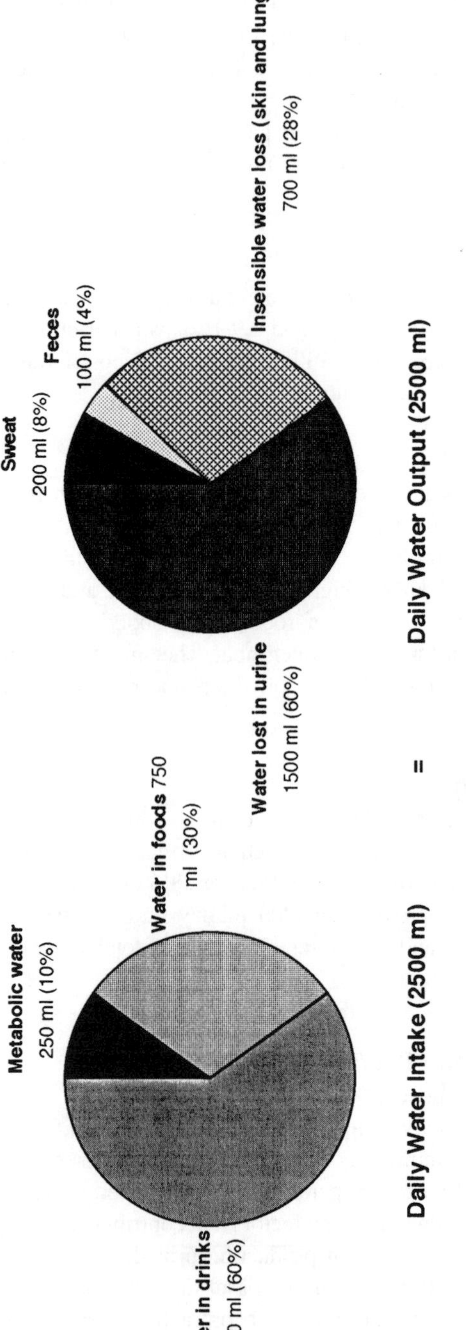

Figure 3. Water balance.

TABLE 1 Physiological Effects of Dehydration

Weight Change (%)	Physiological Change	Health Implications
1.0	+Core temperature	None
2.0	–Plasma volume –Muscle water –Heart stroke volume +Heart rate –Blood pressure	None
3.0	–Blood flow to skin	None
4.1	–Blood flow to muscle	None
5.0	–Sweat rate or heat stroke	+Susceptibility to heat exhaustion
5.8	–Muscle minerals	Spasms, cramping
7.3	+Urine specific gravity +Urine acidity +Protein in urine –Blood flow to kidney	–Nutrient and 0_2 supply to kidney

Water is involved in thermoregulation in a number of ways. During exercise a significant amount of heat is produced as a by-product of the energy metabolism for the contraction and relaxation in active muscle. Nadel[7] found that the rate of heat production by active muscles can be as much as 100 times that of inactive muscles and that if the body stored this heat instead of dissipating it, the internal temperature would rise at a rate of 1°C (1.8°F) every 5 to 8 min during moderate exercise, resulting in hyperthermia (overheating) and collapse within 15 to 20 min.

One response to elevated body temperature is the dilation of skin blood vessels, which increases blood flow to the skin, increasing skin temperature, where it can then be transferred by radiation and convection from the skin to the environment.[7] Of most significance to the athlete is the dissipation of heat by the evaporation of sweat. As sweat evaporates, heat energy is taken from the skin, cooling it in the process.[8] The evaporation of 1 g of water from the skin surface as sweat removes approximately 0.6 kcal of heat.[7]

Sweating has a cooling effect only if the sweat evaporates. In humid, hot environments sweat does not evaporate well because of the moisture content of the surrounding air. Body heat will continue to rise, which, in turn, increases sweat production. This could lead to a serious elevation in the core temperature, with excessive fluid and electrolyte loss. Adequate hydration must be maintained during exercise under these conditions to prevent the serious consequences of dehydration.

2. Physiological Changes Associated with Dehydration

Among the most common causes of dehydration are fluid loss due to exercise, heat exposure, fluid and food restriction, disease, injury, and the use of diuretic drugs. The adverse physiological effects of dehydration are shown in Table 1, as outlined by Horswill.[9]

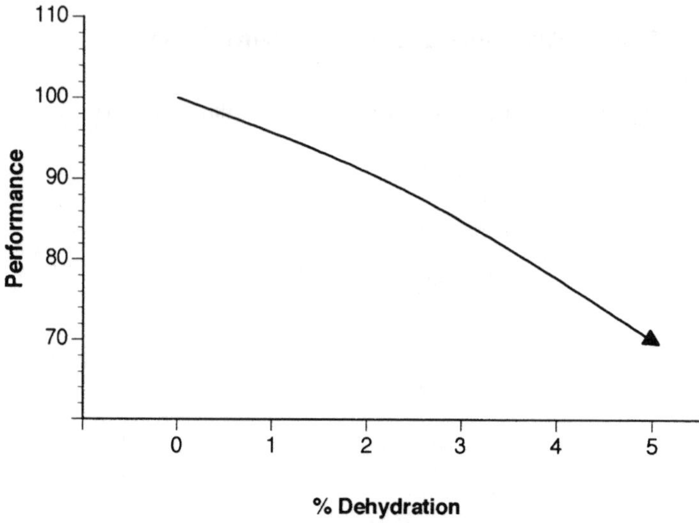

Figure 4. The effect of dehydration on exercise performance.

Thirst is the body's first reaction to dehydration, and occurs when water loss reaches about 1% of body weight. The mouth feels dry as the result of decreased saliva production. Slight increases in body temperature and heart rate during exercise also occurs at this time[10] because of decreased plasma volume and reduced cardiac output. When water loss reaches 3 to 4% of body weight, blood flow to the kidneys, skin, and muscles is decreased with a corresponding decrease in urinary output. At a 5% weight change, the sweat rate is decreased and the capacity for prolonged activity is reduced by 20 to 30%.[11] The impact of dehydration on physical performance is illustrated in Figure 4. The symptoms associated with continued water loss include: difficulty in concentrating; headache; sleepiness; increased pulse and respiratory rate; dizziness; mental confusion; spastic muscles; delirium; circulatory insufficiency; renal failure; and eventual death.[12]

3. Heat Injuries

Any athlete who exercises in a hot environment is vulnerable to heat injury or heat illness. Increased core temperature, loss of body fluids, and loss of electrolytes are among the factors related to the development of a heat injury. It is important that athletes recognize the symptoms of the various heat injuries and the appropriate treatment. Table 2 presents the symptoms, causes, weight loss, and treatment of the major heat injuries.

Heat cramps are thought to be caused by profuse sweating with excessive loss of sodium, potassium, and magnesium. Cramps are usually located in the muscles in the calf of the leg or abdomen. Onset of heat cramps may be experienced when there is a 5% loss of body weight as sweat.

When there is a loss of 5 to 10% body weight as sweat, **heat exhaustion** may occur. Symptoms include reduced sweat production, dizziness, headache, shortness

TABLE 2 Heat Injuries: Diagnosis and Treatment

Heat Injury	Symptoms	Cause	Weight loss	Treatment
Heat cramps	• Thirst • Chills • Clammy skin • Throbbing heart beat • Nausea	Excessive loss of electrolytes in sweat/inadequate salt intake	A loss of up to 5% of body weight as sweat	• Drink 1/2 cup water every 10–15 min • Electrolyte replacement drinks and adequate daily salt intake may prevent difficulties
Heat exhaustion	• Reduced sweating • Dizziness • Headache • Shortness of breath • Weak, rapid pulse • Lack of saliva • Extreme fatigue	Inadequate fluid intake/excessive loss of sweat	A loss of 5–10% of body weight as sweat	• Stop exercise and move to cool environment • Drink 2 cups of cool water for every pound lost • Take off wet clothing and sit on a chair in a cold shower • Place bag of ice on head
Heat stroke	• Lack of sweat • Dry, hot skin • Lack of urine • Hallucinations • Swollen tongue • Deafness • Visual disturbance • Aggression • Unsteady walking • Excessive high body temperature	Elevated body temperature	A loss of 10% of body weight as sweat	• Call for medical assistance immediately • Cool body with ice packs • Drink cool beverage containing glucose, if coherent

of breath, weak rapid pulse, lack of saliva, and extreme fatigue. This condition is frequently observed in athletes who are not conditioned to exercise in heat or athletes who have failed to replace salt losses.[13] The athlete should stop exercising when the first symptoms appear and start rehydrating immediately.

Heat stroke is the most serious of the heat injuries, and can be fatal if not treated in time. It occurs when over 10% of the body weight as sweat has been lost. Symptoms include lack of sweat, hot skin, lack of urine, hallucinations, and an excessively high core body temperature (over 105.8°F or 41°C).[13] The athlete should be cooled down with ice packs and offered a cool beverage containing glucose until medical assistance arrives.

III. RECOMMENDATIONS FOR FLUID REPLACEMENT

A. WATER REQUIREMENTS FOR THE RECREATIONAL ATHLETE

1. Thirst

Thirst is an unreliable indicator of fluid needs after exercise, partly because the intake of water quickly dulls the thirst sensation.[14] Relying on thirst alone might take up to 48 h to replenish fluid lost by some athletes.[15] Thirst lags behind water lack, so by the time the thirst mechanism is initiated, partial dehydration has already occurred. Athletes often do not feel thirst, or ignore it, due to the strain and excitement of the their physical activity, even when dehydrated. Therefore, athletes may need to be reminded and encouraged to drink during vigorous exercise, whether they are thirsty or not.

2. Hydration Requirements

To ensure that the fluid lost during physical activity is replaced, body weight should be measured before and after exercise. Each pound (0.45 kg) lost should be replaced with 2 cups (474 ml) of fluid. If weight is not within 1 to 2 lb of the previous day's pre-exercise weight, additional fluids should be consumed before exercising again.[16]

B. FLUID REPLACEMENT CONSIDERATIONS

For exercise requiring less than 30 min of exertion, replacement of the water lost in sweat is of greater concern than are losses of body carbohydrate stores and electrolytes (sodium, potassium, chloride, and other minerals), which are not usually too severe in such activities.[17] The electrolytes that are lost in sweat can easily be replaced by eating a normal diet.

To rehydrate an athlete following fluid loss, it is essential that fluids be absorbed as rapidly as possible. Fluids must be emptied from the stomach before being absorbed in the small intestines. Gastric emptying time is affected by fluid volume, temperature, and carbohydrate content.

1. Volume

Large amounts of fluid (up to 20 oz or 2.5 cups) empty more quickly from the stomach than small amounts. Normally, up to 1 liter of water can be emptied from the stomach and absorbed from the intestine in 1 h.[18] Costill and Saltin[19] found that exercise intensities up to 70% of maximal oxygen consumption have little or no effect on the emptying and absorption of water. This minimum quantity of fluid must, therefore, be consumed each hour during exercise to help maintain normal hydration and prevent heat injury. Athletes may find it uncomfortable to exercise with a full stomach, because it interferes with breathing. By consuming moderate portions of 100 to 200 ml every 10 to 15 min, fluid needs can be met without feeling bloated.

2. Temperature

Cold fluids are emptied from the stomach at a faster rate than warm fluids. Although fluids at refrigerator temperatures of 3 to 4°C reduce the temperature of the stomach from 37 to 10°C, they do not appear to cause stomach cramps.[20] Consuming unusually large volumes of fluid is the more probable cause of stomach distress.

3. Carbohydrate

As the carbohydrate content of a beverage increases, its osmolality increases, reducing its rate of gastric emptying. Consequently, the rate of fluid repletion decreases.[21] The carbohydrate in beverages is of little value to the athlete if it slows gastric emptying time or restricts the movement of water out of the intestines. Coyle et al.[22] found that a solution containing 4.6 g of carbohydrate (sucrose and glucose) per 100 ml emptied from the stomach at a rate 35% slower than that of water.

The use of glucose polymers (molecules of glucose linked together in short chains) instead of simple sugars in fluid replacement beverages offers the advantage of reduced osmolality with the same caloric content of simple sugars. Glucose polymers were first thought to empty the stomach faster than beverages containing glucose. However, Costill[23] found that there was little difference in the stomach emptying times between beverages containing glucose polymers and those containing simple sugars such as glucose or sucrose as long as the concentrations of carbohydrate are in the 5 to 8% range.

Beverages that contain fructose as the primary carbohydrate source may cause gastric distress in some athletes and are known to require more time before they can be used by muscles as a fuel because of the necessary conversion of fructose to glucose.[24] Drinks that exceed 10% carbohydrate (soft drinks and undiluted fruit juices) can cause cramps, nausea, and diarrhea as well as taking longer to be absorbed. If these beverages are used during athletic performance, they should be diluted.

4. Caffeine/Alcohol/Carbonated Beverages

Caffeine is used by some athletes to increase endurance time. Caffeine enhances the release of fatty acids from adipose tissue, and when used as a fuel source, glycogen is spared and the onset of fatigue is delayed.[25] Dodd et al.[26] found caffeine to be most ergogenic during prolonged, moderate-intensity exercise. Caffeine acts as a diuretic and may impair performance in some athletes by increasing water load in the urine, leading to dehydration or by causing gastrointestinal upset. The International Olympic Committee will not let athletes with urine caffeine levels of 12 mg per ml or greater compete because of its role as a stimulant.

Alcohol is inappropriate as a fluid replacement, as it too is a diuretic. It stimulates the excretion of water; of the vitamins thiamine, riboflavin, and folate; and electrolytes such as calcium, magnesium, and potassium, all important for fluid balance. Alcohol has a negative effect on performance by impairing temperature regulation, making one more prone to thermal injury.

Carbonated beverages are often avoided by athletes or "de-gassed" before drinking. It is generally felt that the ingestion of a carbonated beverage during exercise will induce feelings of gastrointestinal distress either resulting from or inducing poor gastric emptying. However, recent work by Zachwieja et al.[27] who tested this concept showed that the ingestion of carbonated beverages did not affect the rate of gastric emptying nor did it increase perceptions of gastrointestinal distress in subjects while exercising.

C. SCHEDULE FOR FLUID REPLACEMENT

1. Hyperhydration (Pre-Exercise/Competition)

The purpose of pre-exercise/competition hydration is to provide fluid support to the athlete during the upcoming event. This practice is particularly important for recreational athletes participating in endurance events or in hot climates. Hyperhydration is the voluntary ingestion of water or other beverages for the purpose of increasing body fluids. The consumption of "extra" water before exercise helps the recreational athlete to maintain fluid balance during exercise and enhance performance. Hyperhydration can actually begin the day before the event by drinking fluids freely. Hyperhydration should continue throughout the next day with 2 cups of cool water ingested 30 min prior to the event and fluids containing small amounts of carbohydrate (approximately 5 to 8%), as tolerated, taken 5 to 10 min before the activity. A schedule for fluid replacement is shown in Table 3.

2. During Exercise/Competition

During exercise/competition, fluids containing small amounts (4 to 6 oz) of carbohydrate or a glucose-electrolyte beverage should be ingested every 10 to 15 min, regardless of thirst. At this rate, approximately 1 L/h will be consumed. This may be sufficient to offset sweat loss under moderate conditions. The goal of fluid replacement during exercise is to replace at least 50% of fluid losses.[28] It is important to remember that the sensation of thirst is dulled by exercise.

3. After Exercise/Competition

Immediately after the exercise/competition, each pound of body weight lost should be replaced with 2 cups (16 oz) of water or carbohydrate beverage. The

TABLE 3 Recommendations for Fluid Replacement

Time	Amount
Pre-exercise/competition	
• Day before	• Drink fluids freely
• Pre-event meal	• 2–3 Cups water
• 1–2 h before	• 2 Cups cool water
• 30 min before	• 2 Cups cool water
• 5–10 min before	• Fluids containing small amounts of carbohydrate or glucose-electrolyte beverages may be consumed as tolerated
During exercise/competition	
• Every 10–15 min	• 1/2–3/4 Cup cool water, fluids containing small amounts of carbohydrate, or glucose-electrolyte beverages
After exercise/competition	
• Immediately	• Drink 2 cups water or carbohydrate beverage for each pound of body weight loss
Next day	• Drink fluids liberally
	• May take up to 36 h to completely rehydrate

athlete must be weighed before and after the event to calculate his fluid replacement needs. Since complete rehydration may take up to 36 h, fluids should be encouraged into the following day.

4. Sports Drinks

There are a number of commercial sports beverages available for use during exercise to help replace fluids and electrolytes and to supply energy to replace muscle glycogen stores. The nutrient composition of some of the more popular sports drinks, such as Gatorade®, 10-K®, Exceed®, and Body Fuel 450®, is shown in Table 4.

Replacement solutions are most effective when used during events lasting 60 min or more.[29] For activities lasting 1 h or less in moderate temperature conditions, the most appropriate fluid replacement is cool water.

Electrolytes that are lost in sweat are often added to sports drinks, such as sodium, chloride, potassium, calcium, and magnesium. This seems to be unnecessary since the small amount of electrolytes lost to sweat can be easily replaced by eating a balanced diet. The combination of sodium and glucose in sports drinks has, however, been found to improve fluid absorption in the small intestine.[30]

To be effective, sports beverages should taste good to promote consumption, provide a carbohydrate source that enhances performance during endurance activities, and optimize the rate of fluid absorption.

IV. SUMMARY

For the recreational athlete, water is the single most important requirement in sports nutrition. Proper fluid replacement before, during, and after physical activity positively influences an athlete's performance. Dehydration impairs

TABLE 4 Nutrient Comparison of Selected Sports Drinks

Beverage (8 oz)	Carbohydrate (%)	Carbohydrate Source	Calories (kcal)	Sodium (mg)	Potassium (mg)	Other Nutrients
Body Fuel 450®	4.2	Glucose polymers/ fructose	40	80	20	Chloride; iron; phosphorus; vitamins A, C, and B complex
Quickick®	4.7	Fructose/sucrose	44	116	23	Calcium; chloride; phosphorus
Gatorade®	6	Sucrose/glucose	56	110	25	Chloride; phosphorus
PowerBurst®	6	Fructose	56	35	56	Biotin; calcium; chloride; folic acid; magnesium; pantothenic acid; vitamins C, A, E, and B-complex
10-K®	6.3	Sucrose/glucose/ fructose	60	52	26	Chloride; phosphorus; vitamin C
Squincher the Activity Drink®	6.8	Glucose/fructose	64	60	36	Calcium; chloride; magnesium; phosphorus; vitamin C
Exceed®	7	Glucose polymers/ fructose	68	50	45	Calcium; chloride; magnesium; phosphorus

thermoregulation, leading to decreased endurance and decreased performance. As the thirst mechanism is blunted with exercise, it is important for athletes to monitor and meet their fluid needs by implementing the fluid replacement guidelines presented in this chapter, appropriate to their exercise needs. By doing so, the health risks of dehydration can be avoided, allowing warm weather exercise to be enjoyable.

REFERENCES

1. American Dietetic Association, Position of the American Dietetic Association: Nutrition for physical fitness and athletic performance for adults, *J. Am. Diet. Assoc.*, 87, 937, 1987.
2. **Holt, W. S.,** Nutrition and athletes, *Am. Fam. Physician*, 47, 1757, 1993.
3. National Research Council, *Recommended Dietary Allowances*, 10th ed., National Academy Press, Washington D.C., 1989, 249.
4. **Robinson, C. H., Lawler, M. R., Chenoweth, W. L., and Garwick, A. E.,** *Normal and Therapeutic Nutrition*, Macmillian, New York, 1986, 138.
5. **Horne, M. M. and Swearingen, P. L.,** *Pocket Guide to Fluids and Electrolytes*, C. V. Mosby, St. Louis, 1989, 1.
6. **Williams, M. H.,** *Nutritional Aspects of Human Physical and Athletic Performance*, Charles C Thomas, Springfield, IL, 1976, 174.
7. **Nadel, E. R.,** New ideas for rehydration during and after exercise in hot weather, *Sports Sci. Exch.*, 1, 3, 1988.
8. **Greenleaf, J. E.,** Problem: thirst, drinking, behavior, and involuntary dehydration, *Med. Sci. Sports Exerc.*, 24, 645, 1993.
9. **Horswill, C. A.,** Does rapid weight loss by dehydration adversely affect high power performance?, *Sports Sci. Exch.*, 3, 30, 1991.
10. **Ekblom, B., Greenleaf, C. J., Greenleaf, J. E., and Hermansen, L.,** Temperature regulation during exercise dehydration in man, *Acta Physiol. Scand.*, 79, 475, 1970.
11. **Olsson, K. E. and Saltin, B.,** Diet and fluids in training and competition, *Scand. J. Rehab. Med.*, 3, 31, 1971.
12. **Hasket, W., Scala, J., and Whittam, J.,** *Nutrition and Athletic Performance: Nutritional Determinants in Athletic Performance*, Bull Pub. Co., Palo Alto, CA, 1982, 46.
13. **Williams, M. H.,** *Nutrition for Fitness and Sport*, William Brown Pub., Dubuque, IA, 1992, 208.
14. **Wheeler, K. B.,** Water and carbohydrate needs of endurance athletes, *Medical Coverage of Endurance Athletic Events*, Ross Laboratories, Columbus, 1987, 89.
15. **Lamb, D. R. and Wardlow, G. M.,** *Sport Nutrition-Nutri-News*, Mosby-Year Book, Inc., St. Louis, 1991, 13,.
16. **Wardlaw, G. M., Insel, P. M., and Seyler, M. F.,** Athletics and fitness, in *Contemporary Nutrition*, 2nd ed., C.V. Mosby, St. Louis, 1994, 369.
17. **Gisolfi, D. V. and Duchman, S. M.,** Guidelines for optimal replacement beverages for different athletic events, *Med. Sci. Sports Exerc.*, 24, 679, 1992.
18. **Davenport, H. W.,** Digestion and absorption, in *Physiology of the Digestive Tract*, 4th ed., Year Book Medical Publishers, Chicago, 1990, 187.
19. **Costill, D. L. and Saltin, B.,** Factors limiting gastric emptying during rest and exercise, *J. Appl. Physiol.*, 37, 679, 1974.
20. **Wilmore, J. J. and Costill, D. L.,** Nutrition and human performance, in *Eating, Body Weight and Performance in Athletes*, Lea & Febiger, Philadelphia, 71, 1992.
21. **McSwiney, B. A. and Spurrel, W. R.,** Influence of osmotic pressure upon the emptying time of the stomach, *J. Physiol.*, 79, 437, 1933.

22. **Coyle, E. F., Costill, D. L., and Fink, W. J.,** Gastric emptying characteristics of commercial hydration solutions, *Res. Q.*, 49, 119, 1978.
23. **Costill, D. L.,** Carbohydrate for exercise: dietary demands for optimal performance, *Int. J. Sports Med.*, 9, 1, 1988.
24. **Fruth, J. M. and Gisolfi, C. V.,** Effect of carbohydrate consumption on endurance performance: fructose versus glucose, *Nutrition Utilization During Exercise*, Ross Laboratories, Columbus, 1983, 24.
25. **Tarnopolsky, M. A., Atkinson, S. A., and MacDougall, J. D.,** Physiological responses to caffeine during endurance running in habitual caffeine users, *Med. Sci. Sports Exerc.*, 21, 418, 1989.
26. **Dodd, S. L., Herb, R. A., and Powers, S. K.,** Caffeine and exercise performance: an update, *Sports Med.*, 15, 14, 1993.
27. **Zachwieja, J. J., Costill, D. L., Widrick, J. J., Anderson, D. E., and McConell, G. K.,** Effects of drink carbonation on the gastric emptying characteristics of water and flavored water, *Int. J. Sports Med.*, 45, 51, 1991.
28. **Lyle, B. J. and Forgac, T.,** Hydration and Fluid Replacement, in *Sports Nutrition for the 90's, The Health Professional's Handbook*, Aspen Pub., Gaithersburg, MD, 1991, 183.
29. **Placido, V. J., Macaraeg, J. R., and Santos, C. A.,** The effect of glucose polymer-electrolyte solution on exercise duration, in *Proceedings of Australian Sports Medicine Federation: Medical and Scientific Aspects of Elitism in Sport and Science*, 1984, 8.
30. **Murray, R.,** The effects of consuming carbohydrate-electrolyte beverages on gastric emptying and fluid absorption during and following exercise, *Sports Med.*, 4, 322, 1987.

Appendix A

TABLES OF VARIABLES IN SPORTS AND ACTIVITIES

The following tables have been created to illustrate the relationships between variables discussed in Chapter 1 for activities played by adults in America, both team and individual. The values awarded are of an arbitrary nature chosen by the author with the value of "1" being the least while "5" is to be considered the strongest value. The values do not mean that more or fewer people play a particular sport.

Table 1 and Table 5 illustrate motivational factors in team and individual (Table 1) and non-competitive sports (Table 5). Table 1 shows that the team sports are rather equal in nature for motivation factors except it is felt that slow-pitch softball tends to be played by more people for a social experience while fast-pitch softball is the result of a more competitive nature. Individual sports are more diverse in their respective motivational factors. The major difference when comparing the individual sport to the team sport must appear in the area of occupational motivation. Few companies support a sport such as tennis or golf as a company competition, whereas many companies do support softball, basketball, and volleyball teams in the community setting. Individual sports are possibly more useful for wellness than are team sports. Swimming just by its physical nature — in the water — tends to be the least social of the sports.

Table 2 for team and individual sports and Table 6 for noncompetitive sports illustrate the required physical aspects of the various sports. The physical aspects of strength are quite equal in both the team and the individual sports except running, swimming, and biking, while speed is not really an important factor in golf and bowling. The need for agility is also necessary in both team and individual sports with the exceptions of golf and bowling. The major aspect of note is that of endurance. Basketball, tennis, running, swimming, and biking require a great deal of endurance capability, while the need in baseball is for the positions of pitching and catching.

Table 3 for team and individual sports and Table 7 for noncompetitive sports show the types of activities which are most common. Table 4 for team and individual sports and Table 8 for noncompetitive sports illustrate the age groups of participation.

0-8493-7914-8/95/$0.00+$.50

TABLE 1 Matrix of Team and Individual Sports Illustrating Motivation

	Social	Competition	Wellness	Occupational	Fun
Team Sports					
Baseball	3	4	2	3	3
Basketball	4	4	4	4	4
Fast pitch softball	4	5	3	4	3
Slow pitch softball	5	4	3	4	4
Volleyball	4	4	4	4	4
Touch football	3	4	3	4	3
Soccer	4	4	4	3	4
Hockey	3	4	4	3	4
Individual Sports					
Tennis	4	4	4	2	4
Golf	4	3	2	2	4
Racquetball	4	4	4	2	3
Running	3	3	5	1	3
Swimming	2	3	4	1	3
Skiing	3	3	3	1	4
Bowling	4	4	4	4	4
Biking	3	3	5	1	4

TABLE 2 Matrix of Team and Individual Sports Illustrating Physical Aspects

	Strength	Speed	Agility	Endurance Capacity
Team Sports				
Baseball	3	3	3	2
Basketball	3	4	4	5
Fast pitch softball	3	4	4	3
Slow pitch softball	3	4	4	3
Volleyball	3	4	4	3
Touch football	3	4	4	4
Soccer	3	4	4	5
Hockey	3	4	4	4
Individual Sports				
Tennis	3	4	4	5
Golf	3	1	2	3
Racquetball	3	4	4	4
Running	3	3	3	5
Swimming	4	3	3	5
Skiing	4	3	4	4
Bowling	3	1	2	3
Biking	3	3	3	5

TABLE 3 Matrix of Team and Individual Sports Illustrating Types of Activities

	Instruction	Tournaments	Leagues	Meets	Special Events	Open Play
Team Sports						
Baseball	2	3	3	N/A	3	1
Basketball	2	4	4	N/A	4	3
Fast pitch softball	2	3	3	N/A	3	1
Slow pitch softball	2	5	5	N/A	5	3
Volleyball	2	4	4	N/A	4	3
Touch football	1	1	2	N/A	2	2
Soccer	2	2	3	N/A	3	2
Hockey	2	2	3	N/A	3	2
Individual Sports						
Tennis	4	4	2	N/A	3	4
Golf	3	3	3	N/A	3	5
Racquetball	2	3	2	N/A	3	4
Running	1	N/A	N/A	4	4	4
Swimming	3	N/A	N/A	3	3	4
Skiing	4	N/A	N/A	2	2	5
Bowling	3	4	5	N/A	4	3
Biking	2	N/A	N/A	2	2	4

TABLE 4 Matrix of Team and Individual Sports Illustrating Age Groups

	30 and Under	40 and Under	50 and Under	60 and Under	Over 60
Team Sports					
Baseball	3	2	1	1	1
Basketball	4	3	2	2	1
Fast pitch softball	4	2	2	2	1
Slow pitch softball	5	3	2	2	1
Volleyball	4	3	2	2	1
Touch football	3	2	1	1	1
Soccer	3	2	1	1	1
Hockey	3	2	1	1	1
Individual Sports					
Tennis	4	3	3	2	2
Golf	4	4	3	3	3
Racquetball	4	4	3	2	2
Running	4	4	3	3	2
Swimming	4	4	3	3	2
Skiing	4	4	3	3	2
Bowling	4	4	4	3	2
Biking	4	4	3	3	2

TABLE 5 Matrix of Noncompetitive Sports Illustrating Motivation

	Social	Competition	Wellness	Occupational	Fun
Swimming	2	1	4	1	4
Scuba	1	1	4	1	4
Downhill skiing	3	2	3	2	4
Cross-country skiing	4	1	4	1	4
Running	3	1	4	1	3
Biking	3	1	4	1	4
Hiking	2	1	3	1	4
Weight lifting	3	1	4	1	3
Aerobics	4	1	5	1	4
Exercise machine use	3	1	4	1	4
Volkssports	4	1	4	1	5

TABLE 6 Matrix of Noncompetitive Sports Illustrating Physical Aspects

	Strength	Speed	Agility	Endurance Capacity
Swimming	4	2	2	4
Scuba	4	3	3	4
Downhill skiing	4	2	4	4
Cross-country skiing	4	2	3	4
Running	4	2	2	4
Biking	4	3	2	4
Hiking	4	2	3	4
Weight lifting	5	2	3	4
Aerobics	4	2	3	5
Exercise machine use	4	2	2	4
Volkssports	3	2	2	4

TABLE 7 Matrix of Noncompetitive Sports Illustrating Types of Activities

	Instruction	Tournaments	Leagues	Meets	Special Events	Open Play
Swimming	4	N/A	N/A	2	2	5
Scuba	5	N/A	N/A	2	2	4
Downhill skiing	5	N/A	N/A	2	2	4
Cross-country skiing	3	N/A	N/A	1	1	4
Running	2	N/A	N/A	3	3	3
Biking	2	N/A	N/A	2	2	4
Hiking	2	N/A	N/A	N/A	1	4
Weight lifting	3	N/A	N/A	1	1	4
Aerobics	4	N/A	N/A	1	1	3
Exercise machine use	4	N/A	N/A	N/A	N/A	4
Volkssports	1	N/A	N/A	3	3	3

TABLE 8 Matrix of Noncompetitive Sports Illustrating Age Groups

	30 and Under	40 and Under	50 and Under	60 and Under	Over 60
Swimming	4	4	3	2	2
Scuba	3	3	2	2	1
Downhill skiing	4	4	3	2	1
Cross-country skiing	3	3	3	2	1
Running	4	4	3	2	1
Biking	4	4	3	2	2
Hiking	4	4	3	2	2
Weight lifting	4	3	2	1	1
Aerobics	4	4	3	2	1
Exercise machine use	4	3	2	2	1
Volkssports	4	4	3	3	2

Appendix B

AMERICAN COLLEGE OF SPORTS MEDICINE POSITION STAND ON PROPER AND IMPROPER WEIGHT LOSS PROGRAMS*

Millions of individuals are involved in weight reduction programs. With the number of undesirable weight loss programs available and a general misconception by many about weight loss, the need for guidelines for proper weight loss programs is apparent.

Based on the existing evidence concerning the effects of weight loss on health status, physiologic processes, and body composition parameters, the American College of Sports Medicine makes the following statements and recommendations for weight loss programs.

For the purposes of this position stand, body weight will be represented by two components, fat and fat-free (water, electrolytes, minerals, glycogen stores, muscular tissue, bone, etc.):

1. Prolonged fasting and diet programs that severely restrict caloric intake are scientifically undesirable and can be medically dangerous.
2. Fasting and diet programs that severely restrict caloric intake result in the loss of large amounts of water, electrolytes, minerals, glycogen stores, and other fat-free tissue (including proteins within fat-free tissues), with minimal amounts of fat loss.
3. Mild calorie restriction (500 to 1000 kcal less than the usual daily intake) results in smaller loss of water, electrolytes, minerals, and other fat-free tissue, and is less likely to cause malnutrition.
4. Dynamic exercise of large muscles helps to maintain fat-free tissue, including muscle mass and bone density, and results in losses of body weight. Weight loss resulting from an increase in energy expenditure is primarily in the form of fat weight.
5. A nutritionally sound diet resulting in mild calorie restriction coupled with an endurance exercise program along with behavioral modification of existing eating habits is recommended for weight reduction. The rate of sustained weight loss should not exceed 1 kg (2 lb) per week.

* Reprinted from *"Proper and Improper Weight-Loss Programs,"* ©1983 American College of Sports Medicine, *MSSE,* 15:1, 1983, pp ix–xiii. With permission of Williams & Wilkins.

6. To maintain proper weight control and optimal body fat levels, a lifetime commitment to proper eating habits and regular physical activity is required.

RESEARCH BACKGROUND FOR THE POSITION STAND

Each year millions of individuals undertake weight loss programs for a variety of reasons. It is well known that obesity is associated with a number of health-related problems.[3,4,57] These problems include impairment of cardiac function due to an increase in the work of the heart[2] and to left ventricular dysfunction;[1,40] hypertension;[6,22,80] diabetes;[83,97] renal disease;[95] gall bladder disease;[55,72] respiratory dysfunction;[19] joint diseases and gout;[90] endometrial cancer;[15] abnormal plasma lipid and lipoprotein concentrations;[56,74] problems in the administration of anesthetics during surgery;[93] and impairment of physical working capacity.[49] As a result, weight reduction is frequently advised by physicians for medical reasons. In addition, there are a vast number of individuals who are on weight reduction programs for aesthetic reasons.

It is estimated that 60 to 70 million American adults and at least 10 million American teenagers are overfat.[49] Because millions of Americans have adopted unsupervised weight loss programs, it is the opinion of the American College of Sports Medicine that guidelines are needed for safe and effective weight loss programs. This position stand deals with desirable and undesirable weight loss programs. Desirable weight loss programs are defined as those that are nutritionally sound and result in maximal losses in fat weight and minimal losses of fat-free tissue. Undesirable weight loss programs are defined as those that are not nutritionally sound, that result in large losses of fat-free tissue, that pose potential serious medical complications, and that cannot be followed for long-term weight maintenance.

Therefore, a desirable weight loss program is one that:

1. Provides a caloric intake not lower than 1200 $kcal \cdot d^{-1}$ for normal adults in order to get a proper blend of foods to meet nutritional requirements. (Note: this requirement may change for children, older individuals, athletes, etc.)
2. Includes foods acceptable to the dieter from the viewpoints of sociocultural background, usual habits, taste, cost, and ease in acquisition and preparation.
3. Provides a negative caloric balance (not to exceed 500 to 1000 $kcal \cdot d^{-1}$ lower than recommended), resulting in gradual weight loss without metabolic derangements. Maximal weight loss should be 1 $kg \cdot week^{-1}$.
4. Includes the use of behavior modification techniques to identify and eliminate dieting habits that contribute to improper nutrition.

5. Includes an endurance exercise program of at least 3 d/week, 20 to 30 min in duration, at a minimum intensity of 60% of maximum heart rate (refer to ACSM Position Stand on the Recommended Quantity and Quality of Exercise for Developing and Maintaining Fitness in Healthy Adults, *Med. Sci. Sports.* 10, vii, 1978).
6. Provides that the new eating and physical activity habits can be continued for life in order to maintain the achieved lower body weight.

1. Since the early work of Keys et al.[50] and Bloom,[16] which indicated that marked reduction in caloric intake or fasting (starvation or semistarvation) rapidly reduced body weight, numerous fasting, modified fasting, and fad diet and weight loss programs have emerged. While these programs promise and generally cause rapid weight loss, they are associated with significant medical risks.

The medical risks associated with these types of diet and weight loss programs are numerous. Blood glucose concentrations have been shown to be markedly reduced in obese subjects who undergo fasting.[18,32,74,84] Further, in obese nondiabetic subjects, fasting may result in impairment of glucose tolerance.[10,52] Ketonuria begins within a few hours after fasting or low-carbohydrate diets are begun[53] and hyperuricemia is common among subjects who fast to reduce body weight.[18] Fasting also results in high serum uric acid levels with decreased urinary output.[59] Fasting and low-calorie diets also result in urinary nitrogen loss and a significant decrease in fat-free tissue[7,11,17,42,101] (see section 2). In comparison to ingestion of a normal diet, fasting substantially elevates urinary excretion of potassium.[10,32,37,52,53,78] This, coupled with the aforementioned nitrogen loss, suggests that the potassium loss is due to a loss of lean tissue.[78] Other electrolytes, including sodium,[32,53] calcium,[30,84] magnesium,[30,84] and phosphate,[84] have been shown to be elevated in urine during prolonged fasting. Reductions in blood volume and body fluids are also common with fasting and fad diets.[18] This can be associated with weakness and fainting.[32] Congestive heart failure and sudden death have been reported in subjects who fasted[48,79,80] or markedly restricted their caloric intake.[79] Myocardial atrophy appears to contribute to sudden death.[79] Sudden death may also occur during refeeding.[25,79] Untreated fasting has also been reported to reduce serum iron binding capacity, resulting in anemia.[47,73,89] Liver glycogen levels are depleted with fasting,[38,60,63] and liver function[29,31,37,75,76,92] and gastrointestinal tract abnormalities[13,32,53,65,85,91] are associated with fasting. While fasting and calorically restricted diets have been shown to lower serum cholesterol levels,[88,96] a large portion of the cholesterol reduction is a result of lowered HDL-cholesterol levels.[88,96] Other risks associated with fasting and low-calorie diets include lactic acidosis,[12,26] alopecia,[73] hypoalaninemia,[34] edema,[23,78] anuria,[101] hypotension,[18,32,78] elevated serum bilirubin,[8,9] nausea and vomiting,[53] alterations in thyroxine metabolism,[71,91] impaired serum triglyceride removal and production,[86] and death.[25,37,48,61,80]

2. The major objective of any weight reduction program is to lose body fat while maintaining fat-free tissue. The vast majority of research reveals that starvation and low-calorie diets result in large losses of water, electrolytes, and other fat-free tissue. One of the best controlled experiments was conducted from 1944 to 1946 at the Laboratory of Physiological Hygiene at the University of Minnesota.[50] In this study, subjects had their baseline caloric intake cut by 45% and body weight and body composition changes were followed for 24 weeks. During the first 12 weeks of semistarvation, body weight declined by 25.4 lb (11.5 kg) with only an 11.6 lb (5.3 kg) decline in body fat. During the second 12-week period, body weight declined an additional 9.1 lb (4.1 kg) with only a 6.1 lb (2.8 kg) decrease in body fat. These data clearly demonstrate that fat-free tissue significantly contributes to weight loss from semistarvation. Similar results have been reported by several other investigators. Buskirk et al.[20] reported that the 13.5 kg weight loss in 6 subjects on a low-calorie mixed diet averaged 76% fat and 24% fat-free tissue. Similarly, Passmore et al.[64] reported results of 78% of weight loss (15.3 kg) as fat and 22% as fat-free tissue in 7 women who consumed a 400 kcal $\cdot$ d^{-1} diet for 45 d. Yang and Van Itallie[101] followed weight loss and body composition changes for the first 5 d of a weight loss program involving subjects consuming an 800 kcal mixed diet, an 800 kcal ketogenic diet, or undergoing starvation. Subjects on the mixed diet lost 1.3 kg of weight (59% fat loss, 3.4% protein loss, 37.6% water loss), subjects on the ketogenic diet lost 2.3 kg of weight (33.2% fat, 3.8% protein, 63.0% water), and subjects on starvation regimens lost 3.8 kg of weight (32.3% fat, 6.5% protein, 61.2% water). Grande[41] and Grande et al.[43] reported similar findings with a 1000 kcal carbohydrate diet. It was further reported that water restriction combined with 1000 kcal $\cdot$ day^{-1} of carbohydrate resulted in greater water loss and less fat loss.

Recently there has been some renewed speculation about the efficacy of the very low-calorie diet (VLCD). Krotkiewski and associates[51] studied the effects on body weight and body composition after 3 weeks on the so-called Cambridge diet. Two groups of obese middle-aged women were studied. One group had a VLCD only, while the second group had a VLCD combined with a 55 min/d, 3 d/week exercise program. The VLCD-only group lost 6.2 kg in 3 weeks, of which only 2.6 kg was fat loss, while the VLCD plus exercise group lost 6.8 kg in 3 weeks with only a 1.9 kg body fat loss. Thus it can be seen that VLCD results in undesirable losses of body fat, and the addition of the normally protective effect of chronic exercise to VLCD does not reduce the catabolism of fat-free tissue. Further, with VLCD, a large reduction (29%) in HDL-cholesterol is seen.[94]

3. Even mild calorie restriction (reduction of 500 to 1000 kcal $\cdot$ d^{-1} from baseline caloric intake), when used alone as a tool for weight loss, results in the loss of moderate amounts of water and other fat-free tissue. In a study by Goldman et al.,[39] 15 female subjects consumed a low-calorie mixed diet for 7 to 8 weeks. Weight loss during this period averaged 6.43 kg (0.85 kg $\cdot$ $week^{-1}$), 88.6% of which was fat. The remaining 11.4% represented water and other fat-free tissue. Zuti and Golding[102] examined the effect of 500 kcal $\cdot$ d^{-1} calorie restriction on body composition changes in adult females. Over a 16-week period, the women lost approximately 5.2 kg; however, 1.1 kg of the weight loss (21%) was due to a loss of water and other fat-free tissue. More recently, Weltman et al.[96] examined the effects of 500 kcal $\cdot$ d^{-1} calorie restriction (from base-line levels) on body composition changes in sedentary middle-aged males. Over a 10-week period, subjects lost 5.95 kg, 4.03 kg (68%) of which was fat loss and 1.92 kg (32%) of which was loss of water and other fat-free tissue. Further, with calorie restriction only, these subjects exhibited a decrease in HDL-cholesterol. In the same study, the two other groups who exercised and/or dieted and exercised were able to maintain their HDL-cholesterol levels. Similar results for females have been presented by Thompson et al.[88] It should be noted that the decrease seen in HDL-cholesterol with weight loss may be an acute effect. There are data that indicate that stable weight loss has a beneficial effect on HDL-cholesterol.[21,24,46,88]

Further, an additional problem associated with calorie restriction alone for effective weight loss is the fact that it is associated with a reduction in basal metabolic rate.[5] Apparently exercise combined with calorie restriction can counter this response.[14]

4. There are several studies that indicate that exercise helps maintain fat-free tissue while promoting fat loss. Total body weight and fat weight are generally reduced with endurance training programs,[70] while fat-free weight remains constant[36,54,69,70,98] or increases slightly.[62,96,102] Programs conducted at least 3 d/week,[66-69,98] of at least 20-min duration[58,69,98] and of sufficient intensity and duration to expend at least 300 kcal per exercise session, have been suggested as a threshold level for total body weight and fat weight reduction.[27,44,69,70] Increasing caloric expenditure above 300 kcal per exercise session and increasing the frequency of exercise sessions will enhance fat weight loss while sparing fat-free tissue.[54,102] Leon et al.[54] had 6 obese male subjects walk vigorously for 90 min, 5 d/week for 16 weeks. Work output progressed weekly to an energy expenditure of 1000 to 1200 kcal per session. At the end of 16 weeks, subjects averaged 5.7 kg of weight loss with a 5.9 kg loss of fat weight and a 0.2 kg gain in fat-free tissue. Similarly, Zuti and Golding[102] followed the progress of adult women who expended 500 kcal per exercise session 5 d/week for 16 weeks of exercise. At the end of 16 weeks, the women lost 5.8 kg of fat and gained 0.9 kg of fat-free tissue.

5. Review of the literature cited above strongly indicates that optimal body composition changes occur with a combination of calorie restriction (while on a well-balanced diet) plus exercise. This combination promotes loss of fat weight while sparing fat-free tissue. Data of Zuti and Golding[102] and Weltman et al.[96] support this contention. Calorie restriction of 500 kcal $\cdot$ d^{-1} combined with 3 to 5 d of exercise requiring 300 to 500 kcal per exercise session results in favorable changes in body composition.[96,102] Therefore, the optimal rate of weight loss should be between 0.45 to 1 kg (1 to 2 lb) per week. This seems especially relevant in light of the data which indicates that rapid weight loss due to low calorie intake can be associated with sudden death.[79] In order to institute a desirable pattern of calorie restriction plus exercise, behavior modification techniques should be incorporated to identify and eliminate habits contributing to obesity and/or overfatness.[28,33,35,81,87,99,100]

6. The problem with losing weight is that, although many individuals succeed in doing so, they invariably put the weight on again.[45] The goal of an effective weight loss regimen is not merely to lose weight. Weight control requires a lifelong commitment, an understanding of our eating habits, and a willingness to change them. Frequent exercise is necessary, and accomplishment must be reinforced to sustain motivation. Crash dieting and other promised weight loss cures are ineffective.[45]

REFERENCES

1. **Alexander, J.K. and J.R. Pettigrove.** Obesity and congestive heart failure. *Geriatrics.* 22:101–108, 1967.
2. **Alexander, J.K. and K.L. Petterson.** Cardiovascular effects of weight reduction. *Circulation.* 45:310–318, 1972.
3. **Angel, A.** Pathophysiologic changes in obesity. *Can. Med. Assoc. J.* 119:1401–1406, 1978.
4. **Angel, A. and D.A.K. Roncari.** Medical complications of obesity. *Can. Med. Assoc. J.* 191:1408–1411, 1978.
5. **Appelbaum, M., J. Bostsarron, and D. Lacatis.** Effect of caloric restriction and excessive caloric intake on energy expenditure. *Am. J. Clin. Nutr.* 24:1405–1409, 1971.
6. **Bachman, L., V. Freschuss, D. Hallberg, and A. Melcher.** Cardiovascular function in extreme obesity. *Acta Med. Scand.* 193:437–446, 1972.
7. **Ball, M.F., J.J. Canary, and L.H. Kyle.** Comparative effects of caloric restrictions and total starvation on body composition in obesity. *Ann. Intern. Med.* 67:60–67, 1967.
8. **Barrett, P.V.D.** Hyperbilirubinemia of fasting. *JAMA.* 217:1349–1353, 1971.
9. **Barrett, P.V.D.** The effect of diet and fasting on the serum bilirubin concentration in the rat. *Gastroenterology.* 60:572–576, 1971.
10. **Beck, P., J.J.T. Koumans, C.A. Winterling, M.F, Stein, W.H. Daughaday, and D.M. Kipinis.** Studies on insulin and growth hormone secretion in human obesity. *J. Lab. Clin. Med.* 64:654–667, 1964.
11. **Benoit, F.L., R.L. Martin, and R.H. Watten.** Changes in body composition during weight reduction in obesity. *Ann. Intern. Med.* 63:604–612, 1965.
12. **Berger, H.** Fatal lactic acidosis during "crash" reducing diet. *N.Y. State J. Med.* 67:2258–2263, 1967.
13. **Billich, C., G. Bray, T.F. Gallagher, A.V. Hoffbrand, and R. Levitan.** Absorptive capacity of the jejunum of obese and lean subjects; effect of fasting. *Arch. Intern. Med.* 130:377–387, 1972.
14. **Bjorntorp, P., L. Sjostrom, and L. Sullivan.** The role of physical exercise in the management of obesity. In: *The Treatment of Obesity.* J.F. Munro (Ed.). Lancaster, England: MTP Press, 1979.
15. **Blitzer, P.H., E. C. Blitzer, and A.A. Rimm.** Association between teenage obesity and cancer in 56,111 women. *Prev. Med.* 5:20–31, 1976.
16. **Bloom, W.L.** Fasting as an introduction to the treatment of obesity. *Metabolism.* 8:214–220, 1959.
17. **Bolinger, R.E., B.P. Lukert, R.W. Brown, L. Guevera, and R. Steinberg.** Metabolic balances of obese subjects during fasting. *Arch. Intern. Med.* 118:3–8, 1966.
18. **Bray, G.A., M.B. Davidson, and E.J. Drenick.** Obesity: a serious symptom. *Ann. Intern. Med.* 77:779–805, 1972.
19. **Burwell, C.S., E.D. Robin, R.D. Whaley, and A.G. Bickel Mann.** Extreme obesity associated with alveolar hypoventilation—a Pickwickian syndrome. *Am. J. Med.* 21:811–818, 1956.
20. **Buskirk, E.R., R.H. Thompson, L. Lutwak, and G.D. Whedon.** Energy balance of obese patients during weight reduction: influence of diet restriction and exercise. *Ann. NY Acad Sci.* 110:918–940, 1963.

21. **Caggiula, A.W., G. Christakis, M. Ferrand, et al.** The multiple risk factors intervention trial. IV Intervention on blood lipids. *Prev. Med.* 10:443–475, 1981.
22. **Chaing, B.M., L.V. Perlman, and F.H. Epstein.** Overweight and hypertension: a review. *Circulation.* 39:403–421, 1969.
23. **Collison, D.R.** Total fasting for up to 249 days. *Lancet.* 1:112, 1967.
24. **Contaldo, F., P. Strazullo, A. Postiglione, et al.** Plasma high density lipoprotein in severe obesity after stable weight loss. *Atherosclerosis.* 37:163–167, 1980.
25. **Cruickshank, E.K.** Protein malnutrition. In: Proceedings of a conference in Jamaica (1953), J.C. Waterlow (Ed.). Cambridge: University Press, 1955, p. 107.
26. **Cubberley, P.T., S.A. Polster, and C.L. Shulman.** Lactic acidosis and death after the treatment of obesity by fasting. *N.Engl. J. Med.* 272:628–633, 1965.
27. **Cureton, T.K.** *The Physiological Effects of Exercise Programs Upon Adults.* Springfield, IL: C. Thomas Company, 1969.
28. **Dahlkoetter, J., E.J. Callahan, and J. Linton.** Obesity and the unbalanced energy equation: exercise versus eating habit change. *J. Consult. Clin. Psychol.* 47:898–905, 1979.
29. **Drenick, E.J.** The relation of BSP retention during prolonged fasts to changes in plasma volume. *Metabolism.* 17:522–527, 1968.
30. **Drenick, E.J., I.F. Hunt, and M.E. Swendseid.** Magnesium depletion during prolonged fasting in obese males. *J. Clin. Endocrinol Metab.* 29:1341–1348, 1969.
31. **Drenick, E.J., F. Simmons, and J.F. Murphy.** Effect on hepatic morphology of treatment of obesity by fasting, reducing diets and small–bowel bypass. *N. Engl. J Med.* 282:829–834, 1970.
32. **Drenick, E.J., M.E. Swendseid, W.H. Blahd, and S.G. Tuttle.** Prolonged starvation as treatment for severe obesity. *JAMA.* 187:100–105, 1964.
33. **Epstein, L.H. and R.R. Wing.** Aerobic exercise and weight. *Addict. Behav.* 5:371–388, 1980.
34. **Felig, P., O.E. Owen, J. Wahren, and G.F. Cahill, Jr.** Amino acid metabolism during prolonged starvation. *J. Clin. Invest.* 48:584–594, 1969.
35. **Ferguson, J.** *Learning to Eat: Behavior Modification for Weight Control.* Palo Alto, CA: Bull Publishing, 1975.
36. **Franklin, B., E. Buskirk, J. Hodgson, H. Gahagan, J. Kollias, and J. Mendez.** Effects of physical conditioning on cardiorespiratory function, body composition and serum lipids in relatively normal–weight and obese middle–aged women. *Int. J. Obesity.* 3:97–109, 1979.
37. **Garnett, E.S., J. Ford, D.L. Barnard, R.A. Goodbody, and M.A. Woodehouse.** Gross fragmentation of cardiac myofibrils after therapeutic starvation for obesity. *Lancet.* 1:914, 1969.
38. **Garrow, J.S.** *Energy Balance and Obesity in Man.* New York: American Elsevier, 1974.
39. **Goldman, R.F., B. Bullen, and C. Seltzer.** Changes in specific gravity and body fat in overweight female adolescents as a result of weight reduction. *Ann. NY Acad Sci.* 110:913–917, 1963.
40. **Gordon, T. and W.B. Kannel.** The effects of overweight on cardiovascular diseases. *Geriatrics.* 28:80–88, 1973.
41. **Grande, F.** Nutrition and energy balance in body composition studies In: *Techniques for Measuring Body Compositions.* J. Brozek and A. Henschel (Eds.). Washington, DC: National Academy of Sciences—National Research Council, 1961. (Reprinted by the Office of Technical Services, U.S. Department of Commerce, Washington, DC as U.S. Government Research Report AD286, 1963, 560.)
42. **Grande, F.** Energy balance and body composition changes. *Ann. Intern. Med.* 68:467–480, 1968.
43. **Grande, F., H.L. Taylor, J.T. Anderson, E. Buskirk, and A. Keys.** Water exchange in men on a restricted water intake and a low calorie carbohydrate diet accompanied by physical work. *J. Appl. Physiol.* 12:202–210, 1958.
44. **Gwinup, G.** Effect of exercise alone on the weight of obese women. *Arch. Intern. Med.* 135:676–680, 1975.

45. **Hafen, B.A.** *Nutrition, Food and Weight Control.* Boston: Allyn and Bacon. 1981, pp. 271–289.
46. **Hulley, S.B., R. Cohen, and G. Widdowson.** Plasma high density lipoprotein cholesterol level: influence of risk factor intervention. *JAMA.* 238:2269–2271, 1977.
47. **Jagenburg, R and A. Svanborg.** Self-induced protein-calorie malnutrition in a healthy adult male. *Acta Med. Scad.* 183:67–71, 1968.
48. **Kahan, A.** Death during therapeutic starvation. *Lancet.* 1:1378–1379, 1968.
49. **Katch, F.I. and W.B. Mcardle.** *Nutrition, Weight Control and Exercise.* Boston: Houghton Mifflin, 1977.
50. **Keys, A., J. Brozek, A. Henshel, O. Mickelson, and H.L. Taylor.** *The Biology of Human Starvation.* Minneapolis: University of Minnesota Press, 1950.
51. **Krotkiewski, M., L. Toss, P. Bjorntorp, and G. Holm.** The effect of a very low–calorie diet with and without chronic exercise on thyroid and sex hormones, plasma proteins, oxygen uptake, insulin and c peptide concentrations in obese women. *Int. J. Obes.* 5:287–293, 1981.
52. **Laszlo, J., R.F. Klein, and M.D. Bogdonoff.** Prolonged starvation in obese patients, in vitro and in vivo effects. *Clin. Res.* 9:183, 1961. (Abstract).
53. **Lawlor, T. and D.G. Wells.** Metabolic hazards of fasting. *Am. J. Clin. Nutr.* 22:1142–1149, 1969.
54. **Leon, A.S., J. Conrad, D.M. Hunninghake, and R. Serfass.** Effects of a vigorous walking program on body composition, and carbohydrate and lipid metabolism of obese young men. *Am. J. Clin. Nutr.* 32:1776–1787, 1979.
55. **Mabee, F.M., P. Meyer, L. Denbesten, and E.E. Mason.** The mechanism of increased gallstone formation on obese human subjects. *Surgery.* 79:460–468, 1978.
56. **Matter, S., A. Weltman, and B.A. Stamford.** Body fat content and serum lipid levels. *J Am. Diet. Assoc.* 77:149–152, 1980.
57. **Mcardle, W.D., F.l. Katch, and V.L. Katch.** *Exercise Physiology: Energy, Nutrition and Human Performance.* Philadelphia: Lea and Febiger, 1981.
58. **Milesis, C.A., M.L. Pollock, M.D. Bah, J.J. Ayres, A. Ward and A.C. Linnerud.** Effects of different durations of training on cardiorespiratory function, body composition and serum lipids. *Res. Q.* 47:716–725, 1976.
59. **Murphy, R. and K. H.** Shipman. Hyperuricemia during total fasting. *Arch. Intern. Med.* 112:954–959, 1963.
60. **Nilsson, L.H. and E. Hultman.** Total starvation or a carbohydrate-poor diet followed by carbohydrate refeeding. *Scand. J. Clin. Lab. Invest.* 32:325–330, 1973.
61. **Norbury, F.B.** Contraindication of long term fasting. *JAMA.* 188:88, 1964.
62. **O Hara, W., C. Allen, and R.J. Shepard.** Loss of body weight and fat during exercise in a cold chamber. *Eur. J. Appl. Physiol.* 37:205–218, 1977.
63. **Oyama, J., J.A. Thomas, and R.L. Brant.** Effect of starvation on glucose tolerance and serum insulin–like activity of Osborne Mendel rats. *Diabetes.* 12:332–334, 1963.
64. **Passmore, R., J.A. Strong, and F.J. Ritchie.** The chemical composition of the tissue lost by obese patients on a reducing regimen. *Br. J. Nutri.* 12:113–122, 1958.
65. **Pittman, F.E.** Primary malabsorption following extreme attempts to lose weight. *Gut.* 7:154–158, 1966.
66. **Pollock, M.L., T.K. Cureton, and L. Greninger.** Effects of frequency of training on working capacity, cardiovascular function and body composition of adult men. *Med. Sci. Sports.* I:70–74, 1969.
67. **Pollock, M.L., J. Tiffany, L. Gettman, R. Janeway, and H. Lofland.** Effects of frequency of training on serum lipids, cardiovascular function and body composition. In: *Exercise and Fitness*, B.D. Franks (Ed.). Chicago: Athletic Institute, 1969, pp. 161–178.
68. **Pollock, M.L., J. Broida, Z. Kendrick, H.S. Miller, JR., R. Janeway, and A.C. Linnerud.** Effects of training two days per week at different intensities on middle aged men. *Med. Sci. Sports.* 4:192–197, 1972.
69. **Pollock, M L.** The quantification of endurance training programs. *Exercise and Sports Sciences Reviews*, J. Wilmore (Ed.). New York: Academic Press, 1973, pp. 155–188.

70. **Pollock, M.L. and A. Jackson.** Body composition: measurement and changes resulting from physical training. In: *Proceedings National College Physical Education Association for Men and Women*, 1977, pp. 123–137.
71. **Portnay, G.I., J.T. O'brian, J. Bush, et al.** The effect of starvation on the concentration and binding of thyroxine and triiodothyronine in serum and on the response to TRH. *J. Clin. Endocrinol. Metab.* 39:191–194, 1974.
72. **Rimm, A.A., L.H. Werner, R. Bernstein, and B. Van Yserloo.** Disease and obesity in 73,532 women. *Obesity Bariatric Med.* 1:77–84, 1972.
73. **Rooth, G. and S. Carlstrom.** Therapeutic fasting. *Acta Med. Scand.* 187:455–463, 1970.
74. **Rossner, S. and D. Hallberg.** Serum lipoproteins in massive obesity. *Acta Med Scand.* 204:103–110, 1978.
75. **Rozental, P., C. Biara, H. Spencer, and H.J. Zimmerman.** Liver morphology and function tests in obesity and during starvation. *Am. J. Dig. Dis.* 12:198–208, 1967.
76. **Runcie, J.** Urinary sodium and potassium excretion in fasting obese subjects. *Br. Med. J.* 3:432–435, 1970.
77. **Runcie, J. and T.J. Thomson.** Total fasting, hyperuricemia and gout. *Postgrad. Med. J.* 45:251–254, 1969.
78. **Runcie, J. and T.J. Thomson.** Prolonged starvation—a dangerous procedure? *Br. Med. J.* 3:432–435, 1970.
79. **Sours, H.E., V.P. Frattali, C.D. Brand, et al.** Sudden death associated with very low calorie weight reduction regimens. *Am. J. Clin. Nutri.* 34:453–461, 1981.
80. **Spencer, I.O.B.** Death during therapeutic starvation for obesity. *Lancet.* 2:679–680, 1968.
81. **Stalonas, P.M., W.G. Johnson, and M. Christ.** Behavior modification for obesity: the evaluation of exercise, contingency, management, and program behavior. *J. Consult. Clin. Psychol.* 46:463–467, 1978.
82. **Stamler, R., J. Stamler, W.F. Riedlinger, G. Algera, and R.H. Roberts.** Weight and blood pressure. Findings in hypertension screening of 1 million Americans. *JAMA.* 240:1607–1610, 1978.
83. **Stein, J.S. and J. Hirsch.** Obesity and pancreatic function. In: *Handbook of physiology, Section 1. Endocrinology.* Vol. 1, D. Steener and N. Frankel (Eds.). Washington, DC: American Physiological Society, 1972.
84. **Stewart, W.K. and L.W. Fleming.** Features of a successful therapeutic fast of 382 days duration. *Postgrad. Med. J.* 49:203–209, 1973.
85. **Stewart, J.S., D.L. Pollock, A.V. Hoffbrand, D.L. Mollin, and C.C. Booth.** A study of proximal and distal intestinal structure and absorptive function in idiopathic steatorrhea. *Q. J. Med.* 36:425–444, 1967.
86. **Streja, D.A., E.B. Marliss, and G. Steiner.** The effects of prolonged fasting on plasma triglyceride kinetics in man. *Metabolism.* 26:505–516, 1977.
87. **Stuart, R.B. and B. Davis.** *Slim Chance in a Fat World. Behavioral Control of Obesity.* Champaign, IL: Research Press, 1972.
88. **Thompson, P.D., R.W. Jeffrey, R.R. Wing, and P.D. Wood.** Unexpected decrease in plasma high density lipoprotein cholesterol with weight loss. *Am. J. Clin. Nutr.* 32:2016–2021, 1979.
89. **Thomson, T.J., J . Runcie, and V. Miller.** Treatment of obesity by total fasting up to 249 days. *Lancet.* 2:992–996, 1966.
90. **Thorn, G.W., M.M. Wintrobe, R.D. Adams, E. Braunwald, K.J. Isselbacher, and R.G. Petersdorf.** *Harrisons Principles of Internal Medicine, 8th Edition.* New York: McGraw–Hill, 1977.
91. **Vegenakis, A.G., A. Burger, G.I. Portnay, et al.** Diversion of peripheral thyroxine metabolism from activating to inactivating pathways during complete fasting. *J. Clin. Endocrinol. Metab.* 41:191–194, 1975.
92. **Verdy, M. B.S.P.** Retention during total fasting. *Metabolism.* 15:769, 1966.
93. **Warner, W.A. and L.P. Garrett.** The obese patient and anesthesia. *JAMA.* 205:102–103 1968.

94. **Wechsler, J.G., V. Hutt, H. Wenzel, H. Klor, and H. Ditschuneit.** Lipids and lipoproteins during a very-low-calorie diet. *Int. J. Obes.* 5:325–331, 1981.
95. **Weisinger, J.R., A. Seeman, M.G. Herrera, J.P. Assal, J.S. Soeldner, and R.E. Gleason.** The nephrotic syndrome: a complication of massive obesity. *Ann. Intern. Med.* 80:332–341, 1974.
96. **Weltman, A., S. Matter, and B.A. Stamford.** Caloric restriction and/or mild exercise: effects on serum lipids and body composition. *Am. J. Clin. Nutr.* 33:1002–1009, 1980.
97. **West, K.** *Epidemiology of Diabetes and its Vascular Lesions.* New York: Elsevier, 1978.
98. **Wilmore, J.H., J. Royce, R.N. Girandola, F.I. Katch, and V. L. Katch.** Body composition changes with a 10 week jogging program. *Med. Sci. Sports.* 2:113–117, 1970.
99. **Wilson, G.T.** Behavior modification and the treatment of obesity. In: *Obesity.* A.J. Stunkard (Ed.). Philadelphia: W.B. Saunders, 1980.
100. **Wooley, S.C., O.W. Wooley, and S.R. Dyrenforth.** Theoretical practical and social issues in behavioral treatments of obesity. J. *Appl. Behav. Anal.* 12:3–25, 1979.
101. **Yang, M. and T.B. Van Itallie.** Metabolic responses of obese subjects to starvation and low calorie ketogenic and nonketogenic diets. *J. Clin. Invest.* 58:722–730, 1976.
102. **Zuti, W.B. and L.A. Golding.** Comparing diet and exercise as weight reduction tools. *Phys. Sportsmed.* 4(1):49–53, 1976.

Appendix C

AMERICAN COLLEGE OF SPORTS MEDICINE POSITION STAND ON THE RECOMMENDED QUANTITY AND QUALITY OF EXERCISE FOR DEVELOPING AND MAINTAINING CARDIORESPIRATORY AND MUSCULAR FITNESS IN HEALTHY ADULTS*

This Position Stand replaces the 1978 ACSM position paper, "The Recommended Quantity and Quality of Exercise for Developing and Maintaining Fitness in Healthy Adults."

Increasing numbers of persons are becoming involved in endurance training and other forms of physical activity, and, thus, the need for guidelines for exercise prescription is apparent. Based on the existing evidence concerning exercise prescription for healthy adults and the need for guidelines, the American College of Sports Medicine (ACSM) makes the following recommendations for the quantity and quality of training for developing and maintaining cardiorespiratory fitness, body composition, and muscular strength and endurance in the healthy adult:

1. Frequency of training: 3 to 5 d · week^{-1}.
2. Intensity of training: 60 to 90% of maximum heart rate (HR_{max}), or 50 to 85% of maximum oxygen uptake ($\dot{V}O_2max$) or HR_{max} reserve.**
3. Duration of training: 20 to 60 min of continuous aerobic activity. Duration is dependent on the intensity of the activity; thus, lower

* Reprinted from *"The Recommended Quantity and Quality of Exercise for Developing and Maintaining Cardiorespiratory and Muscular Fitness in Healthy Adults."* ©1990 American College of Sports Medicine, (*MSSE*, 22:2, 1990, pp. 265–274. With permission of Williams & Wilkins.

** Maximum heart rate reserve is calculated from the difference between resting and maximum heart rate. To estimate training intensity, a percentage of this value is added to the resting heart rate and is expressed as a percentage of HR_{max} reserve.[85]

intensity activity should be conducted over a longer period of time. Because of the importance of "total fitness" and the fact that it is more readily attained in longer duration programs, and because of the potential hazards and compliance problems associated with high intensity activity, lower to moderate intensity activity of longer duration is recommended for the nonathletic adult.

4. Mode of activity: any activity that uses large muscle groups, can be maintained continuously, and is rhythmical and aerobic in nature, e.g., walking-hiking, running, jogging, cycling-bicycling, cross-country skiing, dancing, rope skipping, rowing, stair climbing, swimming, skating, and various endurance game activities.
5. Resistance training: Strength training of a moderate intensity, sufficient to develop and maintain fat-free weight (FFW), should be an integral part of an adult fitness program. One set of 8 to 12 repetitions of 8 to 10 exercises that condition the major muscle groups at least 2 $d \cdot week^{-1}$ is the recommended minimum.

RATIONALE AND RESEARCH BACKGROUND

INTRODUCTION

The questions "How much exercise is enough?" and "What type of exercise is best for developing and maintaining fitness?" are frequently asked. It is recognized that the term "physical fitness" is composed of a variety of characteristics included in the broad categories of cardiovascular-respiratory fitness, body composition, muscular strength and endurance, and flexibility. In this context, fitness is defined as the ability to perform moderate to vigorous levels of physical activity without undue fatigue and the capability of maintaining such ability throughout life.[167] It is also recognized that the adaptive response to training is complex and includes peripheral, central, structural, and functional factors.[5,172] Although many such variables and their adaptive response to training have been documented, the lack of sufficient in-depth and comparative data relative to frequency, intensity, and duration of training makes them inadequate to use as comparative models. Thus, in respect to the above questions, fitness is limited mainly to changes in $\dot{V}O_2max$, muscular strength and endurance, and body composition, which includes total body mass, fat weight (FW), and FFW. Further, the rationale and research background used for this position stand will be divided into programs for cardiorespiratory fitness and weight control and programs for muscular strength and endurance.

Fitness Vs. Health Benefits of Exercise

Since the original position statement was published in 1978, an important distinction has been made between physical activity as it relates to health vs. fitness. It has been pointed out that the quantity and quality of exercise needed to attain health-related benefits may differ from what is recommended for fitness benefits. It is now clear that lower levels of physical activity than recommended by this position statement may reduce the risk for certain chronic degenerative diseases and yet may not be of sufficient quantity or quality to improve $\dot{V}O_2$max.[71,72,98,167] ACSM recognizes the potential health benefits of regular exercise performed more frequently and for a longer duration, but at lower intensities than prescribed in this position statement.[13A,71,100,120,160] ACSM will address the issue concerning the proper amount of physical activity necessary to derive health benefits in another statement.

Need for Standardization of Procedures and Reporting Results

Despite an abundance of information available concerning the training of the human organism, the lack of standardization of testing protocols and procedures, of methodology in relation to training procedures and experimental design, and of a preciseness in the documentation and reporting of the quantity and quality of training prescribed make interpretation difficult.[123,133,139,164,167] Interpretation and comparison of results are also dependent on the initial level of fitness,[42,43,58,114,148,151,156] length of time of the training experiment,[17,45,125,128,139,145,150] and specificity of the testing and training.[5,43,130,139,145A,172] For example, data from training studies using subjects with varied levels of $\dot{V}O_2$max, total body mass, and FW have found changes to occur in relation to their initial values;[14,33,109,112,113,148,151] i.e., the lower the initial $\dot{V}O_2$max the larger the percentage of improvement found, and the higher the FW the greater the reduction. Also, data evaluating trainability with age, comparison of the different magnitudes and quantities of effort, and comparison of the trainability of men and women may have been influenced by the initial fitness levels.

In view of the fact that improvement in the fitness variables discussed in this position statement continues over many months of training,[27,86,139,145,150] it is reasonable to believe that short-term studies conducted over a few weeks have certain limitations. Middle-aged sedentary and older participants may take several weeks to adapt to the initial rigors of training, and thus need a longer adaptation period to get the full benefit from a program. For example, Seals et al.[150] exercise trained 60 to 69-year-olds for 12 months. Their subjects showed a 12% improvement in $\dot{V}O_2$max after 6 months of moderate intensity walking training. A further 18% increase in $\dot{V}O_2$max occurred during the next 6 months of training when jogging was introduced. How long a training experiment should be conducted is difficult to determine, but 15 to 20 weeks may be a good minimum standard. Although it is difficult to control exercise training experiments for more than 1 year, there is a need to study this effect. As stated earlier, lower doses of exercise may improve $\dot{V}O_2$max and control or maintain body composition, but at a slower rate.

Although most of the information concerning training described in this position statement has been conducted on men, the available evidence indicates that women tend to adapt to endurance training in the same manner as men.[19,38,46,47,49,62,65,68,90,92,122,166]

EXERCISE PRESCRIPTION FOR CARDIORESPIRATORY FITNESS AND WEIGHT CONTROL

Exercise prescription is based upon the frequency, intensity, and duration of training, the mode of activity (aerobic in nature, e.g., listed under No. 4 above), and the initial level of fitness. In evaluating these factors, the following observations have been derived from studies conducted for up to 6 to 12 months with endurance training programs.

Improvement in $\dot{V}O_2$max is directly related to frequency,[3,6,50,75-77,125,126,152,154,164] intensity,[3,6,26,29,58,61,75-77,80,85,93,118,152,164] and duration[3,29,60,61,70,75-77,101,109,118,152,162,164,168] of training. Depending upon the quantity and quality of training, improvement in $\dot{V}O_{22}$max ranges from 5 to 30%.[8,29,30,48,59,61,65,67,69,75-77,82,84,96,99,101,102,111,115,119,123,127,139,141,143,149,150,152,153,158,164,168,173] These studies show that a minimum increase in $\dot{V}O_2$max of 15% is generally attained in programs that meet the above stated guidelines. Although changes in $\dot{V}O_2$max greater than 30% have been shown, they are usually associated with large total body mass and FW loss, in cardiac patients, or in persons with a very low initial level of fitness. Also, as a result of leg fatigue or a lack of motivation, persons with low initial fitness may have spuriously low initial $\dot{V}O_2$max values. Klissouras[94A] and Bouchard[16A] have shown that human variation in the trainability of $\dot{V}O_2$max is important and related to current phenotype level. That is, there is a genetically determined pretraining status of the trait and capacity to adapt to physical training. Thus, physiological results should be interpreted with respect to both genetic variation and the quality and quantity of training performed.

Intensity-Duration

Intensity and duration of training are interrelated, with total amount of work accomplished being an important factor in improvement in fitness.[12,20,27,48,90,92,123,127,128,136,149,151,164] Although more comprehensive inquiry is necessary, present evidence suggests that, when exercise is performed above the minimum intensity threshold, the total amount of work accomplished is an important factor in fitness development[19,27,126,127,149,151] and maintenance.[134] That is, improvement will be similar for activities performed at a lower intensity-longer duration compared to higher intensity-shorter duration if the total energy costs of the activities are equal. Higher intensity exercise is associated with greater cardiovascular risk,[156A] orthopedic injury,[124,139] and lower compliance to training than lower intensity exercise.[36,105,124,146] Therefore, programs emphasizing low to moderate intensity training with longer duration are recommended for most adults.

The minimal training intensity threshold for improvement in $\dot{V}O_2$max is approximately 60% of the HR_{max} (50% of $\dot{V}O_2$max or HR_{max} reserve).[80,85] The 50% of HR_{max} reserve represents a heart rate of approximately 130 to 135 beats · min^{-1} for young persons. As a result of the age-related change in maximum heart rate, the absolute heart rate to achieve this threshold is inversely related to age and can be as low as 105 to 115 beats · min^{-1} for older persons.[35,65,150] Patients who are taking beta-adrenergic blocking drugs may have significantly lower heart rate values.[171] Initial level of fitness is another important consideration in prescribing exercise.[26,90,104,148,151] The person with a low fitness level can achieve a significant training effect with a sustained training heart rate as low as 40 to 50% of HR_{max} reserve, while persons with higher fitness levels require a higher training stimulus.[35,58,152,164]

Classification of Exercise Intensity

The classification of exercise intensity and its standardization for exercise prescription based on a 20 to 60-min training session has been confusing, misinterpreted, and often taken out of context. The most quoted exercise classification system is based on the energy expenditure (kcal · min^{-1} · kg^{-1}) of industrial tasks.[40,89] The original data for this classification system were published by Christensen[24] in 1953 and were based on the energy expenditure of working in the steel mill for an 8-h day. The classification of industrial and leisure-time tasks by using absolute values of energy expenditure has been valuable for use in the occupational and nutritional setting. Although this classification system has broad application in medicine and, in particular, in making recommendations for weight control and job placement, it has little or no meaning for preventive and rehabilitation exercise training programs. To extrapolate absolute values of energy expenditure for completing an industrial task based on an 8-h work day to 20 to 60-min regimens of exercise training does not make sense. For example, walking and jogging/running can be accomplished at a wide range of speeds; thus, the relative intensity becomes important under these conditions. Because the endurance training regimens recommended by ACSM for nonathletic adults are geared for 60 min or less of physical activity, the system of classification of exercise training intensity shown in Table 1 is recommended.[139] The use of a realistic time period for training and an individual's relative exercise intensity makes this system amenable to young, middle-aged, and elderly participants, as well as patients with a limited exercise capacity.[3,137,139]

Table 1 also describes the relationship between relative intensity based on percent HR_{max}, percentage of HR_{max} reserve or percentage of $\dot{V}O_2max$, and the rating of perceived exertion (RPE).[15,16,137] The use of heart rate as an estimate of intensity of training is the common standard.[3,139]

The use of RPE has become a valid tool in the monitoring of intensity in exercise training programs.[11,37,137,139] It is generally considered an adjunct to heart rate in monitoring relative exercise intensity, but once the relationship between heart rate and RPE is known, RPE can be used in place of heart rate.[23,139] This would not be the case in certain patient populations where a more precise knowledge of heart rate may be critical to the safety of the program.

Frequency

The amount of improvement in $\dot{V}O_2max$ tends to plateau when frequency of training is increased above 3 d · $week^{-1}$.[50,123,139] The value of the added improvement found with training more than 5 d · $week^{-1}$ is small to not apparent in regard

TABLE 1 Classification of Intensity of Exercise Based on 20–60 Min of Endurance Training

Relative Intensity (%)		Rating of Perceived Exertion	Classification of Intensity
HR_{max}[a]	$\dot{V}O_2max$ or HR_{max} Reserve		
<35	<30	<10	Very light
35–59	30–49	10–11	Light
60–79	50–74	12–13	Moderate (somewhat hard)
80–89	75–84	14–16	Heavy
≥90	≥85	>16	Very heavy

Table from Pollock, M.L. and J.H. Wilmore, *Exercise in Health and Disease: Evaluation and Prescription for Prevention and Rehabilitation,* 2nd ed., W.B. Saunders, Philadelphia, 1990. Published with permission.

* HR_{max} = maximum heart rate; $\dot{V}O_2max$ = maximum oxygen uptake.

to improvement in $\dot{V}O_2max$.[75-77,106,123] Training of less than 2 d · week^{-1} does not generally show a meaningful change in $\dot{V}O_2max$.[29,50,118,123,152,164]

Mode

If frequency, intensity, and duration of training are similar (total kcal expenditure), the training adaptations appear to be independent of the mode of aerobic activity.[101A,118,130] Therefore, a variety of endurance activities, e.g., those listed above, may be used to derive the same training effect.

Endurance activities that require running and jumping are considered high impact types of activity and generally cause significantly more debilitating injuries to beginning as well as long-term exercisers than do low impact and nonweight bearing-type activities.[13,93,117,124,127,135,140,142] This is particularly evident in the elderly.[139] Beginning joggers have increased foot, leg, and knee injuries when training is performed more than 3 d · week^{-1} and longer than 30 min duration per exercise session.[135] High intensity interval training (run-walk) compared to continuous jogging training was also associated with a higher incidence of injury.[124,136] Thus, caution should be taken when recommending the type of activity and exercise prescription for the beginning exerciser. Orthopedic injuries as related to overuse increase linearly in runners/joggers when performing these activities.[13,140] Thus, there is a need for more inquiry into the effect that different types of activities and the quantity and quality of training has on injuries over short-term and long-term participation.

An activity such as weight training should not be considered as a means of training for developing $\dot{V}O_2max$, but it has significant value for increasing muscular strength and endurance and FFW.[32,54,107,110,165] Studies evaluating circuit weight training (weight training conducted almost continuously with moderate weights, using 10 to 15 repetitions per exercise session with 15 to 30 s rest between bouts of activity) show an average improvement in $\dot{V}O_2max$ of 6%.[1,51-54,83,94,108,170] Thus, circuit weight training is not recommended as the only activity used in exercise programs for developing $\dot{V}O_2max$.

Age

Age in itself does not appear to be a deterrent to endurance training. Although some earlier studies showed a lower training effect with middle-aged or elderly participants,[9,34,79,157,168] more recent studies show the relative change in $\dot{V}O_2max$ to be similar to younger age groups.[7,8,65,132,150,161,163] Although more investigation is necessary concerning the rate of improvement in $\dot{V}O_2max$ with training at various ages, at present it appears that elderly participants need longer periods of time to adapt.[34,132,150] Earlier studies showing moderate to no improvement in $\dot{V}O_2max$ were conducted over a short time span,[9] or exercise was conducted at a moderate to low intensity,[34] thus making the interpretation of the results difficult.

Although $\dot{V}O_2max$ decreases with age and total body mass and FW increase with age, evidence suggests that this trend can be altered with endurance training.[22,27,86-88,139] A 9% reduction in $\dot{V}O_2max$ per decade for sedentary adults after age 25 has been shown,[31,73] but for active individuals the reduction may be less than 5% per decade.[21,31,39,73] Ten or more year follow-up studies where participants continued training at a similar level showed maintenance of cardiorespiratory fitness.[4,87,88,138] A cross-sectional study of older competitive runners showed progressively lower values in $\dot{V}O_2max$ from the fourth to seventh decades of life, but also showed less training in the older groups.[129] More recent 10-year follow-up data on these same athletes (50 to 82 years of age) showed $\dot{V}O_2max$ to be unchanged when training quantity and quality remained unchanged.[138] Thus, lifestyle plays a significant role in the maintenance of fitness. More inquiry into the relationship of long-term training (quantity and quality), for both competitors and noncompetitors, and physiological function with increasing age is necessary before more definitive statements can be made.

Maintenance of Training Effect

In order to maintain the training effect, exercise must be continued on a regular basis.[18,25,28,47,97,111,144,147] A significant reduction in cardiorespiratory fitness occurs after 2 weeks of detraining,[25,144] with participants returning to near pretraining levels of fitness after 10 weeks[47] to 8 months of detraining.[97] A loss of 50% of their initial improvement in $\dot{V}O_2max$ has been shown after 4 to 12 weeks of detraining.[47,91,144] Those individuals who have undergone years of continuous training maintain some benefits for longer periods of detraining than subjects from short-term training studies.[25] While stopping training shows dramatic reductions in $\dot{V}O_2max$, reduced training shows modest to no reductions for periods of 5 to 15 weeks.[18,75-77,144] Hickson et al., in a series of experiments where frequency,[75] duration,[76] or intensity[77] of training were manipulated, found that, if intensity of training remained unchanged, $\dot{V}O_2max$ was maintained for up to 15 weeks when frequency and duration of training were reduced by as much as 2/3. When frequency and duration of training remained constant and intensity of training was reduced by 1/3 or 2/3, $\dot{V}O_2max$ was significantly reduced. Similar findings were found in regards to reduced strength training exercise. When strength training exercise was reduced from 3 or 2 d · week^{-1} to at least 1 d · week^{-1}, strength was maintained for 12 weeks of reduced training.[62] Thus, it appears that missing an exercise session periodically or reducing training for up to 15 weeks will not adversely affect $\dot{V}O_2max$ or muscular strength and endurance as long as training intensity is maintained.

Even though many new studies have given added insight into the proper amount of exercise, investigation is necessary to evaluate the rate of increase and decrease of fitness when varying training loads and reduction in training in relation to level of fitness, age, and length of time in training. Also, more information is needed to better identify the minimal level of exercise necessary to maintain fitness.

Weight Control and Body Composition

Although there is variability in human response to body composition change with exercise, total body mass and FW are generally reduced with endurance training programs,[133,139,171A] while FFW remains constant[123,133,139,169] or increases slightly.[116,174] For example, Wilmore[171A] reported the results of 32 studies that met the criteria for developing cardiorespiratory fitness that are outlined in this position stand and found an average loss in total body mass of 1.5 kg and percent fat of 2.2%. Weight loss programs using dietary manipulation that result in a more dramatic decrease in total body mass show reductions in both FW and FFW.[2,78,174] When these programs are conducted in conjunction with exercise training, FFW loss is more modest than in programs using diet alone.[78,121] Programs that are conducted at least 3 d · week^{-1},[123,125,126,128,169] of at least 20-min duration,[109,123,169] and of sufficient intensity to expend approximately 300 kcal per exercise session (75-kg person)* are suggested as a threshold level for total body mass and FW loss.[27,64,77,123,133,139] An expenditure of 200 kcal per session has also been shown to be useful in weight reduction if the exercise frequency is at least 4 d · week^{-1}.[155] If the primary purpose of the training program is for weight loss, then regimens of greater frequency and duration of training and low to moderate intensity are recommended.[2,139] Programs with less participation generally show little or no change in body composition.[44,57,93,123,133,159,162,169] Significant increases in $\dot{V}O_2max$ have been shown with 10 to 15 min of high intensity training;[6,79,109,118,123,152,153] thus, if total body mass and FW reduction are not considerations, then shorter duration, higher intensity programs may be recommended for healthy individuals at low risk for cardiovascular disease and orthopedic injury.

* Haskell and Haskell et al.[71,72] have suggested the use of 4 kcal kg^{-1} of body weight of energy expenditure per day for a minimum standard for use in exercise programs.

EXERCISE PRESCRIPTION FOR MUSCULAR STRENGTH AND ENDURANCE

The addition of resistance/strength training to the position statement results from the need for a well rounded program that exercises all the major muscle groups of the body. Thus, the inclusion of resistance training in adult fitness programs should be effective in the development and maintenance of FFW. The effect of exercise training is specific to the area of the body being trained.[5,43,145A,172] For example, training the legs will have little or no effect on the arms, shoulders, and trunk muscles. A 10-year follow-up of master runners who continued their training regimen, but did no upper body exercise, showed maintenance of $\dot{V}O_2max$ and a 2-kg reduction in FFW.[138] Their leg circumference remained unchanged, but arm circumference was significantly lower. These data indicate a loss of muscle mass in the untrained areas. Three of the athletes who practiced weight training exercise for the upper body and trunk muscles maintained their FFW. A comprehensive review by Sale[145A] carefully documents available information on specificity of training.

Specificity of training was further addressed by Graves et al.[63] Using a bilateral knee extension exercise, they trained four groups: group A, first 1/2 of the range of motion; group B, second 1/2 of the range of motion; group AB, full range of motion; and a control group that did not train. The results clearly showed that the training result was specific to the range of motion trained, with group AB getting the best full range effect. Thus, resistance training should be performed through a full range of motion for maximum benefit.[63, 95]

Muscular strength and endurance are developed by the overload principle, i.e., by increasing more than normal the resistance to movement or frequency and duration of activity.[32,41,43,74,145] Muscular strength is best developed by using heavy weights (that require maximum or nearly maximum tension development) with few repetitions, and muscular endurance is best developed by using lighter weights with a greater number of repetitions.[10,41,43,145] To some extent, both muscular strength and endurance are developed under each condition, but each system favors a more specific type of development.[43,145] Thus, to elicit improvement in both muscular strength and endurance, most experts recommend 8 to 12 repetitions per bout of exercise.

Any magnitude of overload will result in strength development, but higher intensity effort at or near maximal effort will give a significantly greater effect.[43,74,101B,103,145,172] The intensity of resistance training can be manipulated by varying the weight load, repetitions, rest interval between exercises, and number of sets completed.[43] Caution is advised for training that emphasizes lengthening (eccentric) contractions, compared to shortening (concentric) or isometric contractions, as the potential for skeletal muscle soreness and injury is accentuated.[3A,84A]

Muscular strength and endurance can be developed by means of static (isometric) or dynamic (isotonic or isokinetic) exercises. Although each type of training has its favorable and weak points, for healthy adults, dynamic resistance exercises are recommended. Resistance training for the average participant should be rhythmical, performed at a moderate to slow speed, move through a full range of motion, and not impede normal forced breathing. Heavy resistance exercise can cause a dramatic acute increase in both systolic and diastolic blood pressure.[100A,101C]

The expected improvement in strength from resistance training is difficult to assess because increases in strength are affected by the participants' initial level of strength and their potential for improvement.[43,66,74,114,172] For example, Mueller and Rohmert[114] found increases in strength ranging from two to 9% per week depending on initial strength levels. Although the literature reflects a wide range of improvement in strength with resistance training programs, the average improvement for sedentary young and middle-aged men and women for up to 6 months of training is 25 to 30%. Fleck and Kraemer,[43] in a review of 13 studies representing various forms of isotonic training, showed an average improvement in bench press strength of 23.3% when subjects were tested on the equipment with which they were trained and 16.5% when tested on special isotonic or isokinetic ergometers (6 studies). Fleck and Kraemer[43] also reported an average increase in leg strength of 26.6% when subjects were tested with the equipment that they trained on (6 studies) and 21.2 % when tested with special isotonic or isokinetic ergometers (5 studies). Results of improvement in strength resulting from isometric training have been of the same magnitude as found with isotonic training.[17,43,62,63]

In light of the information reported above, the following guidelines for resistance training are recommended for the average healthy adult. A minimum of 8 to 10 exercises involving the major muscle groups should be performed a minimum of 2 times per week. A minimum of 1 set of 8 to 12 repetitions to near fatigue should be completed. These minimal standards for resistance training are based on two factors. First, the time it takes to complete a comprehensive, well-rounded exercise program is important. Programs lasting more than 60 min per session are associated with higher dropout rates.[124] Second, although greater frequencies of training[17,43,56] and additional sets or combinations of sets and repetitions elicit larger strength gains,[10,32,43,74,145,172] the magnitude of difference is usually small. For example, Braith et al.[17] compared training $2 \text{ d} \cdot \text{week}^{-1}$ with $3 \text{ d} \cdot \text{week}^{-1}$ for 18 weeks. The subjects performed one set of seven to ten repetitions to fatigue. The $2 \text{ d} \cdot \text{week}^{-1}$ group showed a 21% increase in strength compared to 28% in the $3 \text{ d} \cdot \text{week}^{-1}$ group. In other words, 75% of what could be attained in a $3 \text{ d} \cdot \text{week}^{-1}$ program was attained in $2 \text{ d} \cdot \text{week}^{-1}$. Also, the 21% improvement in strength found by the $2 \text{ d} \cdot \text{week}^{-1}$ regimen is 70 to 80% of the improvement reported by other programs using additional frequencies of training and combinations of sets and repetitions.[43] Graves et al.,[62,63] Gettman et al.,[55] Hurley et al.,[83] and Braith et al.[17] found that programs using 1 set to fatigue showed a greater than 25% increase in strength. Although resistance training equipment may provide a better graduated and quantitative stimulus for overload than traditional calisthenic exercises, calisthenics and other resistance types of exercise can still be effective in improving and maintaining strength.

SUMMARY

The combination of frequency, intensity, and duration of chronic exercise has been found to be effective for producing a training effect. The interaction of these factors provides the overload stimulus. In general, the lower the stimulus the lower the training effect, and the greater the stimulus the greater the effect. As a result of specificity of training and the need for maintaining muscular strength and endurance, and flexibility of the major muscle groups, a well-rounded training program including resistance training and flexibility exercises is recommended. Although age in itself is not a limiting factor to exercise training, a more gradual approach in applying the prescription at older ages seems prudent. It has also been shown that endurance training of fewer than 2 $d \cdot week^{-1}$, at less than 50% of maximum oxygen uptake and for less than 10 $min \cdot d^{-1}$, is inadequate for developing and maintaining fitness for healthy adults.

In the interpretation of this position statement, it must be recognized that the recommendations should be used in the context of participants' needs, goals, and initial abilities. In this regard, a sliding scale as to the amount of time allotted and intensity of effort should be carefully gauged for both the cardiorespiratory and muscular strength and endurance components of the program. An appropriate warm-up and cool-down, which would include flexibility exercises, is also recommended. The important factor is to design a program for the individual to provide the proper amount of physical activity to attain maximal benefit at the lowest risk. Emphasis should be placed on factors that result in permanent lifestyle change and encourage a lifetime of physical activity.

REFERENCES

1. **Allen, T.E., R.J. Byrd, and D.P. Smith.** Hemodynamic consequences of circuit weight training. *Res. Q.* 43:299–306, 1976.
2. American College Of Sports Medicine. Proper and improper weight loss programs. *Med. Sci. Sports Exerc.* 15:ix–xiii, 1983.
3. American College Of Sports Medicine. *Guidelines for Graded Exercise Testing and Exercise Prescription*, 3rd Ed. Philadelphia: Lea and Febiger, 1986.

3A. **Armstrong, R.B.** Mechanisms of exercise-induced delayed onset muscular soreness: a brief review. *Med. Sci. Sports Exerc.* 16:529–538, 1984.

4. **Astrand, P.O.** Exercise physiology of the mature athlete. In: *Sports Medicine for the Mature Athlete*, J. R. Sutton and R. M. Brock (Eds.). Indianapolis, IN: Benchmark Press, Inc., 1986, pp. 3–16.
5. **Astrand, P.O. and K. Rodahl.** Textbook of Work Physiology, 3rd Ed. New York: McGraw-Hill, 1986, pp. 412–485.
6. **Atomi, Y., K. Ito, H. Iwasaski, and M. Miyashita.** Effects of intensity and frequency of training on aerobic work capacity of young females. *J. Sports Med.* 18:3–9, 1978.
7. **Badenhop, D.T., P.A. Cleary, S.F. Schaal, E.L. Fox, and R.L. Bartels.** Physiological adjustments to higher- or lower-intensity exercise in elders. *Med. Sci. Sports Exerc.* 15 :496–502, 1983.

8. **Barry, A.J., J.W. Daly, E.D.R. Pruett, et al.** The effects of physical conditioning on older individuals. I. Work capacity, circulatory-respiratory function, and work electrocardiogram. *J. Gerontol.* 21:182–191, 1966.
9. **Benestad, A.M.** Trainability of old men. *Acta Med. Scand.* 178:321–327, 1965.
10. **Berger, R.A.** Effect of varied weight training programs on strength. *Res. Q.* 33:168–181, 1962.
11. **Birk, T.J. and C.A. Birk.** Use of ratings of perceived exertion for exercise prescription. *Sports Med.* 4:1–8, 1987.
12. **Blair, S.N., J.V. Chandler, D.B. Ellisor, and J. Langley.** Improving physical fitness by exercise training programs. *South. Med. J.* 73:1594–1596, 1980.
13. **Blair, S.N., H.W. Kohl, and N.N. Goodyear.** Rates and risks for running and exercise injuries: studies in three populations. *Res. Q. Exerc. Sports.* 58:221–228, 1987.
13A. **Blair, S.N., H.W. Kohl, III, R.S. Paffenbarger, D.G. Clark, K.H. Cooper, and L.H. Gibbons.** Physical fitness and all-cause mortality. A prospective study of healthy men and women. *J.A.M.A* . 262:2395–2401, 1989.
14. **Boileau, R.A., E.R. Buskirk, D.H. Horstman, J. Mendez, and W. Nicholas.** Body composition changes in obese and lean men during physical conditioning. *Med. Sci. Sports.* 3:183–189, 1971.
15. **Borg, G.A.V.** Psychophysical bases of perceived exertion. *Med. Sci. Sports Exerc.* 14:377–381, 1982.
16. **Borg, G. and D. Ottoson (Eds.).** *The Perception of Exertion in Physical Work.* London, England: The MacMillan Press, Ltd., 1986, pp. 4–7.
16A. **Bouchard, C.** Gene-environment interaction in human adaptability. In: *The Academy Papers*, R.B. Malina and H.M. Eckert (Eds.). Champaign, IL: Human Kinetics Publishers, 1988, pp. 56 -66.
17. **Braith, R.W., J.E. Graves, M.L. Pollock, S.L. Leggett, D.M. Carpenter, and A.B. Colvin.** Comparison of two versus three days per week of variable resistance training during 10 and 18 week programs. *Int. J. Sports Med.* 10:450–454, 1989.
18. **Brynteson, P. and W.E. Sinning.** The effects of training frequencies on the retention of cardiovascular fitness. *Med. Sci. Sports.* 5:29–33, 1973.
19. **Burke, E.J.** Physiological effects of similar training programs in males and females. *Res. Q.* 48:510–517, 1977.
20. **Burke, E.J. and B.D. Franks.** Changes in $\dot{V}O_2$max resulting from bicycle training at different intensities holding total mechanical work constant. *Res. Q.* 46:31–37, 1975.
21. **Buskirk, E.R. and J.L. Hodgson.** Age and aerobic power: the rate of change in men and women. *Fed. Proc.* 46:1824–1829, 1987.
22. **Carter, J.E.L. and W.H. Phillips.** Structural changes in exercising middle-aged males during a 2-year period. *J. Appl. Physiol.* 27:787–794, 1969.
23. **Chow, J. R. and J.H. Wilmore.** The regulation of exercise intensity by ratings of perceived exertion. *J. Cardiac Rehabil.* 4:382–387, 1984.
24. **Christensen, E.H.** Physiological evaluation of work in the Nykroppa iron works. In: *Ergonomics Society Symposium on Fatigue*, W.F. Floyd and A. T. Welford (Eds.). London, England: Lewis, 1953, pp. 93–108.
25. **Coyle, E.F., W.H. Martin, D.R. Sinacore, M.J. Joyner, J. M. Hagberg, and J.O. Holloszy.** Time course of loss of adaptation after stopping prolonged intense endurance training. *J. Appl. Physiol.* 57:1857–1864, 1984.
26. **Crews, T.R. and J.A. Roberts.** Effects of interaction of frequency and intensity of training. *Res. Q.* 47:48–55, 1976.
27. **Cureton, T.K.** *The Physiological Effects of Exercise Programs Upon Adults.* Springfield, IL: Charles C. Thomas Co., 1969, pp. 3–6, 33–77.
28. **Cureton, T.K. and E.E. Phillips.** Physical fitness changes in middle-aged men attributable to equal eight-week periods of training, non-training and retraining. *J. Sports Med. Phys. Fitness.* 4:1–7, 1964.

29. **Davies, C.T.M. and A.V. Knibbs.** The training stimulus, the effects of intensity, duration and frequency of effort on maximum aerobic power output. *Int. Z. Angew. Physiol.* 29:299–305, 1971.
30. **Davis, J.A., M.H. Frank, B.J. Whipp, and K. Wasserman.** Anaerobic threshold alterations caused by endurance training in middle-aged men. *J. Appl. Physiol.* 46:1039–1049, 1979.
31. **Dehn, M. M. and R. A. Bruce.** Longitudinal variations in maximal oxygen intake with age and activity. *J. Appl. Physiol.* 33:805-807, 1972.
32. **Delorme, T.L.** Restoration of muscle power by heavy resistance exercise. *J. Bone Joint Surg.* 27:645–667, 1945.
33. **Dempsey, J.A.** Anthropometrical observations on obese and nonobese young men undergoing a program of vigorous physical exercise. *Res. Q.* 35:275–287, 1964.
34. **Devries, H.A.** Physiological effects of an exercise training regimen upon men aged 52 to 88. *J. Gerontol.* 24:325–336, 1970.
35. **Devries, H.A.** Exercise intensity threshold for improvement of cardiovascular-respiratory function in older men. *Geriatrics.* 26:94–101, 1971.
36. **Dishman, R.K., J. Sallis, and D. Orenstein.** The determinants of physical activity and exercise. *Public Health Rep.* 100:158-180, 1985.
37. **Dishman, R.K., R.W. Patton, J. Smith, R. Weinberg, and A. Jackson.** Using perceived exertion to prescribe and monitor exercise training heart rate. *Int. J. Sports Med.* 8:208–213, 1987.
38. **Drinkwater, B.L.** Physiological responses of women to exercise. In: *Exercise and Sports Sciences Reviews*, Vol. 1, J.H. Wilmore (Ed.). New York: Academic Press, 1973, pp. 126–154.
39. **Drinkwater, B.L., S.M. Horvath, and C.L. Wells.** Aerobic power of females, ages 10 to 68. *J. Gerontol.* 30:385–394, 1975.
40. **Durnin, J.V.G.A. and R. Passmore.** *Energy, Work and Leisure*. London, England: Heinemann Educational Books, Ltd., 1967, pp. 47–82.
41. **Edstrom, L. and L. Grimby.** Effect of exercise on the motor unit. *Muscle Nerve.* 9: 104–126, 1986.
42. **Ekblom, B., P.O. Astrand, B. Saltin, J. Stenberg, and B. Wallstrom.** Effect of training on circulatory response to exercise. *J. Appl. Physiol.* 24:518–528, 1968.
43. **Fleck, S.J. and W.J. Kraemer.** *Designing Resistance Training Programs*. Champaign, IL: Human Kinetics Books, 1987, pp. 15–46, 161–162.
44. **Flint, M.M., B.L. Drinkwater, and S.M. Horvath.** Effects of training on women's response to submaximal exercise. *Med. Sci. Sports.* 6:89–94, 1974.
45. **Fox, E.L., R.L. Bartels, C.E. Billings, R. O'Brien, R. Bason, and D.K. Mathews.** Frequency and duration of interval training programs and changes in aerobic power. *J. Appl. Physiol.* 38:481–484, 1975.
46. **Franklin, B., E. Buskirk, J. Hodgson, H. Gahagan, J. Kollias, and J. Mendez.** Effects of physical conditioning on cardiorespiratory function, body composition and serum lipids in relatively normal weight and obese middle-age women. *Int. J. Obes.* 3:97–109, 1979.
47. **Fringer, M.N. and A.G. Stull.** Changes in cardiorespiratory parameters during periods of training and detraining in young female adults. *Med. Sci. Sports.* 6:20–25, 1974.
48. **Gaesser, G.A. and R.G. Rich.** Effects of high- and low intensity exercise training on aerobic capacity and blood lipids. *Med. Sci. Sports Exerc.* 16:269–274, 1984.
49. **Getchell, L.H. and J.C. Moore.** Physical training: comparative responses of middle-aged adults. *Arch. Phys. Med. Rehabil.* 56:250–254, 1975.
50. **Gettman, L.R., M.L. Pollock, J.L. Durstine, A. Ward, J. Ayres, and A.C. Linnerud.** Physiological responses of men to 1,3, and 5 day per week training programs. *Res. Q.* 47:638–646, 1976.
51. **Gettman, L.R., J.J. Ayres, M.L. Pollock, and A. Jackson.** The effect of circuit weight training on strength, cardiorespiratory function, and body composition of adult men. *Med. Sci. Sports.* 10:171–176, 1978.
52. **Gettman, L.R., J. Ayres, M.L. Pollock, J.L. Durstine, and W. Grantham.** Physiological effects of circuit strength training and jogging. *Arch. Phys. Med. Rehabil.* 60:115–120, 1979.

53. **Gettman, L.R., L.A. Culter, and T. Strathman.** Physiologic changes after 20 weeks of isotonic vs. isokinetic circuit training. *J. Sports Med. Phys. Fitness.* 20:265–274, 1980.
54. **Gettman, L.R. and M.L. Pollock.** Circuit weight training: a critical review of its physiological benefits. *Phys. Sports Med.* 9:44–60, 1981.
55. **Gettman, L.R., P. Ward, and R.D. Hagman.** A comparison of combined running and weight training with circuit weight training. *Med. Sci. Sports Exerc.* 14:229–234, 1982.
56. **Gillam, G.M.** Effects of frequency of weight training on muscle strength enhancement. *J. Sports Med.* 21:432–436, 1981.
57. **Girandola, R.N.** Body composition changes in women: effects of high and low exercise intensity. *Arch. Phys. Med. Rehabil.* 57:297–300, 1976.
58. **Gledhill, N. and R.B. Eynon.** The intensity of training. In: *Training Scientific Basis and Application*, A. W. Taylor and M.L. Howell (Eds.). Springfield, IL: Charles C Thomas Co., 1972, pp. 97–102.
59. **Golding, L.** Effects of physical training upon total serum cholesterol levels. *Res. Q.* 32:499–505, 1961.
60. **Goode, R.C., A. Virgin, T.T. Romet, et al.** Effects of a short period of physical activity in adolescent boys and girls. *Can. J. Appl. Sports Sci.* 1:241–250, 1976.
61. **Gossard, D., W.L. Haskell, B. Taylor, et al.** Effects of low and high-intensity home-based exercise training on functional capacity in healthy middle-age men. *Am. J. Cardiol.* 57:446–449, 1986.
62. **Graves, J.E., M.L. Pollock, S.H. Leggett, R.W. Braith, D.M. Carpenter, and L.E. Bishop.** Effect of reduced training frequency on muscular strength. *Int. J. Sports Med.* 9:316–319, 1988.
63. **Graves, J.E., M.L. Pollock, A.E. Jones, A.B. Colvin, and S.H. Leggett.** Specificity of limited range of motion variable resistance training. *Med. Sci. Sports Exerc.* 21:84–89, 1989.
64. **Gwinup, G.** Effect of exercise alone on the weight of obese women. *Arch. Int. Med.* 135:676–680, 1975.
65. **Hagberg, J.M., J.E. Graves, M. Limacher, et al.** Cardiovascular responses of 70–79 year old men and women to exercise training. *J. Appl. Physiol.* 66:2589–2594, 1989.
66. **Hakkinen, K.** Factors influencing trainability of muscular strength during short term and prolonged training. *Natl. Strength Cond. Assoc. J.* 7:32–34, 1985.
67. **Hanson, J.S., B.S. Tabakin, A.M. Levy, and W. Nedde.** Long-term physical training and cardiovascular dynamics in middle-aged men. *Circulation.* 38:783–799, 1968.
68. **Hanson, J.S. and W.H. Nedde.** Long-term physical training effect in sedentary females. J. *Appl. Physiol.* 37:112–116, 1974.
69. **Hartley, L.H., G. Grimby, A. Kilbom, et al.** Physical training in sedentary middle-aged and older men. *Scand. J. Clin. Lab. Invest.* 24:335–344, 1969.
70. **Hartung, G.H., M.H. Smolensky, R.B. Harrist, and R. Runge.** Effects of varied durations of training on improvement in cardiorespiratory endurance. *J. Hum. Ergol.* 6:61–68, 1977.
71. **Haskell, W.L.** Physical activity and health: need to define the required stimulus. *Am. J. Cardiol.* 55:4D–9D, 1985.
72. **Haskell, W.L., H.J. Montoye, and D. Orenstein.** Physical activity and exercise to achieve health-related physical fitness components. *Public Health Rep.* 100:202–212, 1985.
73. **Heath, G.W., J.M. Hagberg, A.A. Ehsani, and J.O. Holloszy.** A physiological comparison of young and older endurance athletes. *J. Appl. Physiol.* 51:634 - 640, 1981.
74. **Hettinger, T.** *Physiology of Strength.* Springfield, IL: C.C. Thomas Publisher, 1961, pp. 18–40.
75. **Hickson, R.C. and M.A. Rosenkoetter.** Reduced training frequencies and maintenance of increased aerobic power. *Med. Sci. Sports Exerc.* 13:13–16, 1981.
76. **Hickson, R.C., C. Kanakis, J.R. Davis, A.M. Moore, and S. Rich.** Reduced training duration effects on aerobic power, endurance, and cardiac growth. *J. Appl. Physiol.* 53:225–229, 1982.

77. **Hickson, R.C., C. Foster, M.L. Pollock, T.M. Galassi, and S. Rich.** Reduced training intensities and loss of aerobic power, endurance, and cardiac growth. *J. Appl. Physiol.* 58:492–499, 1985.
78. **Hill, J.O., P.B. Sparling, T.W. Shields, and P.A. Heller.** Effects of exercise and food restriction on body composition and metabolic rate in obese women. *Am. J. Clin. Nutr.* 46:622–630, 1987.
79. **Hollmann, W.** *Changes in the Capacity for Maximal and Continuous Effort in Relation to Age. Int. Res. Sports Phys. Ed,* E. Jokl and E. Simon (Eds.). Springfield, IL: Charles C Thomas Co., 1964, pp. 369–371.
80. **Hollmann, W. and H. Venrath.** Die Beinflussung von Herzgrösse, maximaler O_2—Aufnahme und Ausdauergranze durchein Ausdauertraining mittlerer und hoher Intensitat. *Der Sportarzt.* 9:189–193, 1963.
81. No reference 81 due to renumbering in proof.
82. **Huibregtse, W.H., H.H. Hartley, L.R. Jones, W.D. Doolittle, and T.L. Criblez.** Improvement of aerobic work capacity following non-strenuous exercise. *Arch. Environ. Health.* 27:12–15, 1973.
83. **Hurley, B.F., D.R. Seals, A.A. Ehsani, et al.** Effects of high intensity strength training on cardiovascular function. *Med. Sci. Sports Exerc.* 16:483–488, 1984.
84. **Ismail, A.H., D. Corrigan, and D.F. McLeod.** Effect of an eight-month exercise program on selected physiological, biochemical, and audiological variables in adult men. *Br. J. Sports Med.* 7:230–240, 1973.

84A. **Jones, D.A., D.J. Newman, J.M. Round, and S.E.L. Tolfree.** Experimental human muscle damage: morphological changes in relation to other indices of damage. *J. Physiol. (Lond)* 375:435–438, 1986.

85. **Karvonen, M., K. Kentala, and O. Mustala.** The effects of training heart rate: a longitudinal study. *Ann. Med. Exp. Biol. Fenn.* 35:307–315, 1957.
86. **Kasch, F.W., W.H. Phillips, J.E.L. Carter, and J.L. Boyer.** Cardiovascular changes in middle-aged men during two years of training. *J. Appl. Physiol.* 314:53–57, 1972.
87. **Kasch, F.W. and J.P. Wallace.** Physiological variables during 10 years of endurance exercise. *Med. Sci. Sports.* 8:5–8, 1976.
88. **Kasch, F.W., J.P. Wallace, and S.P. Van Camp.** Effects of 18 years of endurance exercise on physical work capacity of older men. *J. Cardiopulmonary Rehabil.* 5:308–312, 1985.
89. **Katch, F.I. and W.D. McArdle.** *Nutrition, Weight Control and Exercise*, 3rd Ed. Philadelphia: Lea and Febiger, 1988, pp. 110–112.
90. **Kearney, J.T., A.G. Stull, J.L. Ewing, and J.W. Strein.** Cardiorespiratory responses of sedentary college women as a function of training intensity. *J. Appl. Physiol.* 41:822–825, 1976.
91. **Kendrick, Z.B., M.L. Pollock, T.N. Hickman, and H.S. Miller.** Effects of training and detraining on cardiovascular efficiency. *Am. Corr. Ther. J.* 25:79–83, 1971.
92. **Kilbom, A.** Physical training in women. *Scand. J. Clin. Lab. Invest.* 119 (Suppl.):1–34, 1971.
93. **Kilbom, A., L. Hartley, B. Saltin, J. Bjure, G. Grimby, and I. Åstrand.** Physical training in sedentary middle-aged and older men. *Scand. J. Clin. Lab. Invest.* 24:315–322, 1969.
94. **Kimura, Y., H. Itow, and S. Yamazakie.** The effects of circuit weight training on $\dot{V}O_2$max and body composition of trained and untrained college men. *J. Physiol Soc. Jpn.* 43:593–596, 1981.

94A. **Klissouras, V., F. Pirnay, and J. Petit.** Adaptation to maximal effort: genetics and age. *J. Appl. Physiol.* 35:288–293, 1973.

95. **Knapik, J.J., R.H. Maudsley, and N.V. Rammos.** Angular specificity and test mode specificity of isometric and isokinetic strength training. *J. Orthop. Sports Phys. Ther.* 5:58–65, 1983.
96. **Knehr, C.A., D.B. Dill, and W. Neufeld.** Training and its effect on man at rest and at work. *Am. J. Physiol.* 136:148–156, 1942.

97. **Knuttgen, H.G., L O. Nordesjo, B. Ollander, and B. Saltin.** Physical conditioning through interval training with young male adults. *Med. Sci. Sports.* 5:220–226, 1973.
98. **Laporte, R.E., L.L. Adams, D.D. Savage, G. and Brenes, S. Dearwater, and T. Cook. The** spectrum of physical activity, cardiovascular disease and health: an epidemiologic perspective. *Am. J. Epidemiol.* 120:507–517, 1984.
99. **Leon, A.S., J. Conrad, D.B. Hunninghake, and R. Serfass.** Effects of a vigorous walking program on body composition, and carbohydrate and lipid metabolism of obese young men. *Am. J. Clin. Nutr.* 32:1776–1787, 1979.
100. **Leon, A.S., J. Connett, D.R. Jacobs, and R. Rauramaa.** Leisure-time physical activity levels and risk of coronary heart disease and death: the multiple risk of coronary heart disease and death: the multiple risk factor intervention trial. *JAMA.* 258:2388–2395, 1987.
100A. **Lewis, S.F., W.F. Taylor, R.M. Graham, W.A. Pettinger, J.E. Shutte, and C.G. Blomqvist.** Cardiovascular responses to exercise as functions of absolute and relative work load. *J. Appl. Physiol.* 54:1314–1323, 1983.
101. **Liang, M.T., J.F. Alexander, H.L. Taylor, R.C. Serfrass, A.S. Leon, and G.A. Stull.** Aerobic training threshold, intensity duration, and frequency of exercise. *Scand. J. Sports Sci.* 4:5–8, 1982.
101A. **Lieber, D.C., R.L. Lieber, and W.C. Adams.** Effects of run training and swim-training at similar absolute intensities on treadmill $\dot{V}O_2$max. *Med. Sci. Sports Exerc.* 21:655–661, 1989.
101B. **MacDougall, J.D., G.R Ward, D.G. Sale, and J.R. Sutton.** Biochemical adaptation of human skeletal muscle to heavy resistance training and immobilization. *J. Appl. Physiol.* 43:700–703, 1977.
101C. **MacDougall, J.D., D. Tuxen, D.G. Sale, J.R. Moroz, and J.R. Sutton.** Arterial blood pressure response to heavy resistance training. *J. Appl Physiol.* 58:785–790, 1985.
102. **Mann, G.V., L.H. Garrett, and A. Farhi, et al.** Exercise to prevent coronary heart disease. *Am. J. Med.* 46:12–27, 1969.
103. **Marcinik, E.J., J.A. Hodgdon, U. Mittleman, and J.J. O'Brien.** Aerobic/calisthenic and aerobic/circuit weight training programs for Navy men: a comparative study. *Med. Sci. Sports Exerc.* 17:482–487, 1985.
104. **Marigold, E.A.** The effect of training at predetermined heart rate levels for sedentary college women. *Med. Sci. Sports.* 6:14–19, 1974.
105. **Martin, J.E. and P.M. Dubbert.** Adherence to exercise. In: *Exercise and Sports Sciences Reviews*, Vol. 13, R.L. Terjung (Ed.). New York: MacMillan Publishing Co., 1985, pp. 137–167.
106. **Martin, W.H., J. Montgomery, P.G. Snell, et al.** Cardiovascular adaptations to intense swim training in sedentary middle-aged men and women. *Circulation.* 75:323–330, 1987.
107. **Mayhew, J.L. and P.M. Gross.** Body composition changes in young women with high resistance weight training. *Res. Q.* 45:433–439, 1974.
108. **Messier, J.P. and M. Dill.** Alterations in strength and maximal oxygen uptake consequent to Nautilus circuit weight training. *Res. Q. Exerc. Sport.* 56:345–351, 1985.
109. **Milesis, C.A., M.L. Pollock, M.D. Bah, J.J. Ayres, A. Ward, and A.C. Linnerud.** Effects of different durations of training on cardiorespiratory function, body composition and serum lipids. *Res. Q.* 47:716–725, 1976.
110. **Misner, J.E., R.A. Boileau, B.H. Massey, and J.H. Mayhew.** Alterations in body composition of adult men during selected physical training programs. *J. Am. Geriatr. Soc.* 22:33–38, 1974.
111. **Miyashita, M., S. Haga, and T. Mitzuta.** Training and detraining effects on aerobic power in middle-aged and older men. *J. Sports Med.* 18:131–137, 1978.
112. **Moody, D.L., J. Kollias, and E.R. Buskirk.** The effect of a moderate exercise program on body weight and skinfold thickness in overweight college women. *Med. Sci. Sports.* 1:75–80, 1969.
113. **Moody, D.L., J.H. Wilmore, R.N. Girandola, and J.P. Royce.** The effects of a jogging program on the body composition of normal and obese high school girls. *Med. Sci. Sports.* 4:210–213, 1972.

114. **Mueller, E.A. and W. Rohmert.** Die geschwindigkeit der muskelkraft zunahme bein isometrischen training. *Int. Z. Angew. Physiol.* 19:403–419, 1963.
115. **Naughton, J. and F. Nagle.** Peak oxygen intake during physical fitness program for middle-aged men. *JAMA* 191:899–901, 1965.
116. **O'Hara, W., C. Allen, and R.J. Shephard.** Loss of body weight and fat during exercise in a cold chamber. *Eur. J. Appl. Physiol.* 37:205–218, 1977.
117. **Oja, P., P. Teraslinna, T. Partanen, and R. Karava.** Feasibility of an 18 months' physical training program for middle-aged men and its effect on physical fitness. *Am. J. Public Health.* 64:459–465, 1975.
118. **Olree, H.D., B. Corbin, J. Penrod, and C. Smith.** Methods of achieving and maintaining physical fitness for prolonged space flight. Final Progress Rep. to NASA, Grant No. NGR-04-002-004, 1969.
119. **Oscai, L.B., T. Williams, and B. Hertig.** Effects of exercise on blood volume. *J. Appl. Physiol.* 24:622–624, 1968.
120. **Paffenbarger, R.S., R.T. Hyde, A.L. Wing, and C. Hsieh.** Physical activity and all-cause mortality, and longevity of college alumni. *N. Engl. J. Med.* 314:605–613, 1986.
121. **Pavlou, K.N., W.P. Steffee, R.H. Learman, and B.A. Burrows.** Effects of dieting and exercise on lean body mass, oxygen uptake, and strength. *Med. Sci. Sports Exerc.* 17:466–471, 1985.
122. **Pels, A.E., M.L. Pollock, T.E. Dohmeier, K.A. Lemberger, and B. F. Oehrlein.** Effects of leg press training on cycling, leg press, and running peak cardiorespiratory measures. *Med. Sci. Sports Exerc.* 19:66–70, 1987.
123. **Pollock, M.L.** The quantification of endurance training programs. In: *Exercise and Sport Sciences Reviews*, J. H. Wilmore (Ed.). New York: Academic Press, 1973, pp. 155–188.
124. **Pollock, M.L.** Prescribing exercise for fitness and adherence. In: *Exercise Adherence: Its Impact on Public Health,* R. K. Dishman (Ed.). Champaign, IL: Human Kinetics Books, 1988, pp. 259–277.
125. **Pollock, M.L., T.K. Cureton, and L. Greninger.** Effects of frequency of training on working capacity, cardiovascular function, and body composition of adult men. *Med. Sci. Sports.* 1:70–74, 1969.
126. **Pollock, M.L., J. Tiffany, L. Gettman, R. Janeway, and H. Lofland.** Effects of frequency of training on serum lipids, cardiovascular function, and body composition. In: *Exercise and Fitness*, B.D. Franks (Ed.). Chicago: Athletic Institute, 1969, pp. 161–178.
127. **Pollock, M.L., H. Miller, R. Janeway, A.C. Linnerud, B. Robertson, and R. Valentino.** Effects of walking on body composition and cardiovascular function of middle-aged men. *J. Appl. Physiol.* 30:126–130, 1971.
128. **Pollock, M.L., J. Broida, Z. Kendrick, H.S. Miller, R. Janeway, and A.C. Linnerud.** Effects of training two days per week at different intensities on middle-aged men. *Med. Sci. Sports.* 4:192–197, 1972.
129. **Pollock, M.L., H.S. Miller, Jr., and J. Wilmore.** Physiological characteristics of champion American track athletes 40 to 70 years of age. *J. Gerontol.* 29:645–649, 1974.
130. **Pollock, M.L., J. Dimmick, H.S. Miller, Z. Kendrick, and A.C. Linnerud.** Effects of mode of training on cardiovascular function and body composition of middle-aged men. *Med. Sci. Sports.* 7:139–145, 1975.
131. No reference 131 due to renumbering in proof.
132. **Pollock, M.L., G.A. Dawson, H.S. Miller, Jr., et al.** Physiologic response of men 49 to 65 years of age to endurance training. *J. Am. Geriatr. Soc.* 24:97–104, 1976.
133. **Pollock, M.L. and A. Jackson.** Body composition: measurement and changes resulting from physical training. Proceedings National College Physical Education Association for Men and Women, January, 1977, pp. 125–137.
134. **Pollock, M.L., J. Ayres, and A. Ward.** Cardiorespiratory fitness: response to differing intensities and durations of training. *Arch. Phys. Med. Rehabil.* 58:467–473, 1977.

135. **Pollock, M.L., R. Gettman, C A. Milesis, M.D. Bah, J.L. Durstine, and R.B. Johnson.** Effects of frequency and duration of training on attrition and incidence of injury. *Med. Sci. Sports.* 9:31–36, 1977.
136. **Pollock, M.L., L.R. Gettman, P.B. Raven, J. Ayres, M. Bah, and A. Ward.** Physiological comparison of the effects of aerobic and anaerobic training. In: *Physical Fitness Programs for Law Enforcement Officers: A Manual for Police Administrators*, C. S. Price, M.L. Pollock, L.R. Gettman, and D.A. KENT (Eds.). Washington, D.C.: U. S. Government Printing Office, No. 027-000-00671-0, 1978, pp. 89–96.
137. **Pollock, M.L., A.S. Jackson, and C. Foster.** The use of the perception scale for exercise prescription. In: *The Perception of Exertion in Physical Work*, G. Borg and D. Ottoson (Eds.). London, England: The MacMillan Press, Ltd., 1986, pp. 161–176.
138. **Pollock, M.L., C. Foster, D. Knapp, J.S. Rod, and D.H. Schmidt.** Effect of age and training on aerobic capacity and body composition of master athletes. *J. Appl. Physiol.* 62:725–731, 1987.
139. **Pollock, M.L. and J.H. Wilmore.** *Exercise in Health and Disease. Evaluation and Prescription for Prevention and Rehabilitation*, 2nd Ed. Philadelphia: W.B. Saunders, Co., 1990.
140. **Powell, K.E., H.W. Kohl, C.J. Caspersen, and S.N. Blair.** An epidemiological perspective of the causes of running injuries. *Phys. Sportsmed.* 14:100–114, 1986.
141. **Ribisl, P.M.** Effects of training upon the maximal oxygen uptake of middle-aged men. *Int. Z. Angew. Physiol.* 26:272–278, 1969.
142. **Richie, D.H., S.F. Kelso, and P.A. Bellucci.** Aerobic dance injuries: a retrospective study of instructors and participants. *Phys. Sportsmed.* 13:130-140, 1985.
143. **Robinson, S. and P.M. Harmon.** Lactic acid mechanism and certain properties of blood in relation to training. *Am. J. Physiol.* 132:757–769, 1941.
144. **Roskamm, H.** Optimum patterns of exercise for healthy adults. *Can. Med. Assoc. J.* 96:895–899, 1967.
145. **Sale, D.G.** Influence of exercise and training on motor unit activation. In: *Exercise and Sport Sciences Reviews*, K.B. Pandolf (Ed.). New York: MacMillan Publishing Co., 1987, pp. 95–152.
145A. **Sale, D.G.** Neural adaptation to resistance training. *Med. Sci. SportsExerc.* 20:S135–S145, 1988.
146. **Sallis, J.F., W.L. Haskell, S.P. Fortman, K.M. Vranizan,C.B. Taylor, and D.S. Soloman.** Predictors of adoption and maintenance of physical activity in a community sample. *Prev. Med.* 15:131–141, 1986.
147. **Saltin, B., G. Blomqvist, J. Mitchell, R.L. Johnson, K. Wildenthal, and C.B. Chapman.** Response to exercise after bed rest and after training. *Circulation.* 37, 38(Suppl. 7):1–78, 1968.
148. **Saltin, B., L. Hartley, A. Kilbom, and I. Åstrand.** Physical training in sedentary middle-aged and older men. *Scand. J. Clin. Lab. Invest.* 24:323–334, 1969.
149. **Santigo, M.C., J.F. Alexander, G.A. Stull, R.C. Serfrass, A.M. Hayday, and A.S. Leon.** Physiological responses of sedentary women to a 20-week conditioning program of walking or jogging. *Scand. J. Sports Sci.* 9:33–39, 1987.
150. **Seals, D.R., J.M. Hagberg, B.F. Hurley, A.A. Ehsani, and J.O. Holloszy.** Endurance training in older men and women. I. Cardiovascular responses to exercise. *J. Appl. Physiol.* 57:1024–1029, 1984.
151. **Sharkey, B.J.** Intensity and duration of training and the development of cardiorespiratory endurance. *Med. Sci. Sports.* 2:197–202, 1970.
152. **Shephard, R.J.** Intensity, duration, and frequency of exercise as determinants of the response to a training regime. *Int. Z. Angew. Physiol.* 26:272–278, 1969.
153. **Shephard, R.J.** Future research on the quantifying of endurance training. *J. Hum. Ergol.* 3:163–181, 1975.
154. **Sidney, K.H., R.B. Eynon, and D A. Cunningham.** Effect of frequency of training of exercise upon physical working performance and selected variables representative of cardiorespiratory fitness. In: *Training Scientific Basis and Application*, A. W. Taylor (Ed.). Springfield, IL: Charles C Thomas Co., 1972, pp. 144–188.

155. **Sidney, K.H., R.J. Shephard, and J. Harrison.** Endurance training and body composition of the elderly. *Am. J. Clin. Nutr.* 30:326–333, 1977.
156. **Siegel, W., G. Blomqvist, and J.H. Mitchell.** Effects of a quantitated physical training program on middle-aged sedentary males. *Circulation.* 41:19–29, 1970.

156A. **Siscovick, D.S., N.S. Weiss, R.H. Fletcher, and T. Lasky.** The incidence of primary cardiac arrest during vigorous exercise. *N. Engl. J. Med.* 311:874–877, 1984.

157. **Skinner, J.** The cardiovascular system with aging and exercise. In: *Physical Activity and Aging*, D. Brunner and E. Jokl (Eds.). Baltimore: University Park Press, 1970, pp. 100–108.
158. **Skinner, J., J. Holloszy, and T. Cureton.** Effects of a program of endurance exercise on physical work capacity and anthropometric measurements of fifteen middle-aged men. *Am. J. Cardiol.* 14:747–752, 1964.
159. **Smith, D.P. and F.W. Stransky.** The effect of training and detraining on the body composition and cardiovascular response of young women to exercise. *J. Sports Med.* 16:112–120, 1976.
160. **Smith, E.L., W. Reddan, and P.E. Smith.** Physical activity and calcium modalities for bone mineral increase in aged women. *Med. Sci. Sports Exerc.* 13:60–64, 1981.
161. **Suominen, H., E. Heikkinen, and T. Tarkatti.** Effect of eight weeks physical training on muscle and connective tissue of the m. vastus lateralis in 69-year-old men and women. *J. Gerontol.* 32:33–37, 1977.
162. **Terjung, R.L., K.M. Baldwin, J. Cooksey, B. Samson, and R.A. Sutter.** Cardiovascular adaptation to twelve minutes of mild daily exercise in middle-aged sedentary men. *J. Am. Geriatr. Soc.* 21:164–168, 1973.
163. **Thomas, S.G., D.A. Cunningham, P.A. Rechnitzer, A.P. Donner, and J.H. Howard.** Determinants of the training response in elderly men. *Med. Sci. Sports Exerc.* 17:667–672, 1985.
164. **Wenger, H.A. and G.J. Bell.** The interactions of intensity, frequency, and duration of exercise training in altering cardiorespiratory fitness. *Sports Med.* 3:346–356, 1986.
165. **Wilmore, J.H.** Alterations in strength, body composition, and anthropometric measurements consequent to a 10-week weight training program. *Med. Sci. Sports.* 6:133–138, 1974.
166. **Wilmore, J.** Inferiority of female athletes: myth or reality. *J. Sports Med.* 3:1–6, 1974.
167. **Wilmore, J.H.** Design issues and alternatives in assessing physical fitness among apparently healthy adults in a health examination survey of the general population. In: *Assessing Physical Fitness and Activity in General Population Studies*, T.F. Drury (Ed.). Washington, D.C.: U.S. Public Health Service, National Center for Health Statistics, 1988 (in press).
168. **Wilmore, J.H., J. Royce, R.N. Girandola, F.I. Katch, and V.L. Katch.** Physiological alternatives resulting from a 10 week jogging program. *Med. Sci. Sports.* 2:7–14, 1970.
169. **Wilmore, J.H., J. Royce, R.N. Girandola, F.I. Katch, and V.L. Katch.** Body composition changes with a 10-week jogging program. *Med. Sci. Sports.* 2:113–117, 1970.
170. **Wilmore, J., R.B. Parr, P.A. Vodak, et al.** Strength, endurance, BMR, and body composition changes with circuit weight training. *Med. Sci. Sports.* 8:58–60, 1976.
171. **Wilmore, J.H., G.A. Ewy, A.R. Mortan, et al.** The effect of beta-adrenergic blockade on submaximal and maximal exercise performance. *J. Cardiac Rehabil.* 3:30–36, 1983.

171A. **Wilmore, J.H.** Body composition in sport and exercise: directions for future research. *Med. Sci. Sports Exerc.* 15:21–31, 1983.

172. **Wilmore, J.H. and D.L. Costill.** *Training for Sport and Activity. The Physiological Basis of the Conditioning Process*, 3rd Ed. Dubuque, IA: Wm. C. Brown, 1988, pp. 113 - 212.
173. **Wood, P.D., W.L. Haskell, S.N. Blair,** et al. Increased exercise level and plasma lipoprotein concentrations: a one year, randomized, controlled study in sedentary, middle-aged men. *Metabolism.* 32:31–39, 1983.
174. **Zuti, W.B. and L.A. Golding.** Comparing diet and exercise as weight reduction tools. *Phys. Sports Med.* 4:49–53, 1976.

Appendix D

AMERICAN COLLEGE OF SPORTS MEDICINE POSITION STAND ON PHYSICAL ACTIVITY, PHYSICAL FITNESS, AND HYPERTENSION*

SUMMARY

Hypertension is present in epidemic proportions in adults of industrialized societies and is associated with a markedly increased risk of developing numerous cardiovascular pathologies. There is a continuing debate as to the efficacy of aggressive pharmacological therapy in individuals with mild to moderate elevations in blood pressure. This has led to a search for nonpharmacological therapies such as exercise training for these individuals. The available evidence indicates that endurance exercise training by individuals at high risk for developing hypertension will reduce the rise in blood pressure that occurs with time. Thus, it is the position of the American College of Sports Medicine that endurance exercise training is recommended as a nonpharmacological strategy to reduce the incidence of hypertension in susceptible individuals. A large number of studies indicate that endurance exercise training will elicit a 10 mmHg average reduction in both systolic and diastolic blood pressures in individuals with mild essential hypertension (blood pressures 140 to 180/90 to 105 mmHg). Endurance exercise training also has the capacity to improve other risk factors for cardiovascular disease in hypertensive individuals. Endurance exercise training appears to elicit even greater reductions in blood pressure in patients with secondary hypertension due to renal dysfunction. The mode (large muscle activities), frequency (3 to 5 $d \cdot week^{-1}$), duration (20 to 60 min), and intensity (50 to 85% of maximal oxygen uptake) of the exercise recommended to achieve this effect are generally the same as those prescribed for developing and maintaining cardiovascular fitness in healthy adults. Exercise training at somewhat lower intensities (40 to 70% $\dot{V}O_2max$) appears to lower blood pressure as much or more than exercise at higher intensities, which may be important in specific hypertensive populations. Physically active and fit individuals with hypertension have markedly lower rates of mortality than sedentary, unfit hypertensive individuals. Thus, it seems reasonable to

* Reprinted from *"Physical Activity, Physical Fitness, and Hypertension,"* ©1993 American College of Sports Medicine, *MSSE,* 25:10, 1993, pp i–x. With permission of Williams & Wilkins.

recommend exercise as the initial treatment strategy for individuals with mild to moderate essential hypertension. A follow-up period should assess the efficacy of the patient's exercise program, and adjunct therapies should be implemented according to the individual patient's blood pressure and CAD risk factor goals. Individuals with more marked elevations in blood pressure (>180/105 mmHg) should add endurance exercise training to their treatment regimen only after initiating pharmacologic therapy. Resistive, or strength, exercise training is not recommended to lower blood pressure in individuals with hypertension when done as their only form of exercise training. It is recommended when included as one component of a well-rounded fitness program, such as circuit training done in conjunction with endurance exercise training. Exercise testing is not advocated to determine normotensive individuals with an exaggerated exercise blood pressure response who might be at high risk of developing hypertension in the future. However, if exercise test results are available, they can be used to provide some indication of risk stratification and the need for appropriate lifestyle behavior counseling that might ameliorate this risk.

INTRODUCTION

Hypertension, defined as a blood pressure above 140/90 mmHg, is present in 17% of adults according to the National Health and Nutrition Examination Survey.[94] However, hypertension prevalence rates rise sharply with age and are also generally higher in men than in women and in blacks than in whites.[59] At least 90% and probably as much as 95% of all hypertension is of unknown cause, i.e., primary or essential.[59] Despite tremendous increases in the recognition and treatment of hypertension over the past 25 years,[9,25] the incidence of hypertension has not decreased.[26] This Position Stand primarily addresses the effect of exercise training on individuals with hypertension and on those individuals at an increased risk of developing hypertension. In addition, this Position Stand also addresses the role of exercise testing in predicting those individuals at higher risk of developing hypertension in the future.

HYPERTENSION AND PREMATURE MORTALITY AND MORBIDITY

Men and women with blood pressures exceeding 160/95 mmHg have a 150 to 300% higher annual incidence rate for coronary artery disease (CAD), congestive heart failure, intermittent claudication, and stroke than their normotensive peers.[58] Women appear to tolerate increased blood pressures better than men as they have substantially lower incidence rates for these four cardiovascular pathologies than men with comparable blood pressures.[58] On the other hand, black hypertensives have higher death rates than whites with the same blood pressure.[59]

Older individuals also have a substantially greater risk of a cardiovascular event than younger persons with the same elevation in blood pressure,[59] indicating that an increase in blood pressure should not be accepted as an inconsequential concomitant of the aging process.

The dramatic benefits derived from aggressive pharmacological therapy for individuals with marked elevations in blood pressure were first demonstrated over 20 years ago in the Veterans Administration Cooperative Study of individuals with diastolic blood pressures of 115 to 129 mmHg,[115] where 40% of patients receiving a placebo experienced a cardiovascular event compared with only 3% of patients receiving antihypertensive medications over the same time period. Numerous other trials have continued to demonstrate the dramatic benefits of pharmacological therapy in individuals with marked elevations in blood pressure.[59]

Individuals with mild hypertension (140 to 160/90 to 105 mmHg) are also at a greater risk of developing future cardiovascular morbidity.[58] However, there is a continuing debate as to the efficacy of aggressive pharmacological therapy to reduce their cardiovascular risks, perhaps because of deleterious side effects of medications on other risk factors for CAD.[59,68] This debate has led to a search for nonpharmacological therapies such as exercise training for individuals with mild hypertension. Exercise training has also been proposed as a strategy to reduce the likelihood of a high-risk individual developing hypertension and to reduce mortality in individuals initiating an exercise program even if they remain hypertensive. In addition, exercise testing has been advocated as a means to identify normotensive individuals who may have a greater risk for developing hypertension in the future.

EXERCISE TESTING AND THE PREDICTION OF THE DEVELOPMENT OF HYPERTENSION

Over 50 years ago the blood pressure responses of prehypertensive individuals to local cold[51] and mental tests[70] were found to be higher than those of individuals at lower risk for the future development of hypertension. Although most studies have shown that normotensive individuals with a family history of hypertension have more marked pressor responses to dynamic and isometric exercise than individuals without such a history,[10,76,119] other studies have not reported such differences (cf., References 106, 107). Several longitudinal studies indicate that normotensive individuals with a hypertensive response to exercise have an increased risk of developing hypertension in the future.[20,54,69,73,103] These reports vary in the type of population studied, the mode of exercise testing, the definition of a hypertensive response to exercise, and the length of follow-up. Nevertheless, results are consistent with a two- to threefold increase in risk for developing hypertension in individuals with an exaggerated blood pressure response to exercise. The sensitivity and specificity of exercise hypertension to predict future hypertension at rest are modest,[10] but these terms are usually discussed in reference to a diagnostic test where high values are required to have confidence in a definitive diagnosis. Screening tests to predict future disease or death have lower sensitivity and specificity than diagnostic tests, but screening is still useful to identify groups at risk. Thus, mass exercise testing is not recommended to indicate future hypertensive individuals. However, if exercise test results are available, individuals with exercise blood pressure responses above the 85th or 90th percentile should be counseled about their increased risk for developing hypertension at rest in the future and given appropriate advice regarding health habits that might ameliorate that increased risk.

EXERCISE AND PREVENTION OF HYPERTENSION

STUDIES IN ANIMALS

In animal models it is important to differentiate those animals that become hypertensive because of genetic influences — spontaneously hypertensive (SH) rats — from those that become hypertensive as a result of interventions such as hormonal injections (deoxycorticosterone), salt intake, or arterial constriction (two kidney-one clip). In the former, blood pressure is elevated because of interactions between genetic factors and the maturation process; whereas, in the latter it is generally the magnitude and duration of the intervention that determines the rise in pressure. In general, the rise in blood pressure seen over time in SH rats is attenuated when they undergo exercise training during maturation, although the attenuation will not maintain their resting blood pressures within the normotensive range.[108] This effect of training is seldom found in rat models of renal hypertension and is variable in salt-sensitive rats.[106,107] However, in these animal models, the peripheral vasculature and renal structural changes that develop with hypertension are major and may totally eliminate the possibility of any physiological intervention maintaining a normotensive state.

Training intensity also appears to be an important consideration in SH rats because when the intensity exceeds 75% of their maximal oxygen consumption ($\dot{V}O_2max$), higher rather than lower resting systolic blood pressure result.[108,113] On the other hand, when exercise intensity is 40 to 70% $\dot{V}O_2max$, lower resting pressures are found for trained SH rats.[108,109]

STUDIES IN HUMANS

Six of thirteen epidemiological studies reviewed in 1972 showed somewhat lower blood pressures in active compared with sedentary individuals.[77] The remaining seven cross-sectional studies in this review by Montoye et a1.[77] generally found no differences in blood pressure between active individuals and their less active peers. Reaven et al.[90] recently reported that in women a significant inverse relationship exists between physical activity and blood pressure, that the most active women had systolic and diastolic blood pressures 9 to 24 and 3 to 13 mmHg lower, respectively, than the lowest active women, and that this relationship persisted after correcting for differences in body mass index. In the Tecumseh Community Health Study,[77] the blood pressure of adult males was inversely related to occupational and leisure physical activity habits; however, the absolute difference in blood pressure was only 2 to 3 mmHg between the most and least active men.

In more recent longitudinal studies, University of Pennsylvania alumni who played intramural sports less than 5 h · week^{-1} were found to be 32% more likely to develop hypertension during 22 to 31 years of follow-up than those who played sports more than 5 h · week^{-1}; similar results were evident when athletes and nonathletes were compared.[81] Follow-up surveys of this population indicated that participation in light or moderate activity later in life did not alter the incidence of hypertension, but alumni who had subsequently engaged in vigorous activity had a 19 to 29% lower rate of developing hypertension.[83] Harvard alumni who did not participate in vigorous sports had a 35% higher incidence of hypertension during a 6 to 10-year follow-up period.[84] At the Institute for Aerobic Research in Dallas, physically unfit individuals, assessed by the results of treadmill exercise tests relative to age- and sex-specific norms, were 52% more likely than fit individuals to develop hypertension during a 4-year follow-up period.[13]

The first and only long-term primary prevention trial found that 75% of hypertension-prone men and women 30 to 44 years of age in an exercise and dietary intervention program increased their reported physical activity, and improved their exercise tolerance more than hypertension-prone controls.[101] The incidence of new hypertension in this intervention group (8.8%) was 54% lower than the incidence in the control group (19.2%) over the 5-year duration of the trial. However, since this trial combined several interventions it was not possible to assess the independent contribution of exercise toward lowering the incidence of hypertension.

Thus, recent large, long-term studies that allow for control of potentially confounding variables support the concepts that regular exercise and increased aerobic fitness levels ($\dot{V}O_2max$) reduce an individual's risk of developing hypertension. However, most of these investigations studied white, middle-class males and little information is available for women, minorities, and other demographic groups.

EFFECT OF EXERCISE ON INDIVIDUALS WITH HYPERTENSION

STUDIES IN ANIMALS

There have been very few studies in which hypertension was established before the animals began training. In SH rats older than 40 weeks of age, moderate intensity exercise training for several months maintained resting blood pressure at their initial value, whereas SH rats not undergoing training exhibited a gradual increase in pressure over the same time.[117] However, the available data on exercise training in animals do not convincingly support the concept that exercise training will lower blood pressures in those with established hypertension.

STUDIES IN HUMANS

Forty studies published prior to 1992 in the English literature have assessed the blood pressure-lowering effects of endurance exercise training on individuals with essential hypertension.[2,5,7,8,14-16,18,19,22-24,27,29,32,36,38,44,47,49,50,55,56,62,64,66,67,74,78,79,92,93,95-97,102,114,116-188] All 1574 subjects enrolled in these studies initially had systolic hypertension (systolic blood pressure ≥140 mmHg) while 755 subjects (48%) initially also had diastolic hypertension (diastolic blood pressure ≥90 mmHg). Seventy-two percent of the groups in these studies that initially had systolic hypertension elicited significant decreases in systolic blood pressure as a result of endurance exercise training. Their training-induced reduction in systolic blood pressure averaged approximately 11 mmHg. Seventy-seven percent of the groups that initially had diastolic hypertension in these studies reduced their diastolic pressure significantly with endurance exercise training. Their reduction in diastolic blood pressure with exercise training averaged approximately 9 mmHg from an initial value of 99 mmHg. Thus, these data indicate that endurance exercise training lowers causal systolic and diastolic blood pressure measured in the laboratory or in a clinic setting by approximately 10 mmHg in the large majority of individuals with mild elevations in blood pressure.

Four studies in individuals with hypertension have assessed the impact of exercise training on the ambulatory blood pressures measured while they took part in their usual daily activities.[14,36,98,100] Two of these studies found no changes in either casual or ambulatory pressures as a result of endurance exercise training.[14,36] The two remaining studies[98,100] reported significant reductions in both casual and ambulatory blood pressures with exercise training in individuals with hypertension. However, the significant reduction in ambulatory blood pressure was generally only evident during the daytime hours, and the magnitude of the reduction was generally less than that observed in casual blood pressure. Thus, future studies must continue to assess the impact of exercise training on ambulatory blood pressure in individuals with hypertension, especially in light of the fact that ambulatory blood pressure is more indicative of their future prognosis.[89]

Roughly half of the 40 investigations that have assessed the impact of endurance exercise training on individuals with hypertension studied only men and only 2 studies reported data from women separately. However, no studies that have compared men and women have found gender-related differences in the blood pressure changes elicited with exercise training.[32,44,47,97,116] This would also appear to be the case in numerous other studies that include hypertensive men and women and made no specific mention of gender-related differences in blood pressure reductions elicited by endurance exercise training.[2,7,8,14,18,23,24,27,36,38,64,66,78,79,114,117,118]

The subjects in these 40 studies ranged in age from 15 to 79 years. The one study in adolescent hypertensives reported reductions in systolic blood pressure, and in diastolic blood pressure in those with diastolic hypertension,[44] that approximated 10 mmHg, even though their initial pressures were lower than those in older hypertensives. Studies that have assessed the blood pressure-lowering effects of endurance exercise training programs longer than 3 months in hypertensive men and women over the age of 60 years generally report reductions in blood pressure similar in magnitude to those elicited in younger hypertensives.[18,24,32,47] The only races studied extensively have been Caucasians and Asians.

The few studies that are available generally indicate that the blood pressure-lowering effect of exercise training is also evident and quantitatively similar in patients taking antihypertensive medications;[2,19,24,47,62] rat models of hypertension undergoing exercise training generally require less than normal amounts of antihypertensive medications.[108] Thus, although the data support the general conclusion that endurance exercise training lowers blood pressure in individuals with essential hypertension, extrapolations of this conclusion to specific hypertensive populations and situations are, except for white middle-aged men and women, almost universally based on results of single, or at best, very few studies.

A number of studies[24,47,55,64,66,93,97,114] have reported that training at 40 to 70% $\dot{V}O_2max$ had the same, or greater, blood pressure-lowering effect as higher intensity training. Along these lines, it has also been shown that SH rats had lower blood pressures than nonexercising age-matched controls only if they trained at 40–70% $\dot{V}O_2max$.[108,109] Thus, it appears that moderate-intensity training may elicit as great or greater reductions in blood pressure as higher intensity training; this may be especially important in specific populations of hypertensive individuals, such as the elderly, as acute cardiovascular and musculoskeletal risk will be reduced.

Most studies have found that blood pressure was reduced early (3 weeks to 3 months) after the initiation of exercise training, and that up to 9 months of additional training failed to elicit further reductions in blood pressure.[66,93,114] However, it was recently reported that older hypertensives who decreased their blood pressure significantly with 3 months of moderate-intensity training reduced both their systolic and diastolic blood pressures further with an additional 6 months of training.[47] In a previous review,[41] the reduction in diastolic blood pressure was found to be related to the length of the training, whereas the reduction in systolic pressure was not. Thus, although it appears that blood pressure may be reduced early after the initiation of an endurance exercise training program, it does not appear that prolonging such training beyond 3 months will result in further decrease in blood pressure, though this may not be the case with more moderate training intensities. However, those investigations that have had individuals with hypertension stop training indicate that their blood pressure returned to initial untrained levels.[44,93,100] Thus, although more prolonged training may not bring about further reductions in blood pressure in individuals with hypertension, the blood pressure-lowering effect of exercise training is evident only as long as a regular endurance exercise training program is maintained.

It has been proposed that some specific subsets of hypertensive individuals might not lower their blood pressure in response to endurance exercise training. Recent studies and reviews have reported that overweight hypertensives,[41] those with high initial plasma renin levels,[66,114] low norepinephrine levels,[29] high cardiac output,[64] high serum sodium to potassium ratios,[64] or those taking nonselective beta-blockade medications[2] show either no, or attenuated, blood pressure-lowering responses to endurance exercise training. However, this attenuated blood pressure-lowering response is not consistent in other studies that have investigated these specific subgroups of hypertensives.[24,44,47,62] A recent study reported that hypertensive subjects with hypertensive exercise blood pressure responses did not change their systolic blood pressure and actually increased their diastolic blood pressure significantly (from 87 to 92 mmHg) in response to exercise training.[5] However, in the same study,[5] hypertensives with normal blood pressure responses to exercise decreased their systolic and diastolic blood pressure significantly. This is the only study to report a significant increase in resting blood pressure in a group of hypertensive individuals as a result of exercise training. Finally, a recent review[41] indicated that in previous studies the magnitude of the reductions in systolic and diastolic blood pressure elicited with endurance exercise training was somewhat correlated to the initial diastolic blood pressure ($r = 0.34$ and 0.46, respectively) but not to the initial systolic blood pressure.

Thus, there is minimal definitive evidence to support the conclusion that certain subsets of individuals with essential hypertension do not lower their blood pressure in response to endurance exercise training. However, in view of the recent report of strikingly different blood pressure responses to exercise training between hypertensives with normal vs. exaggerated blood pressure responses to maximal exercise, further investigation is warranted.

Another important consideration for hypertensive individuals is the possibility that endurance exercise training may elicit other potential benefits in addition to lowering their blood pressure. The incidence of other modifiable CAD risk factors, including obesity, abnormal plasma lipoprotein-lipid profiles, insulin resistance, and glucose intolerance, is also more prevalent in hypertensive individuals.[60,104] Endurance exercise training, in addition to reducing blood pressure in hypertensive individuals, also improves glucose intolerance and insulin resistance,[52] obesity and caloric balance,[17] and plasma lipoprotein-lipid profiles[121] in healthy individuals. Furthermore, some of these beneficial training-induced adaptations have also already been demonstrated in individuals with essential hypertension.[15,38,62,97,102,116,118] These positive effects of exercise training are in contrast to the known deleterious side effects of many of the antihypertensive medications on CAD risk factors.[58] Preliminary research suggests that certain antihypertensive drug therapies such as beta-blockers may offset or negate the exercise training-induced increase in HDL-cholesterol levels.[30] However, the interactive effects of exercise and specific drug therapies on other CAD risk factors are largely unknown.

STUDIES IN HUMANS WITH SECONDARY HYPERTENSION

Few studies have assessed the impact of exercise training on patients with secondary hypertension, probably because most of these patients have an underlying etiology that should be treated directly by standard medical, pharmacological, and surgical interventions. However, some patients with end-stage renal disease have endocrine abnormalities that maintain or exacerbate their hypertension even after their excess fluid volume is removed by dialysis. Two studies have reported that exercise training in end-stage renal disease patients decreases their systolic and diastolic blood pressures 2 to 3 times more than the reductions generally achieved in patients with essential hypertension, i.e., 20 to 30 mmHg, and results in substantial reductions in the required dosages of their antihypertensive medications.[43,85] Another study also found that a small number of patients with hypertension secondary to renal dysfunction decreased their blood pressures with exercise training to a greater extent than those with essential hypertension.[19] Therefore, it appears that patients with secondary forms of hypertension related to renal dysfunction can also reduce their blood pressure with endurance exercise training, and to an even greater extent than individuals with essential hypertension.

DEATH RATES, FITNESS, AND HYPERTENSION

A strong inverse gradient for age-adjusted all-cause mortality exists across physical activity strata in Harvard alumni.[82] Hypertensive University of Pennsylvania alumni who engaged in vigorous sports had a 37% lower age-adjusted all-cause death rate than sedentary hypertensive alumni.[83] Additional studies have shown that morbidity and mortality rates are also inversely related to physical fitness status in hypertensive individuals.[12,53,87] More recently in one study, fit hypertensive individuals were shown to have a 60% lower mortality rate than in their unfit normotensive peers, and that the increased mortality associated with hypertension is completely overcome by fitness.[11] Although more research is clearly needed, especially in women, minorities, and other demographic groups, the existing studies support the conclusion that physical activity, and the resultant increased physical fitness, is an effective secondary intervention therapy in hypertensive individuals.

RELATIVE EFFECTIVENESS OF NONPHARMACOLOGICAL THERAPIES

A review of weight loss studies[59] found average reductions of 15 and 10 mmHg in systolic and diastolic blood pressure, respectively, as a result of a 10 kg average weight loss. A recent review concluded that reducing dietary sodium intake by 80 meq $\cdot$ d^{-1} was associated with a 5 and 3 mmHg reduction in systolic and diastolic blood pressure, respectively, and that increasing dietary potassium intake by the same amount resulted in average reductions of 8 and 4 mmHg for systolic and diastolic blood pressures, respectively.[59] Thus, overweight individuals who undergo a substantial weight loss elicit a reduction in blood pressure only slightly greater than that observed with endurance exercise training. However, altering sodium and potassium intake alone has a smaller effect on blood pressure than endurance exercise training.[59]

The other nonpharmacologic therapies proposed to induce an antihypertensive effect are behavioral modalities, such as relaxation and biofeedback. A review of 15 studies of the effect of biofeedback training, many of which lacked appropriate control groups, indicated that it reduces systolic and diastolic blood pressure by an average of 12 and 5 mmHg, respectively, whereas relaxation techniques may be somewhat more effective with reductions averaging 18 and 11 mmHg for systolic and diastolic blood pressure, respectively.[99] However, the addition of appropriate control groups in recent studies appears to have diminished the favorable effect of relaxation and biofeedback interventions to levels lower than those attained by endurance exercise training.[37,71]

SAFETY OF ENDURANCE EXERCISE

HEMODYNAMIC RESPONSES

In unmedicated hypertensive individuals, acute exercise generally elicits a normal rise in systolic blood pressure from baseline levels, though the response may be exaggerated or diminished in certain patients.[88,120] However, because of their elevated baseline levels, the absolute levels of systolic blood pressure during exercise are usually higher in hypertensive persons. Furthermore, hypertensive persons may not change, or may even slightly increase, their diastolic blood pressure during incremental exercise probably as a result of impaired vasodilatory response.[88] On the other hand, recent studies have demonstrated that individuals with essential hypertension can exhibit 10 to 20 mmHg reductions in systolic blood pressure for 1 to 3 h following 30 to 45 min of moderate intensity exercise.[46,61] There is also some indication that this response may persist for up to 9 h following acute exercise in individuals with hypertension.[86] This response appears to be mediated by a transient decrease in stroke volume and, hence, cardiac output, perhaps due to a decrease in venous return, rather than a peripheral vasodilation that persists after the cessation of exercise.[46,80]

In view of the higher levels of blood pressure induced by exercise in individuals with hypertension, it has been postulated that they are at greater risk for sudden cardiac death or hemorrhagic stroke. However, at present there is no convincing evidence to substantiate this assumption in humans,[35,88] even though in young and mature stroke-prone SH rats, moderate-intensity endurance exercise training increased the incidence of cerebrovascular lesions.[110] Thus, it seems prudent to avoid an excessive rise in blood pressure during exercise training and, in patients with target organ involvement (e.g., left ventricular hypertrophy), to impose some restrictions on participation in vigorous exercise.[35] The facts that high blood pressure is a major risk factor for CAD, which is by far the leading cause of sudden death during exercise, and that the impaired coronary vasodilatory capacity in patients with left ventricular hypertrophy may provoke myocardial ischemia, even in the absence of severe CAD, should also be considered when prescribing exercise for hypertensive patients.

INTERACTION BETWEEN EXERCISE AND MEDICATION

Antihypertensive medications do not preclude participation in endurance exercise. Although most antihypertensive drugs do not substantially alter the blood pressure response to endurance exercise, they do lower resting blood pressure and, thus, the absolute level attained.[21,88] Beta-blockers, however, can attenuate the magnitude of the rise in systolic blood pressure during endurance exercise as well as resting blood pressure. Consequently, they may be considered as the antihypertensive agents of greatest potential benefit to hypertensive persons who have an excessive rise in systolic blood pressure during dynamic exercise. Unfortunately, the usefulness of beta-blockers, especially nonselective ones, is often considerably limited by a concomitant impairment of exercise tolerance in persons without myocardial ischemia[40] and the possibility that they may blunt the exercise training-induced lowering of blood pressure[2] and the exercise training induced increases in HDL-cholesterol[30] in hypertensive individuals. Therefore, unless beta-blocker therapy is specifically indicated, other agents with more favorable side effect profiles should be considered for such patients. In this regard, angiotensin-converting enzyme inhibitors, calcium channel blockers, and alpha-blockers are especially well suited for persons with uncomplicated essential hypertension and physically active lifestyles.[3,40] Irrespective of the drugs prescribed, the physician and patient should be aware of their interactions with exercise and whether any special precautions are needed.[35]

SAFETY AND THE EFFECTS OF RESISTIVE EXERCISE TRAINING

Patients with high blood pressure have traditionally been discouraged from participating in resistive training for fear of precipitating a cerebrovascular event or imposing an excessive demand on an already compromised myocardium. Such fears have arisen largely as a result of the marked pressor response elicited during acute high intensity resistive exercise.[34,72] However, studies investigating the impact of chronic resistive training on resting blood pressure have, in fact, not documented such an adverse effect; on the contrary, although considerable additional research is needed, the results of some,[42,50,62,65] but not all,[6,14,24] studies suggest that resistive training and especially circuit weight training may lower resting blood pressure.

Experimental evidence on the effects of acute and chronic resistive training on the risk for cerebrovascular complications in humans with high blood pressure is not available. Recently stroke-prone hypertensive rats were found to not increase their development of cerebrovascular lesions with long-term resistive exercise training.[111] Although considerable further research is required before these findings can be extrapolated to humans with high blood pressure, they do indicate that resistive training may not necessarily increase the risk for cerebrovascular lesions.

Resistive training produces concentric left ventricular hypertrophy in some individuals. In hypertensive patients, concentric left ventricular hypertrophy is associated with an accentuated risk of cardiovascular events even in the absence of other CAD risk factors.[28] In general, the magnitude of cardiac hypertrophy is smaller than the hypertrophy produced by chronic hypertension, perhaps in part due to the mild to moderate and intermittent nature of the pressure overload associated with resistive training compared with the chronic elevated pressure state associated with hypertension. In fact, resistive training is typically characterized by normal diastolic function, in contrast to what occurs with pathologic concentric hypertrophy. Thus, although the eccentric hypertrophy elicited by endurance training is seemingly more desirable, resistive training does not appear to produce any adverse effects on left ventricular function.[31,39]

POTENTIAL MECHANISMS UNDERLYING THE ANTIHYPERTENSIVE EFFECT OF EXERCISE TRAINING

At present the mechanisms by which exercise training decreases blood pressure in hypertensive individuals are unclear. This effect is probably not mediated by a single mechanism, and, for the different types of hypertension or in heterogeneous hypertensive populations, different mechanisms are possible. The blood pressure-lowering effect of exercise is, however, independent of decreases in body weight and body fat.[2,5,7,15,16,22,24,29,44,55,64,74,78,97,102,114]

In most individuals with long-standing hypertension, total peripheral resistance (TPR) is usually increased at rest.[1] However, in the limited number of studies in humans that have measured cardiovascular hemodynamics, reductions in both cardiac output and TPR have been observed after training.[41,107] Recently, trained SH rats were shown to have a lower cardiac output and blood pressure at rest than their sedentary strain-matched counterparts, although their TPR was actually increased.[109]

The sympathetic nervous system (SNS) is believed to play a central role in essential hypertension,[1,75] and there is evidence that the decrease in pressure with exercise training in some hypertensives is associated with a decrease in plasma norepinephrine levels.[29,47,66,114] This effect may be especially important in hypertensives who have high plasma norepinephrine levels at rest, where the reduction in blood pressure elicited with endurance exercise training was significantly correlated to the changes in plasma norepinephrine levels.[29] In addition, chemically sympathectomized SH rats have been shown to undergo less of a rise in blood pressure with exercise training than their treatment-matched sedentary counterparts.[112] The fact that not all studies have found a decrease in plasma norepinephrine with training[23,24,45] does not rule out SNS involvement, as plasma norepinephrine levels are only an indirect estimate of SNS activity and small but potentially important, training-induced decreases in peripheral SNS activity may not be detectable by measuring plasma norepinephrine levels.[33]

Conversely the lowering of blood pressure with exercise training could be due to an increase in circulating vasodilator substances. However, except for a suggested role for endorphins,[105] there are no consistent data indicating that the blood pressure-lowering effect of exercise training is mediated by compounds such as prostaglandins, kinins, adenosine, dopamine, or atrial natriuretic factor.

Recently, hyperinsulinemia secondary to insulin resistance has been proposed as a potential mechanism responsible for the development of hypertension and the increased incidence of diabetes, upper body obesity, hypertriglyceridemia, and CAD that occur in hypertensive individuals.[91] However, although it is known that exercise training can ameliorate an individual's hyperinsulinemic state,[52] no studies have yet assessed if this mechanism is involved in the blood pressure-lowering effect of endurance exercise training.

The kidney, because of its ability to regulate body sodium, and thus plasma volume and cardiac output, is believed to play a dominant role in maintaining the increased blood pressure in essential hypertension.[48] Thus, exercise training may lower blood pressure by altering renal function.[63] Although acute exercise influences various hormones that may influence renal sodium metabolism (e.g., renin, angiotensin, aldosterone, atrial natriuretic factor, prostaglandins, and insulin[122]), there are no consistent data implicating these compounds in the blood pressure-lowering effect of endurance exercise training.

CONCLUSIONS

The American College of Sports Medicine makes the following recommendations regarding exercise testing and exercise training of persons with hypertension:

1. Mass exercise testing is not advocated to determine those individuals at high risk for developing hypertension at rest in the future as a result of an exaggerated exercise blood pressure response. However, if exercise test results are available and an individual has an exercise blood pressure response above the 85th percentile, this information does provide some indication of risk stratification for that patient and the necessity for appropriate lifestyle behavior counseling to ameliorate this increased risk.
2. Endurance exercise training by individuals who are at high risk for developing hypertension will reduce the rise in blood pressure that occurs with time, thus justifying its use as a nonpharmacological strategy to reduce the incidence of hypertension in susceptible individuals.

3. Endurance exercise training will elicit an average reduction of 10 mmHg for both systolic and diastolic blood pressures in individuals with mild essential hypertension (blood pressures in the range of 140 to 180/90 to 105 mmHg). Endurance exercise training appears to elicit even greater reductions in blood pressure in patients with secondary hypertension due to renal dysfunction. The mode (large muscle activities), frequency (3 to 5 $d \cdot week^{-1}$), duration (20 to 60 min), and intensity of exercise (50 to 85% of maximal oxygen uptake) recommended are generally the same as those outlined in the previous Position Stand of the American College of Sports Medicine entitled "The Recommended Quality and Quantity of Exercise for Developing and Maintaining Cardiorespiratory and Muscular Fitness in Healthy Adults".[4] Exercise training at somewhat lower intensities (40 to 70% $\dot{V}O_2max$) appears to lower blood pressure as much, or more, than exercise at higher intensities, which may be especially important in specific hypertensive populations, such as the elderly. Physically active and aerobically fit patients with hypertension have markedly lower rates of mortality than sedentary, unfit hypertensive individuals, probably because exercise training also improves a number of other cardiovascular disease risk factors. In concurrence with the Joint National Committee's Recommendations for the Treatment of Essential Hypertension[57] and based on the high number of exercise-related health benefits and low risk for morbidity/mortality, it seems reasonable to recommend exercise as part of the initial treatment strategy for individuals with mild to moderate essential hypertension. A follow-up period should assess the efficacy of the patient's exercise program, and adjunct therapies should be implemented according to the individual patient's blood pressure and CAD risk factor goals.
4. Individuals with more marked elevations in blood pressure (>180/105) should add endurance exercise training to their treatment regimen only after initiating pharmacologic therapy, as it may reduce their blood pressure further, allow them to decrease their antihypertensive medications, and attenuate their risk for premature mortality.
5. Resistive, or strength, training is not recommended as the only form of exercise training for hypertensive individuals as, with the exception of circuit weight training, it has not consistently been shown to lower blood pressure. Thus, resistive exercise training is recommended when done as one component of a well-rounded fitness program, but not when done independently.

ACKNOWLEDGMENTS

This pronouncement was written for the American College of Sports Medicine by James M. Hagberg, Ph.D., FACSM (Chair); Steven N. Blair, P.E.D.,

FACSM; Ali A. Ehasani, M.D.; Neil F. Gordon, M.D., Ph.D., FACSM; Norman Kaplan, M.D.; Charles M. Tipton, Ph.D., FACSM; and Edward J. Zambraski, Ph.D., FACSM.

This pronouncement was reviewed for the American College of Sports Medicine by College Members-at-Large; the Pronouncements Committee; and by John J. Duncan, Ph.D.; William L. Haskell, Ph.D., FACSM; Ralph S. Paffenbarger, Jr., M.D., FACSM; and Douglas R. Seals, Ph.D., FACSM.

REFERENCES

1. **Abboud, F.M.** Sympathetic nervous system in hypertension. *Hypertension.* 4(Suppl.11):11208–11225, 1982.
2. **Ades, P.A., P.G.S. Gunther, W.L. Meyer, T.C. Gibson, J. Maddalena, and T. Orfeo.** Cardiac and skeletal muscle adaptations to training in systemic hypertension and effect of beta-blockade (metoprolol or propranolol). *Am. J. Cardiol.* 66:591–596, 1990.
3. American College Of Sports Medicine. *Guidelines for Exercise Testing and Prescription.* Lea and Febiger: Philadelphia, 1991, pp. 150–154.
4. American College Of Sports Medicine Position Stand. The recommended quantity and quality of exercise for developing and maintaining cardiorespiratory and muscular fitness in healthy adults. *Med. Sci. Sports Exercise.* 22:265–274, 1990.
5. **Attina, D.A., G. Giuliano, G. Arcangeli, R. Musante, and V. Cupelli.** Effects of one year of physical training on borderline hypertension: an evaluation by bicycle ergometer exercise testing. *J. Cardiovasc. Pharmacol.* 8(Suppl.5):S145–S147,1986.
6. **Baechle, T.R.** Effects of heavy resistance weight training on arterial biood pressure and other selected measures in normotensive and borderline hypertensive college men. In: *Sports Medicine*, Vol. 5, F. Landry and W.A.R. Orban (Eds.). Miami, FL: Symposia Specialists: 1978, pp. 169–176.
7. **Baglivo, H., G. Fabregues, H. Burrieza, R.C. Esper, M. Talarico, and R.J. Esper.** Effect of moderate physical training on left ventricular mass in mild hypertensive persons. *Hypertension.* 15(Suppl. l):I153–I156, 1990.
8. **Barry, A.C., J.W. Daly, E.D.R. Pruett, et al.** The effects of physical conditioning on older individuals. I. Work capacity, circulatory-respiratory function, and work electrocardiogram. *J. Gerontol.* 21:182–191, 1966.
9. **Baum, C., D.L. Kennedy, M.B. Forbes, and J.K. Jones.** Drug use and expenditures in 1982. *JAMA.* 253:382–386, 1985.
10. **Benbassat, J. and P.F. Froom.** Blood pressure response to exercise as a predictor of hypertension. *Arch. Int. Med.* 146:2053–2055, 1986.
11. **Blair, S.N., H.W. Kohl III, R.S. Paffenbarger Jr., D.G. Clark, K.H. Cooper, and L.W. Gibbons.** Physical fitness and all-cause mortality: a prospective study of healthy men and women. *JAMA.* 262:2395–2401, 1989.
12. **Blair, S.N., H.W. Kohl III, C.E. Barlow, and L.W. Gibbons.** Physical fitness and all-cause mortality in hypertensive men. *Ann. Med.* 23:307–312, 1991.
13. **Blair, S.N., N.N. Goodyear, L.W. Gibbons, and K.H. Cooper.** Physical fitness and incidence of hypertension in healthy normotensive men and women. *JAMA.* 252:487–490, 1984,.
14. **Blumenthal, J.A., W.C. Siegel, and M. Appelbaum.** Failure of exercise to reduce blood pressure in patients with mild hypertension. *JAMA.* 266:2098–2104, 1991.
15. **Bonnano, J.A. and J.E. Lies.** Effects of physical training on coronary risk factors. *Am. J. Cardiol.* 33:760–763, 1974.

16. **Boyer, J.L. and F.W. Kasch.** Exercise therapy in hypertensive men. *JAMA.* 211:1668–1671, 1970.
17. **Bray, G.A.** Exercise and obesity. In: *Exercise, Fitness, and Health.* C. Bouchard, R.J. Shephard, T. Stephens, J.R. Sutton, and B.D. McPherson. (Eds.). Champaign, IL: Human Kinetics Press, 1988, pp. 497–510.
18. **Buccola, V.A. and W.J. Stone.** Effects of jogging and cycling programs on physiological and personality variables in aged men. *Res. Q.* 46:134–139, 1975.
19. **Cade, R., D. Mars, H. Wagemaker, et al.** Effect of aerobic exercise training on patients with systemic arterial hypertension. *Am. J. Med.* 77:785–790, 1984.
20. **Chaney, R.H. and R.K. Eyman.** Blood pressure at rest and maximal dynamic and isometric exercise as predictors of systemichypertension. *Am. J. Cardiol.* 62:1058–1061, 1988.
21. **Chick, T.W., A.K. Halperin, and E.M. Gacek.** Effect of antihypertensive medications on exercise performance: a review. *Med. Sci. Sports Exercise.* 20:447–454, 1988.
22. **Choouette, G. and R.J. Ferguson.** Blood pressure reduction in borderline hypertensives following physical training. *Can. Med. Assoc. J.* 108:699–703, 1973.
23. **Cleroux, J., F. Peronnet, and J. de Champlain.** Effects of exercise training on plasma catecholamines and blood pressure in labile hypertensive subjects. *Eur. J. Appl. Physiol.* 56:550–554, 1987.
24. **Cononie, C.C., J.E. Graves, M.L. Pollock, M.I. Phillips, C. Sumners, and J.M. Hagberg.** Effect of exercise training on blood pressure in 70–79 year old men and women. *Med. Sci. Sports Exerc.* 23:505–511, 1991.
25. **Cypress, B.K.** NCHS Advance Data, No. 80, July 22, 1982, Vital and Health Statistics of the National Center for Health Statistics. U.S. Department of Health and Human Services.
26. **Dannenberg, A.L., R.J. Garrison, and W.B. Kannel.** Incidence of hypertension in the Framingham Study. *Am. J. Public Health.* 78:676–679, 1988.
27. **DePlaen, J.F. and J.M. Detry.** Hemodynamic effects of physical training in established arterial hypertension. *Acta Cardiol.* 35:179–188, 1980.
28. **DiPette, D.J. and E.D. Frohlich.** Cardiac involvement in hypertension. *Am. J. Cardiol.* 61:67H–72H, 1988.
29. **Duncan, J.J., J.E. Farr, J. Upton, R.D. Hagan, M.E. Oglesby, and S.N. Blair.** The effects of aerobic exercise on plasma catecholamines and blood pressure in patients with mild essential hypertension. *J. Am. Med. Assoc.* 254:2609–2613, 1985.
30. **Duncan, J.J., H. Vandrager, J.E Farr, H.W. Kohl, and N.F. Gordon.** Effect of intrinsic sympathomimetic activity on serum lipids during exercise training in hypertensive patients receiving chronic beta-blocker therapy. *J. Cardiopulmon. Rehabil.* 9:110–114, 1989.
31. **Effron, M.D.** Effects of resistive training on left ventricular function. *Med. Sci. Sports Exerc.* 21:694–697, 1989.
32. **Emes, C.G.** The effects of a regular program of light exercise on seniors. *Int. J. Sports Med. Phys. Fitness.* 19:185–190, 1979.
33. **Esler, M., G. Jennings, P. Korner, I. Willett, F. Dudley, G. Hasking, W. anderson, and G. Lambert.** Assessment of human sympathetic nervous system activity from measurements of norepinephrine turnover. *Hypertension* 11:3–20, 1988.
34. **Fleck, S.J.** Cardiovascular adaptations to resistance training. *Med. Sci. Sports Exerc.* 20:S146–S151, 1988.
35. **Frohlich, E.D., D.T. Lowenthal, H.S. Miller, T. Pickering, and W.B. Strong.** Task force IV: systemic arterial hypertension. *J. Am. Coll. Cardiol.* 6:1218–1221, 1985.
36. **Gilders, R.M., C. Voiner, and G.A. Dudley.** Endurance training and blood pressure in normotensive and hypertensive adults. *Med. Sci. Sports Exercise.* 21:629–636, 1989.
37. **Glasgow, M.S., K.R. Gaardner, and B.T. Engel.** Behavioral treatment of high blood pressure. II. Acute and sustained effects of relaxation and systolic blood pressure feedback. *Psychosom. Med.* 44:155–170, 1982.
38. **Gleichmann, U.M., H.-H. Philippi, S.I. Gleichmann, et al.** Group exercise improves patient compliance in mild to moderate hypertension. *J. Hypertens.* 7(Suppl. 3):S77–S80, 1989.

39. **Gordon, N.F., C.B. Scott, W.J. Wilkinson, J.J. Duncan, and S.N. Blair.** Exercise and mild essential hypertension: recommendations for adults. *Sports Med.* 10:390–404, 1990.
40. **Gordon, N.F. and J.J. Duncan.** Effect of beta-blockers on exercise physiology: implications for exercise training. *Med. Sci. Sports Exerc.* 23:668–676, 1991.
41. **Hagberg, J.M.** Exercise, fitness, and hypertension. In: *Exercise, Fitness, and Health*, C. Bouchard, R.J. Shephard, T. Stephens, J.R. Sutton, and B.D. McPherson (Eds.). Champaign, IL: Human Kinetics Press, 1988, pp. 455–466.
42. **Hagberg, J.M., A.A. Ehsani, D. Goldring, A. Hernandez, D. R. Sinacore, and J.O. Holloszy.** Effect of weight training on blood pressure and hemodynamics in hypertensive adolescents. *J. Pediatr.* 104:147–151, 1984.
43. **Hagberg, J.M., A.P. Goldberg, A.A. Ehsani, G.W. Heath, J. A. Delmez, and H.R.** Harter. Exercise training improves hypertension in hemodialysis patients. *Am. J. Nephrol.* 3:209–212, 1983.
44. **Hagberg, J.M., D. Goldring, A.A. Ehsani, et al.** Effect of exercise training on the blood pressure and hemodynamic features of hypertensive adolescents. *Am. J. Cardiol.* 52:763–768, 1983.
45. **Hagberg, J.M., D. Goldring, G.W. Heath, A.A. Ehsani, A. Hernandez, and J.O. Holloszy.** Effect of exercise training on plasma catecholamines and hemodynamics of adolescent hypertensives during rest, submaximal exercise, and orthostatic stress. *Clin. Physiol.* 4: 117–124, 1984.
46. **Hagberg, J.M., S.J. Montain, and W.H. Martin.** Blood pressure and hemodynamic responses after exercise in older hypertensives. *J. Appl. Physiol.* 63:270–276, 1987.
47. **Hagberg, J.M., S.J. Montain, W.H. Martin, and A.A. Ehsani.** Effect of exercise training on 60-69 year old persons with essential hypertension. *Am. J. Cardiol.* 64:348–353, 1989.
48. **Hall, J.E., L. Mizelle, D.A. Hildebrandt, and M.W. Brands.** Abnormal pressure natriuresis: a cause or consequence of hypertension? *Hypertension.* 15:547–559,1990.
49. **Hanson, J.S. and W.H. Nedde.** Preliminary observations on physical training for hypertensive males. *Circ. Res.* 27(Suppl. 1):49–53, 1970.
50. **Harris, K.A. and R.G. Holly.** Physiological response to circuit weight training in borderline hypertensive subjects. *Med. Sci. Sports Exercise.* 19:246–252, 1987.
51. **Hines, E.A.** Significance of vascular hyperreaction as measured by the cold pressor test. *Am. Heart J.* 20:408–416, 1940.
52. **Holloszy, J.O., J. Schultz, J. Kusnierkiewicz, J.M. Hagberg, and A.A. Ehsani.** Effects of exercise on glucose tolerance and insulin resistance. *Acta Med. Scand. Suppl.* 711:55–65, 1987.
53. **Hossack, K.F., R.A. Bruce, and T.A. Derouen.** Evaluation of hypertensive males for primary coronary heart disease events using conventional risk factors and maximal exercise testing. *Clin. Cardiol.* 3:229–235, 1980.
54. **Jackson, A.S., W.G. Squires, G. Grimes, and E.F. Beard.** Prediction of future resting hypertension from exercise blood pressure. *J. Cardiac Rehabil.* 3:263–268, 1983.
55. **Jo, Y., M. Arita, A. Baba, et al.** Blood pressure and sympathetic activity following responses to aerobic exercise in patients with essential hypertension. *Clin. Exp. Hypertens. Theor. Pract.* A11(Suppl. 1):411–417, 1989.
56. **Johnson, W.P. and J.A. Grover.** Hemodynamic and metabolic effects of physical training in four patients with essential hypertension. *Can. Med. Assoc. J.* 96:842–846, 1967.
57. Joint National Committee On Detection, Evaluation, And Treatment Of High Blood Pressure. 1988 REPORT. *Arch. Int. Med* 148:1023–1038, 1988.
58. **Kannel, W.B., J.T. Doyle, A.M. Ostfeld, et al.** Original resources for primary prevention of atherosclerotic diseases. *Circulation.* 70:157A–205A, 1984.
59. **Kaplan, N.** *Clinical Hypertension*, 5th Ed. Baltimore: Williams and Wilkins, 1990, pp. 3–5, 17, 138, 149–153, 165–171.
60. **Kaplan, N.M.** The deadly quartet: upper-body obesity, glucose intolerance, hypertriglyceridemia, and hypertension. *Arch. Intern. Med.* 149:1514–1520, 1989.

61. **Kaufman, F.L., R.L. Hughson, and J.P. Schaman.** Effect of exercise on recovery blood pressure in normotensive and hypertensive subjects. *Med. Sci. Sports Exerc.* 19:17–20, 1987.
62. **Kelemen, M.H., M.B. Effron, S A. Valenti, and K.J. Stewart.** Exercise training combined with antihypertensive drug therapy. *JAMA.* 263:2766–2771, 1990.
63. **Kenney, W.L. and E.J. Zambraski.** Physical activity in human hypertension—a mechanisms approach. *Sports Med.* 1:459–473, 1984.
64. **Kinoshita, A., H. Urata, Y. Tanabe, M. Ikeda, H. Tanaka, M. Shindo, and K. Arakawa.** What types of hypertensives respond better to mild exercise therapy? *J. Hypertens.* 6(Suppl. 4):S631–S633, 1988.
65. **Kiveloff, B. and O. Huber.** Brief maximal isometric exercise in hypertension. *J. Am. Geriatr. Soc.* 19:1006–1009, 1971.
66. **Kiyonaga, A., K. Arakawa, H. Tanaka, and M. Shindo.** Blood pressure and hormonal responses to aerobic exercise. *Hypertension.* 7:125–131, 1985.
67. **Kukkonen, K., R. Rauramaa, E. Voutilainen, and E. Lansimies.** Physical training of middle-aged men with borderline hypertension. *Ann. Clin. Res.* 14(Suppl. 34):139–145, 1982.
68. **Kuller, L.H., S.B. Hulley, J.D. Cohen, and J. Neaton.** Unexpected effects of treating hypertension in men with ECG abnormalities: a critical analysis. *Circulation.* 73:114–123, 1986.
69. **Lauer, R.M., T. L. Burns, L.T. Mahoney, and C.M. Tipton.** Blood pressure in children. In: *Perspectives in Exercise Science and Sports Medicine.* C.V. Gisolfi and D.R. Lamb (Eds.). Indianapolis: Benchmark Press, 2:431–463, 1989.
70. **Levy, R.L., C.C. Hillman, W.D. Stroud, and P.D. White.** Transient hypertension: its significance in terms of later development of sustained hypertension and cardiovascular-renal diseases. *JAMA.* 126:829–833, 1944.
71. **Luborsky, L., P. Crits-Christoph, J.P. Brady, et al.** Behavioral versus pharmacological treatments for essential hypertension—a needed comparison. *Psychosom. Med.* 44:203–213, 1982.
72. **MacDougall, J.D., D. Tuxen, D.G. Sale, J.R. Moroz, and J.R. Sutton.** Arterial blood pressure response to heavy resistance exercise. *J. Appl. Physiol.* 58:785–790, 1985.
73. **Mahoney, L.T., R.M. Scheiken, W.R. Clarke, and R.M. Lauer.** Left ventricular mass and exercise responses predict future blood pressure: the Muscatine study. *Hypertension.* 12:206–213, 1988.
74. **Martin, J.E., P.M. Dubbert, and W.C. Cushman.** Controlled trial of aerobic exercise in hypertension. *Circulation.* 81:1560–1567, 1990.
75. **Michel, M.C., O.E. Brodde, and P.A. Insel.** Peripheral adrenergic receptors in hypertension. *Hypertension.* 16:107–120, 1990.
76. **Molineux, D. and A. Steptoe.** Exaggerated blood pressure responses to submaximal exercise in normotensive adolescents with a family history of hypertension. *J. Hypertens.* 6:261–265, 1988.
77. **Montoye, H.J., H.L. Metzner, and J.B. Keller.** Habitual physical activity and blood pressure. *Med. Sci. Sports.* 4:175–181, 1972.
78. **Nelson, L., M.D. Esler, G.L. Jennings, and P.I. Korner.** Effect of changing levels of physical activity on blood pressure and haemodynamics in essential hypertension. *Lancet.* 2:473–476, 1986.
79. **Nomura, G., E. Kumagai, K. Midorikawa, T. Kitano, H. Tashiro, and H. Toshima.** Physical training in essential hypertension: alone and in combination with dietary salt restriction. *J. Cardiac Rehabil.* 4:469–475, 1984.
80. **Overton, M.J., M.J. Joyner, and C.M. Tipton.** Reductions in blood pressure after acute exercise by hypertensive rats. *J. Appl. Physiol.* 64:742–747, 1988.
81. **Paffenbarger, R.S., Jr.** Energy imbalance and hypertension risk. In: *Diet and Exercise: Synergism in Health Maintenance*, P.L. White and T. Mondeika (Eds.). Chicago: American Medical Association, 1982, pp. 115–125.

82. **Paffenbarger R.S., Jr., R.T. Hyde, A.L. Wing, and C.C. Hsieh.** Physical activity, all-cause mortality, and longevity of college men. *N. Engl. J. Med.* 314:605–613, 1986.
83. **Paffenbarger, R.S., Jr., D.L. Jung, R.W. Leung, and R.T. Hyde.** Physical activity and hypertension: an epidemiological view. *Ann. Med.* 23:319–327, 1991.
84. **Paffenbarger, R.S., Jr., A.L. Wing, R.T. Hyde, and D.L. Jung.** Physical activity and incidence of hypertension in college alumni. *Am. J. Epidemiol.* 117:245–257, 1983.
85. **Painter, P.L., J.N. Nelson-Worrel, M.M. Hill, D.R. Thronbery, W.R. Schelp, A.R. Harrington, and A.B. Weinstein.** Effects of exercise training during hemodialysis. *Nephron.* 43:87–92, 1986.
86. **Pescatello, L.S., A.E. Fargo, C.N. Leach, and H.H. Scherzer.** Short-term effect of dynamic exercise on arterial blood pressure. *Circulation.* 83:1557–1561, 1991.
87. **Peters, R.K., L.D. Cady Jr., D.P. Bischoff, L. Bernstein and M.C. Pike.** Physical fitness and suhsequent myocardial infarction in healthy workers. *JAMA.* 249:3052–3056, 1983.
88. **Pickering, T.G.** Pathophysiology of exercise hypertension. *Herz.* 12:119–124, 1987.
89. **Pickering, T.G. and R.B. Devereux.** Ambulatory monitoring of blood pressure as a predictor of cardiovascular risk. *Am. Heart J.* 114:925–928, 1987.
90. **Reaven, P.D., E. Barrett-Connor, and S. Edelstein.** Relation hetween leisure-time physical activity and blood pressure in older women. *Circulation.* 83:559–565, 1991.
91. **Reaven, G.M.** Role of insulin resistance in human disease. *Diabetes.* 37:1595–1607, 1988.
92. **Ressl, J., J. Chrastek, and R. Jandova.** Haemodynamic effects of physical training in essential hypertension. *Cardiologica.* 32:121–133, 1977.
93. **Roman, O., A. L. Camuzzi, E. Villalon, and C. Klenner.** Physical training program in arterial hypertension: a long-term prospective follow-up. *Cardiology.* 67:230–243, 1981.
94. **Rowland, M. and J. Roberts.** NCHS Advance Data, No. 84, October 8, 1982, Vital and Health Statistics of the National Center for Health Statistics. U.S. Department of Health and Human Services.
95. **Rudd, J.L and W.C. Day.** A physical fitness program for patients with hypertension. *J. Am. Geriatr. Soc.* 15:373–379, 1967.
96. **Sannerstedt, R., H. Wasir, R. Henning, and L. Werko.** Systemic haemodynamics in mild arterial hypertension before and afler physical training. *Clin. Sci. Mol. Med.* 45:145S-149S, 1973.
97. **Sasaki, J., H. Urata, Y. Tanabe, et al.** Mild exercise therapy increases serum high density lipoprotein2 cholesterol levels in patients with essential hypertension. *Am. J. Med. Sci.* 297:220–223, 1989.
98. **Seals, D.R. and M.J. Reiling.** Effect of regular exercise on 24-hr arterial pressure in older hypertensive humans. *Hypertension.* 18:583–592, 1991.
99. **Shapiro, A.P., G.E. Schwartz, D.C.E. Ferguson, D.P. Redmond, and S.M. Weiss.** Behavioral methods in the treatment of hypertension: a review of their clinical status. *Ann. Int. Med.* 86:626–636, 1977.
100. **Somers, V. K., J. Conway, J. Johnston, and P. Sleight.** Effects of endurance exercise training on baroreflex sensitivity and blood pressure in borderline hypertension. *Lancet.* 337: 1363–1368, 1991.
101. **Stamler, R., J. Stamler, F.C. Gosch, J. Civinelli, J. Fishman, A. McDonald, and A.R. Dyer.** Primary prevention of hypertension by nutritional-hygienic means: final report of a randomized clinical trial. *JAMA.* 262:1801–1807, 1989.
102. **Tanabe, Y., J. Sasaki, H. Urata, et al.** Effect of mild aerobic exercise on lipid and apolipoprotein levels in patients with essential hypertension. *Jpn. Heart J.* 29:199–206, 1988.
103. **Tanji, J.L., J.J. Champlin, G.Y. Wong, E.Y. Lew, T.C. Brown, and E. A.** Amsterdam. Blood pressure recovery curves after submaximal exercise: a predictor of hypertension at 10 yr follow-up. *Am. J. Hypertens.* 2:135–138, 1989.
104. **Teuscher, A., M. Egger, and J.B. Herman.** Diabetes and hypertension: blood pressure in clinical diabetic patients and a control population. *Arch. Intern. Med.* 149:1945–1949, 1989.
105. **Thoren, P., J.S. Floras, P. Hoffman, and D.R. Seals.** Endorphins and exercise: physiological mechanisms and clinical implications. *Med. Sci. Sports Exerc.* 22:417–428, 1990.

106. **Tipton, C.M.** Exercise, training, and hypertension. In: *Exercise and Sport Science Reviews*, R Terjung (Ed.). Lexington, MA: DC Health, pp. 245–306, 1984.
107. **Tipton, C.M.** Exercise, training, and hypertension: an update. In: *Exercise and Sport Science Reviews*, Vol. 19, J.O. Holloszy (Ed.). Baltimore: Williams and Wilkins, 1991, pp. 447–505.
108. **Tipton, C.M., R.D. Matthes, K.D. Marcus, K.A. Rowlett, and J.R. Leininger.** Influences of exercise intensity, age, and medication on resting blood pressure in SHR populations. *J. Appl. Physiol.* 55:1305–1310, 1983.
109. **Tipton, C.M., L.A. Sebastian, J.M. Overton, C.R. Woodman, and S.B. Williams.** Chronic exercise and its hemodynamic influences on resting blood pressure of hypertensive rats. *J. Appl. Physiol.* 71:2206–2210, 1991.
110. **Tipton, C.M., S. Mcmahon, J.R. Leininger, E.L. Pauli and C. Lauber.** Exercise training and incidence of cerebrovascular lesions in stroke-prone spontaneously hypertensive rats. *J. Appl. Physiol.* 68:1080–1085,1990.
111. **Tipton, C.M., S. Mcmahon, E.M. Youmans, et al.** Response of hypertensive rats to acute and chronic conditions of static exercise. *Am. J. Physiol.* 254:H592–H598, 1988.
112. **Tipton, C.M., M.S. Sturek, R.A. Oppliger, R.D. Matthes, J. M. Overton, and J.G. Edwards.** Responses of SHR to combinations of chemical sympathectomy, adrenal demedullation, and training. *Am. J. Physiol.* 247:H109–H118, 1984.
113. **Tomanek, R.J., C.V. Gisolfi, C.A. Bauer, and P.J. Palmer.** Coronary vasodilator reserve, capillarity, and mitochondria in trained hypertensive rats. *J. Appl. Physiol.* 64:1170–1185, 1988.
114. **Urata, H., Y. Tanabe, A. Kiyonaga, et al.** Antihypertensive and volume-depleting effects of mild exercise on essential hypertension. *Hypertension.* 9:245–252, 1987.
115. Veterans Administration Cooperative Study Group On Antihypertensive A. Effects of treatment on morbidity in hypertension: results in patients with diastolic blood pressures averaging 115 through 129 mm Hg. *JAMA.* 202:116–122, 1967.
116. **Weber, F., R.J. Barnard, and D. Roy.** Effects of a high complex-carbohydrate, low-fat diet and daily exercise on individuals 70 years and older. *J. Gerontol.* 38:155–161, 1986.
117. **Westheim, A., K. Simonsen, O. Schamaun, E.K. Qvigstad, P. Staff, and P. Teisberg.** Effect of exercise training in patients with essential hypertension. Proceedings of the 10th Scandinavian Congress of Cardiology. *Acta Med. Scand. Suppl.* 712:99–103, 1986.
118. **Westheim, A., K. Simonsen, O. Schamaun, O. Muller, O. Stokke, and P. Teisberg.** Effect of exercise training in patients with essential hypertension. *J. Hypertens.* 3(Suppl. 3):S479–S481, 1985.
119. **Wilson, M.F., B.H. Sung, G.A. Pincomb, and W.R. Lovallo.** Exaggerated pressure response to exercise in men at risk for systemic hypertension. *Am. J. Cardiol.* 66:731–736, 1990.
120. **Wong, H.E., I.S. Kasser, and R.A. Bruce.** Impaired maximal exercise performance with hypertensive cardiovascular disease. *Circulation.* 39:633–638, 1969.
121. **Wood, P.D. and M.L. Stefanick.** Exercise, fitness, and atherosclerosis. In: *Exercise, Fitness, and Health*, C. Bouchard, R.J. Shephard, T. Stephens, J.R. Sutton, and B.D. McPherson (Eds.). Champaign, IL: Human Kinetics Press, 1988, pp. 409–423.
122. **Zambraski, E.J.** Renal regulation of fluid homeostasis during exercise. In: *Perspectives in Exercise Science and Sports Medicine (Vol. 3), Fluid Homeostasis during Exercise*, C.V. Gisolfi and D.R. Lamb (Eds.). Carmel, IN: Benchmark Press, 1990, pp. 247–280.

Appendix E

AMERICAN COLLEGE OF SPORTS MEDICINE POSITION STAND ON THE USE OF ANABOLIC-ANDROGENIC STEROIDS IN SPORTS*

INTRODUCTION

Based on a comprehensive literature survey and a careful analysis of the claims concerning the ergogenic effects and the adverse effects of anabolic-androgenic steroids, it is the position of the American College of Sports Medicine that:

1. Anabolic-androgenic steroids in the presence of an adequate diet can contribute to increases in body weight, often in the lean mass compartment.
2. The gains in muscle strength achieved through high-intensity exercise and proper diet can be increased by the use of anabolic-androgenic steroids in some individuals.
3. Anabolic-androgenic steroids do not increase aerobic power or capacity for muscular exercise.
4. Anabolic-androgenic steroids have been associated with adverse effects on the liver, cardiovascular system, reproductive system, and psychological status in therapeutic trials and in limited research on athletes. Until further research is completed, the potential hazards of the use of the anabolic-androgenic steroids in athletes must include those found in therapeutic trials.
5. The use of anabolic-androgenic steroids by athletes is contrary to the rules and ethical principles of athletic competition as set forth by many of the sports governing bodies. The American College of Sports Medicine supports these ethical principles and deplores the use of anabolic-androgenic steroids by athletes.

* Reprint of *"The Use of Anabolic-Androgenic Steroids in Sports,* ©1984 American College of Sports Medicine, *MSEE,* 19:5, 1987, pp. 534–539. With permission of Williams & Wilkins.

This document is a revision of the 1977 position stand of the American College of Sports Medicine concerning anabolic-androgenic steroids.[4]

BACKGROUND

In 1935 the long-suspected positive effect of androgens on protein anabolism was documented.[56] Subsequently, this effect was confirmed,[53,77] and the development of 19-nortestosterone heralded the synthesis of steroids that have greater anabolic properties than natural testosterone but less of its virilizing effect.[39] The use of androgenic steroids by athletes began in the early 1950s[106] and has increased through the years,[60,62,83,98,104,106] despite warnings about potential adverse reactions[4,83,106,112] and the banning of these substances by sports governing bodies.

ANABOLIC-ANDROGENIC STEROIDS, BODY COMPOSITION AND ATHLETIC PERFORMANCE

BODY COMPOSITION

Animal studies investigating the effect of anabolic-androgenic steroids on body composition have shown increases in lean body mass, nitrogen retention, and muscle growth in castrated males[37,57,58] and normal females.[26,37,71] The effects of anabolic-androgenic steroids on the body weights of normal, untrained male animals,[37,40,71,105,114] treadmill-trained[43,97] or isometrically trained rats,[82] or strength-trained monkeys[80] have been minimal to absent; however, the effects of steroids on animals undergoing heavy resistance training have not been adequately studied. Human males who are deficient in natural androgens by castration or other causes have shown significant increases in nitrogen retention and muscular development with anabolic-androgenic steroid therapy.[23,58,103] Human males and females involved in experimental[38] and therapeutic trials of anabolic steroids[15,16,93] have shown increases in body weight.

The majority of the strength-training studies in which body weight was reported showed greater increases in weight under steroid treatment than under placebo.[17,41,42,50,61,74,94,96,107] Other training studies have reported no significant changes in body weight.[21,27,31,34,100,108] The weight gained was determined to be lean body mass in three studies that made this determination with hydrostatic weighing techniques.[41,42,107] Four other studies found no significant differences in lean body mass between steroid and placebo treatments,[17,21,27,34] but in two of those the mean differences favored the steroid treatment.[21,27] The extent to which increased water retention accounts for steroid-induced changes in body composition is controversial[17,42] and has yet to be resolved.

In summary, anabolic-androgenic steroids can contribute to an increase in body weight in the lean mass compartment of the body. The amount of weight gained in the training studies has been small but statistically significant.

MUSCULAR STRENGTH

Strength is an important factor in many athletic events. The literature concerning the efficacy of anabolic steroids for promoting strength development is controversial. Many factors contribute to the development of strength, including heredity, intensity of training, diet, and the status of the psyche.[112] It is very difficult to control all of these factors in an experimental design. The additional variable of dosage is included when drug research is undertaken. Some athletes claim that doses greater than therapeutic are necessary for strength gains[106] even though positive results have been reported using therapeutic (low-dose) regimens.[50,74,94,107] Double-blind studies using anabolic-androgenic steroids are also difficult to conduct because of the physical and/or psychological effects of the drug that, for example, allowed 100% of the participants in one "double-blind" study to correctly identify the steroid phase of the experiment.[32] The placebo effect has been shown to be a factor in studies of anabolic-androgenic steroids as in all drug studies.[6]

In animal studies, the combination of anabolic-androgenic steroids and overload training has not produced larger gains in force-production than training alone.[80,97] However, steroid-induced gains in strength have been reported in experienced[42,74,94,107] and inexperienced weight trainers[50,51,96] with[50,51,74,94] and without dietary control or supplemental protein.[42,96] In contrast, no positive effect of steroids on gains in strength over those produced by training alone were reported in other studies involving experienced[21,34,54] and inexperienced weight trainers[17,27,31,41,54,61,100,108] with[21,34,61,100] and without dietary control or supplemental protein.[17,27,31,41,54,108] The studies that reported no changes in strength with anabolic-androgenic steroids have been criticized[112] for the use of inexperienced weight trainers, lack of dietary control, low-intensity training,[17,27,31,61] and nonspecific testing of strength.[21] The studies that have shown strength gains with the use of anabolic-androgenic steroids have been criticized[83] for inadequate numbers of subjects,[74,94,107] improper statistical designs, inadequate execution, and the unsatisfactory reporting of experimental results.

There have been no studies of the effects of the massive doses of steroids used by some athletes over periods of several years. Similarly, there have been no studies of the use of anabolic-androgenic steroids and training in women or children. Theoretically, anabolic and androgenic effects would be greater in women and children because they have lower levels of androgens than men.

Three proposed mechanisms for the actions of the anabolic-androgenic steroids for increases in muscle strength are

1. Increase in protein synthesis in the muscle as a direct action of the anabolic-androgenic steroid.[81,82,92]
2. Blocking of the catabolic effect of glucocorticoids after exercise by increasing the amount of anabolic-androgenic hormone available.[1,92,112]
3. Steroid-induced enhancement of aggressive behavior that promotes a greater quantity and quality of weight training.[14]

In spite of the controversial and sometimes contradictory results of the studies in this area, it can be concluded that the use of anabolic-androgenic steroids, especially by experienced weight trainers, can often increase strength gains beyond those seen with training and diet alone. This positive effect on strength is usually small and obviously is not exhibited by all individuals. The explanation for this variability in steroid effects is unclear. When small increments in strength occur, they can be important in athletic competition.

AEROBIC CAPACITY

The effect of anabolic-androgenic steroids on aerobic capacity has also been questioned. The potential of these drugs to increase total blood volume and hemoglobin[88] might suggest a positive effect of steroids on aerobic capacity. However, only three studies indicated positive effects,[3,51,54] and there has been no substantiation of these results in subsequent studies.[27,41,50,52] Thus, the majority of evidence shows no positive effect of anabolic-androgenic steroids on aerobic capacity over aerobic training alone.

ADVERSE EFFECTS

Anabolic-androgenic steroids have been associated with many undesirable or adverse effects in laboratory studies and therapeutic trials. The effects of major concern are those on the liver, cardiovascular, and reproductive systems, and on the psychological status of individuals who are using anabolic-androgenic steroids.

ADVERSE EFFECTS ON THE LIVER

Impaired excretory function of the liver, resulting in jaundice, has been associated with anabolic-androgenic steroids in a number of therapeutic trials.[76,84,90] The possible cause-and-effect nature of this association is strengthened by the observation of jaundice remission after discontinuance of the drug.[76,84] In studies of athletes using anabolic-androgenic steroids (65 athletes tested),[89,98,104] no evidence of cholestasis has been found.

Structural changes in the liver following anabolic steroid treatment have been found in animals[95,101] and in humans.[73,86] Conclusions concerning the clinical significance of these changes on a short- or long-term basis have not been drawn. Investigations in athletes for these changes have not been performed, but there is no reason to believe that the athlete using anabolic-androgenic steroids is immune from these effects of the drugs.

The most serious liver complications associated with anabolic-androgenic steroids are peliosis hepatitis (blood-filled cysts in the liver of unknown etiology) and liver tumors. Cases of peliosis hepatitis have been reported in individuals treated with anabolic-androgenic steroids for various conditions.[7-10,13,35,65,66,70,88,102] Rupture of the cysts or liver failure resulting from the condition was fatal in some individuals.[9,70,102] In other case reports the condition was an incidental finding at autopsy.[8,10,66] The possible cause-and-effect nature of the association between peliosis hepatitis and the use of anabolic-androgenic steroids is strengthened by the observation of improvement in the condition after discontinuation of drug therapy is some cases.[7,35] There are no reported cases of this condition in athletes using anabolic-androgenic steroids, but investigations specific for this disorder have not been performed in athletes.

Liver tumors have been associated with the use of anabolic-androgenic steroids in individuals receiving these drugs as a part of their treatment regimen.[28,29,49,67,69,99,115] These tumors are generally benign,[29,67,69,115] but there have been malignant lesions associated with individuals using these drugs.[28,99,115] The possible cause-and-effect nature of this association between the use of the drug and tumor development is strengthened by a report of tumor regression after cessation of drug treatment.[49] The 17-alpha-alkylated compounds are the specific family of anabolic steroids indicated in the development of liver tumors.[46,49] There is one reported case of a 26-year-old male body builder who died of liver cancer after having abused a variety of anabolic steroids for at least 4 years.[75] The testing necessary for discovery of these tumors is not commonly performed, and it is possible that other tumors associated with steroid use by athletes have gone undetected.

Blood tests of liver function have been reported to be unchanged with steroid use in some training studies[31,41,54,94] and abnormal in other training studies[32,51] and in tests performed on athletes known to be using anabolic-androgenic steroids.[54,89,104] However, the lesions of peliosis hepatitis and liver tumors do not always result in blood test abnormalities,[8,28,29,49,67,115] and some authors state that liver radioisotope scans, ultrasound, or compound tomography scans are needed for diagnosis.[28,29,113]

In summary, liver function tests have been shown to be adversely affected by anabolic-androgenic steroids, especially the 17-alpha-alkylated compounds. The short- and long-term consequences of these changes, though potentially hazardous, have yet to be reported in athletes using these drugs.

ADVERSE EFFECTS ON THE CARDIOVASCULAR SYSTEM

The steroid-induced changes that may affect the development of cardiovascular disease include hyperinsulinism and altered glucose tolerance,[111] decreased high-density lipoprotein cholesterol levels,[72,98] and elevated blood pressure.[68] These effects are variable for different individuals in various clinical situations. Triglycerides are lowered by anabolic-androgenic steroids in certain individuals[24,72] and are increased in others.[18,78] Histological examinations of myofibrils and mitochondria from cardiac tissue obtained from laboratory animals have shown that administration of anabolic steroids leads to pathological alterations in these structures.[5,11,12] The cardiovascular effects of the anabolic-androgenic steroids, though potentially hazardous, need further research before any conclusions can be made.

ADVERSE EFFECTS ON THE MALE REPRODUCTIVE SYSTEM

The effects of the anabolic-androgenic steroids on the male reproductive system are oligospermia (small number of sperm) and azoospermia (lack of sperm in the semen), decreased testicular size, abnormal appearance of testicular biopsy material, and reductions in testosterone and gonadotropic hormones. These effects have been shown in training studies,[19,41,100] studies of normal volunteers,[38] therapeutic trials,[44] and studies of athletes who were using anabolic-androgenic steroids.[55,79,104] In view of the changes shown in the pituitary-gonadal axis, the dysfunction accounting for these abnormalities is believed to be steroid-induced suppression of gonadotropin production.[19,36,38,79] The changes in these hormones are ordinarily reversible after cessation of drug treatment, but the long-term effects of altering the hypothalamic-pituitary-gonadal axis remain unknown. However, there is a report of residual abnormalities in testicular morphology of healthy men 6 months after discontinuing steroid use.[38] It has been reported that the metabolism of androgens to estrogenic compounds may lead to gynecomastia in males.[23,58,98,112]

ADVERSE EFFECTS ON THE FEMALE REPRODUCTIVE SYSTEM

The effects of androgenic steroids on the female reproductive system include reduction in circulating levels of luteinizing hormone, follicle-stimulating hormone, estrogens, and progesterone; inhibition of folliculogenesis and ovulation; and menstrual cycle changes including prolongation of the follicular phase, shortening of the luteal phase, and amenorrhea.[20,63,91]

ADVERSE EFFECTS ON PSYCHOLOGICAL STATUS

In both sexes, psychological effects of anabolic-androgenic steroids include increases or decreases in libido, mood swings, and aggressive behavior,[38,98] which is related to plasma testosterone levels.[25,85] Administration of steroids causes changes in the electroencephalogram similar to those seen with psycho-stimulant drugs.[47,48] The possible ramifications of uncontrollably aggressive and possible hostile behavior should be considered prior to the use of anabolic-androgenic steroids.

OTHER ADVERSE EFFECTS

Other side effects associated with the anabolic-androgenic steroids include: ataxia;[2] premature epiphysial closure in youths;[23,58,64,109,110] virilization in youths and women, including hirsutism,[45] clitoromegaly,[63,112] and irreversible deepening of the voice;[22,33] acne, temporal hair recession; and alopecia.[45] These adverse reactions can occur with the use of anabolic-androgenic steroids and are believed to be dependent on the type of steroid, dosage, and duration of drug use.[58] There is no method for predicting which individuals are more likely to develop these adverse effects, some of which are potentially hazardous.

THE ETHICAL ISSUE

Equitable competition and fair play are the foundation of athletic competition. If competition is to remain on this foundation, rules are necessary. The International Olympic Committee (IOC) has defined "doping" as "the administration of or the use by a competing athlete of any substance foreign to the body or of any physiological substance taken in abnormal quantity or taken by an abnormal route of entry into the body, with the sole intention of increasing in an artificial and unfair manner his performance in competition." Accordingly, the medically unjustified use of anabolic steroids with the intention of gaining an athletic advantage is clearly unethical. Anabolic-androgenic steroids are listed as banned substances by the IOC in accordance with the rules against doping. The American College of Sports Medicine supports the position that the eradication of anabolic-androgenic steroids use by athletes is in the best interest of sport and endorses the development of effective procedures for drug detection and of policies that exclude from competition those athletes who refuse to abide by the rules.

The "win at all cost" attitude that has pervaded society places the athlete in a precarious situation. Testimonial evidence suggests that some athletes would risk serious harm and even death if they could obtain a drug that would ensure their winning an Olympic gold medal. However, the use of anabolic-androgenic steroids by athletes is contrary to the ethical principles of athletic competition and is deplored.

REFERENCES

1. **Aakvaag, A., O. Bentdol, K. Quigstod, P. Walstod, H. Reningen, and F. Fonnum.** Testosterone and testosterone binding globulin (TeBg) in young men during prolonged stress. *Int. J. Androl.* 1:22–31, 1978.
2. **Agrawal, B.L.** Ataxia caused by fluoxymesterone therapy in breast cancer. *Arch. Intern. Med.* 141:953–959, 1981.
3. **Albrecht, H. and E. Albrecht.** Ergometric, rheographic, reflexographic and electropraphic tests at altitude and effects of drugs on human physical performance. *Fed. Proc.* 28:1262–1267, 1969.
4. **American College of Sports Medicine.** Position statement on the use and abuse of anabolic-androgenic steroids in sports. *Med. Sci. Sports.* 9(4):xi–xiii, 1977.
5. **Appell, H.-J., B. Heller-Umpenbach, M. Feraudi, and H. Weicker.** Ultrastructural and morphometric investigations on the effects of training and administration of anabolic steroids on the myocardium of guinea pigs. *Int. J. Sports Med.* 4:268–274, 1983.
6. **Ariel, G. and W. Saville.** Anabolic steroids: the physiological effects of placebos. *Med. Sci. Sports.* 4:124–126, 1972.
7. **Arnold, G.L. and M.M. Kaplan.** Peliosis hepatitis due to oxymetholone-a clinically benign disorder. *Am. J. Gastroenterol.* 71:213–216, 1979.

8. **Asano, A., H. Wakasa, S. Kaise, T. Nishimaki, and R. Kasukawa.** Peliosis hepatitis. Report on two autopsy cases with a review of literature. *Acta Pathol. Jpn.* 32:861–877, 1982.
9. **Bagheri, S. and J. Boyer.** Peliosis hepatitis associated with androgenic-anabolic steroid therapy-a severe form of hepatic injury. *Ann. Intern. Med.* 81:610–618, 1974.
10. **Bank, J.I., D. Lykkebo, and I. Hagerstrand.** Peliosis hepatitis in a child. *Acta Ped. Scand.* 67:105–107, 1978.
11. **Behrendt, H.** Effect of anabolic steroid on rat heart muscle cells I. Intermediate filaments. *Cell Tissue Res.* 180:305–315, 1977.
12. **Behrendt, H. and H. Boffin.** Myocardial cell lesions caused by anabolic hormone. *Cell Tissue Res.* 181:423–426, 1977.
13. **Benjamin, D.C. and B. Shunk.** A fatal case of peliosis of the liver and spleen. *Am. J. Dis. Child.* 132:207–208, 1978.
14. **Brooks, R.V.** Anabolic steroids and athletes. Phys. Sportsmed. 8(3):161–163, 1980.
15. **Buchwald, D., S. Argyers, R.E. Easterling, et al.** Effects of Nandrolone Decanoate on the anemia of chronic hemodialysis patients. *Nephron.* 18:232–238, 1977.
16. **Carter, C.H.** The anabolic steroid, Stanozolol, its evaluation in debilitated children. *Clin. Pediatr.* 4:671–680, 1965.
17. **Casner, S.W., R.G. Early and B.R. Carlson.** Anabolic steroid effects on body composition in normal young men. *J. Sports Med. Phys. Fitness.* 11:98–103, 1971.
18. **Choi, E.S.K., T. Chung, R.S. Morrison, C. Myers, and M.S. Greenberg.** Hypertriglyceridemia in hemodialysis patients during oral dromostanolone therapy for anemia. *Am. J. Clin. Nutr.* 27:901–904, 1974.
19. **Clerico, A., M. Ferdeghini, C. Palombo, et al.** Effects of anabolic treatment on the serum levels of gonadotropins, testosterone, prolactin, thyroid hormones and myoglobin of male athletes under physical training. *J. Nuclear Med. Allied Sci.* 25:79–88, 1981.
20. **Cox, D.W., W.L. Heinrichs, C.A. Paulsen, et al.** Perturbations of the human menstrual cycle by oxymethalone. *Am. J. Obstet. Gynecol.* 121:121–126, 1975.
21. **Crist, D.M., P.J. Stackpole, and G.T. Peake.** Effects of androgenic-anabolic steroids on neuromuscular power and body composition. *J. Appl. Physiol.* 54:366–370, 1983.
22. **Damste, P.H.** Voice changes in adult women caused by virilizing agents. *J. Speech Hear. Disord.* 32:126–132, 1967.
23. **Dorfman, R.I. and R.A. Shipley.** *Androgens: Biochemistry, Physiology and Clinical Significance.* New York: J. Wiley and Sons, 1956.
24. **Doyle, A.E., N.B. Pinkus, and J. Green.** The use of oxandrolone in hyperlipidaemia. *Med. J. Australia.* 1:127–129, 1974.
25. **Ehrenkranz, J., E. Bliss, and M.H. Sheard.** Plasma testosterone correlation with aggressive behavior and social dominance in man. *Psychosom. Med.* 36:469–475, 1974.
26. **Exner, G.U., H.W. Staudte, and D. Pette.** Isometric training of rats-effects upon fast and slow muscle and modification by an anabolic hormone (Nandolone Decanoate) I. Female rats. *Pflügers Arch.* 345:1–14, 1973.
27. **Fahey, T.D. and C.H. Brown.** The effects of an anabolic steroid on the strength, body composition and endurance of college males when accompanied by a weight training program. *Med. Sci. Sports.* 5:272–276, 1973.
28. **Falk, H., L. Thomas, H. Popper, and H.G. Ishak.** Hepatic angiosarcoma associated with androgenic-anabolic steroids. *Lancet.* 2:1120–1123, 1979.
29. **Farrell, G.C., D.E. Joshua, R.F. Uren, P.J. Baird, K.W. Perkins, and H. Kronenberg.** Androgen-induced hepatoma. *Lancet.* 1:430, 1975.
30. **Forsyth, B.T.** The effect of testosterone proprianate at various protein calorie intakes in malnutrition after trauma. *J. Lab. Clin. Med.* 43:732–740, 1954.
31. **Fowler, W.M., Jr., G.W. Gardner, and G.H. Egstrom.** Effect of an anabolic steroid on physical performance in young men. *J. Appl. Physiol.* 20:1038–1040, 1965.
32. **Freed, D.L., A.J. Banks, D. Longson, and D.M. Burley.** Anabolic steroids in athletics: crossover double-blind trial on weightlifters. *Br. Med. J.* 2:471–473, 1975.

33. **Gelder, L.V.** Psychosomatic aspects of endocrine disorders of the voice. *J. Commun. Disord.* 7:257–262, 1974.
34. **Golding, L.A., J.E. Freydinger, and S.S. Fishel.** The effect of an androgenic-anabolic steroid and a protein supplement on size, strength, weight and body composition in athletes. *Phys. Sportsmed.* 2(6):39–45, 1974.
35. **Groos, G., O.H. Arnold, and G. Brittinger.** Peliosis hepatitis after long administration of oxymetholone. *Lancet.* 1:874, 1974.
36. **Harjness, R.A., B.H. Kilshaw, and B.M. Hobson.** Effects of large doses of anabolic steroids. *Br. J. Sports Med.* 9:70–73, 1975.
37. **Heitzman, R.J.** The effectiveness of anabolic agents in increasing rate of growth in farm animals; reports on experiments in cattle. In: *Anabolic Agents in Animal Production*, F.C. Lu and J. Rendel (Eds.). Stuttgart: Georg Thieme Publishers, 1976, pp. 89–98.
38. **Heller, C.G., D.J. Moore, C.A. Paulsen, W.O. Nelson, and W.M. Laidlaw.** Effects of progesterone and synthetic progestins on the reproductive physiology of normal men. *Fed. Proc.* 18:1057–1066, 1959.
39. **Hershberger, J.G., E.G. Shipley, and R.K. Meyer.** Myotrophic activity of 19-nortestosterone and other steroids determined by modified levator ani muscle method. *Proc. Soc. Exper. Biol. Med.* 83:175–180, 1953.
40. **Hervey G.R. and I. Hutchison.** The effects of testosterone on body weight and composition in the rat. *J. Endocrinol.* 57:xxiv–xxv, 1973.
41. **Hervey, G.R., I. Hutchison, A.V. Knibbs, et al.** Anabolic effects of methandienone in men undergoing athletic training. *Lancet.* 2:699–702, 1976.
42. **Hervey, G.R., A.V. Knibbs, L. Burkinshaw, et al.** Effects of methandienone on the performance and body composition of men undergoing athletic training. *Clin. Sci.* 60:457–461, 1981.
43. **Hickson, R.C., W.W. Heusner, W.D. Van Huss, et al.** Effects of Diabanol and high-intensity sprint training on body composition of rats. *Med. Sci. Sports.* 8:191–195, 1976.
44. **Holma, P. and H. Aldercreutz.** Effect of an anabolic steroid (methandienon) on plasma LH, FSH, and testosterone and on the response to intravenous administration of LRH. *Acta Endocrinol.* 83:856–864, 1976.
45. **Houssay, A.B.** Effects of anabolic-androgenic steroids on the skin including hair and sebaceous glands. In: *Anabolic-Androgenic Steroids.* C.D. Kochakan (Ed.). New York: Springer-Verlag, 1976, pp. 155–190.
46. **Ishak, K.G.** Hepatic Lesions caused by anabolic and contraceptive steroids. *Sem. Liver Dis.* 1:116–128, 1981.
47. **Itil, T.M.** Neurophysiological effects of hormones in humans: computer EEG profiles of sex and hypothalamic hormones. In: *Hormones, Behavior and Psychotherapy.* E.J. Sachar (Ed.). New York: Raven Press, 1976, pp. 31–40.
48. **Itil, T.M., R. Cora, S. Akpinar, W.M. Hermann, and C.J. Patterson.** Psychotropic action of sex hormones: computerized EEG in establishing the immediate CNS effects of steroid hormones. *Curr. Ther. Res.* 16:1147–1170, 1974.
49. **Johnson, F.L., K.G. Lerner, M. Siegel, et al.** Association of androgenic-anabolic steroid therapy with development of hepatocellular carcinoma. *Lancet.* 2:1273, 1972.
50. **Johnson, L.C., G. Fisher, L.J. Silvester, and C.C. Hofheins.** Anabolic steroid: effects of strength, body weight, oxygen uptake, and spermatogenesis upon mature males. *Med. Sci. Sports.* 4:43–45, 1972.
51. **Johnson, L.C. and J.P O'Shea.** Anabolic steroid: effects on strength development. *Science.* 164:957–959, 1969.
52. **Johnson, L.C., E.S. Roundy, P.E. Allsen, A.G. Fisher, and L.J. Silvester.** Effect of anabolic steroid treatment on endurance. *Med. Sci. Sports.* 7:287–289, 1975.
53. **Kenyon, A.T., K. Knowlton, and I. Sandiford.** The anabolic effects of the androgens and somatic growth in man. *Ann. Intern. Med.* 20:632–654, 1944.
54. **Keul, J., H. Deus, and W. Kinderman.** Anabole hormone: Schadigung, Leistungsfahigkeit and Stoffwechses. *Med. Klin.* 71:497–503, 1976.

55. **Kilshaw, B.H., R.A. Harkness, B.M. Hobson, and A.W. M. Smith.** The effects of large doses of the anabolic steroid, methandrostenolone, on an athlete. *Clin. Endocrinol.* 4:537–541, 1975.
56. **Kochakian, C.D. and J.R. Murlin.** The effect of male hormones on the protein and energy metabolism of castrate dogs. *J. Nutr.* 10:437–458, 1935.
57. **Kochakian, C.D. and B.R. Endahl.** Changes in body weight of normal and castrated rats by different doses of testosterone propionate. *Proc. Soc. Exper. Biol. Med.* 100:520–522, 1959.
58. **Kruskemper, H.L.** *Anabolic Steroids.* New York: Academic Press, 1968, pp. 128–133, 162-164, 182.
59. **Landau. R.L.** The metabolic effects of anabolic steroids ion man. In: *Anabolic-Androgenic Steroids.* C.D. Kochakian (Ed.). New York: Springer-Verlag, 1976, pp. 45–72.
60. **Ljungqvist, A.** The use of anabolic steroids in top Swedish athletes. *Br. J. Sports Med.* 9:82, 1975.
61. **Loughton, S. J. and R.O. Ruhling.** Human strength and endurance responses to anabolic steroid and training. *J. Sports Med.* 17:285–296, 1977.
62. **MacDougall, J. D., D. G. Sale, G. C. B. Elder, and J. R. Sutton.** Muscle ultrastructural characteristics of elite powerlifters and bodybuilders. *Eur. J. Applied Physiol.* 48:117–126, 1982.
63. **Maher, J. M., E. L. Squires, J. L. Voss, and R. K. Shideler.** Effect of anabolic steroids on reproductive function of young mares. *J. Am. Vet. Med. Assoc.* 183:519–524, 1983.
64. **Mason, A. S.** Male precocity: the clinician's view. In: *The Endocrine Function of the Human Testis,* V. H. T. James, M. Serra, and L. Martini (Eds.). New York: Academic Press, 1974, pp. 131–143.
65. **McDonald, E. C. and C. E. Speicher.** Peliosis hepatis associated with administration of oxymetholone. *JAMA.* 240:243–244, 1978.
66. **McGlven, A. R.** Peliosis hepatis: case report and review of pathogenesis. *J. Pathol.* 101:283–285, 1970.
67. **Meadows, A. T., J. L. Naiman, and M. Valdes-Dapena.** Hepatoma associated with androgen therapy for aplastic anemia. *J. Pediatr.* 85:109–110, 1974.
68. **Messerli, F. H. and E. D. Frohlich.** High blood pressure: a side effect of drugs, poisons, and food. *Arch. Intern. Med.* 139:682–687, 1979.
69. **Mulvihill, J. J., R. L. Ridolfi, F. R. Schultz, M. S. Brozy and P. B. T. Haughton.** Hepatic adenoma in Fanconi anemia treated with oxymetholone. *J. Pediatr.* 87:122–124, 1975.
70. **Nadell, J. and J. Kosek.** Peliosis hepatis. *Arch. Pathol. Lab. Med.* 101:405-410, 1977.
71. **Nesheim, M. C.** Some observations on the effectiveness of anabolic agents in increasing the growth rate of poultry. In: *Anabolic Agents in Animal Production,* F. C. Lu and J. Rendel (Eds.). Stuttgart: Georg Thieme Publishers, 1976, pp. 110–114.
72. **Olsson, A. G., L. Oro, and S. Rossner.** Effects of oxandrolone on plasma lipoproteins and the intravenous fat tolerance in man. *Atherosclerosis.* 19:337–346, 1974.
73. **Orlandi, F., A. Jezequel, and A. Melliti.** The action of some anabolic steroids on the structure and the function of human liver cell. *Tijdschr. Gastro-Enterol.* 7:109–113, 1964.
74. **O'shea, J. P.** The effects of an anabolic steroid on dynamic strength levels of weightlifters. *Nutr. Rep. Int.* 4:363–370, 1971.
75. **Overly, W. L., J. A. Danicoff, B. K. Wang, and U. D. Singh.** Androgens and hepatocellular carcinoma in an athlete. *Ann. Intern. Med.* 100:158–159, 1984.
76. **Palva, I. P. and C. Wasastjerna.** Treatment of aplastic anaemia with methenolone. *Acta Haematol.* 47:13–20, 1972.
77. **Papanicolaou, G. N. and G. A. Falk.** General muscular hypertrophy induced by androgenic hormone. *Science.* 87:238–239, 1938.
78. **Reeves, R. D., M. D. Morris, and G. L. Barbour.** Hyperlipidemia due to oxymetholone therapy. *JAMA.* 236:464–472, 1976.
79. **Remes, K., P. Vuopio, M. Jarvinen, M. Harkonen, and H. Adlercreutz.** Effect of short-term treatment with an anabolic steroid (methandienone) and dehydroepiandrosterone sulphate on plasma hormones, red cell volume and 2,3-diphosphoglycerate in athletes. *Scand. J. Clin. Lab. Invest.* 37:577–586, 1977.

80. **Richardson, J. H.** A comparison of two drugs on strength increase in monkeys. *J. Sports Med. Phys. Fitness.* 17:251–254, 1977.
81. **Rogozkin, V. A.** The role of low molecular weight compounds in the regulation of skeletal muscle genome activity during exercise. *Med. Sci. Sports.* 8:1–4, 1976.
82. **Rogozkin, V. A.** Anabolic steroid metabolism in skeletal muscle. *J. Steroid Biochem.* 11:923–926, 1979.
83. **Ryan, A. J.** Anabolic steroids are fool's gold. *Fed. Proc.* 40:2682–2688, 1981.
84. **Sacks, P., D. Gale, T. H. Bothwell, K. Stevens.** Oxymetholone therapy in aplastic and other refractory anaemias. *S. Afr. Med. J.* 46:1607–1615, 1972.
85. **Scaramella, T. J. and W. A. Brown.** Serum testosterone and aggressiveness in hockey players. *Psychosom. Med.* 40:262–265, 1978.
86. **Schaffner, F., H. Popper, and V. Perez.** Changes in bile canaliculi produced by norethandrolone: electron microscopic study of human and rat liver. *J. Lab. Clin. Med.* 56:623–628, 1960.
87. **Shahidi, N. T.** Androgens and erythropoeisis. *N. Engl. J. Med.* 289:72–80, 1973.
88. **Shapiro, P., R. M. Ikedo, B. H. Ruebner, M. H. Conners, C. C. Halsted, and C. F. Abildgaard.** Multiple hepatic tumors and peliosis hepatitis in Fanconi's anemia treated with androgens. *Am. J. Dis. Child.* 131: 1104–1106, 1977.
89. **Shephard, R. J., D. Killinger, and T. Fried.** Responses to sustained use of anabolic steroid. *Br. J. Sports Med.* 11:170–173, 1977.
90. **Skarberg, K. O., L. Engstedt, S. Jameson, et al.** Oxymetholone treatment in hypoproliferative anaemia. *Acta Haematol.* 49:321–330, 1973.
91. **Smith, K. D., L. J. Rodrlguez-Rigau, R. K. Tcholakian, and E. Steinberg.** The relation between plasma testosterone levels and the lengths of phases of the menstrual cycle. *Fertil. Steril.* 32:403–407, 1979.
92. **Snochowski, M., E. Dahlberg, E. Eriksson, and J. A. Gustafsson.** Androgen and glucocorticoid receptors in human skeletal muscle cytosol. *J. Steroid Biochem.* 14:765–771, 1981.
93. **Spiers, A. S. D., S. F. Devita, M. J. Allar, S. Richards, and N. Sedransk.** Beneficial effects of an anabolic steroid during cytotoxic chemotherapy for metastatic cancer. *J. Med.* 12:433–445, 1981.
94. **Stamford, B. A. and R. Moffatt.** Anabolic steroid: effectiveness as an ergogenic aid to experienced weight trainers. *J. Sports Med. Phys. Fitness* .14:191–197, 1974.
95. **Stang-Voss, C. and H-J. Appel.** Structural alterations of liver parenchyma induced by anabolic steroids. *Int. J. Sports Med.* 2:101–105, 1981.
96. **Steinbach, M.** Uber den Einfluss Anaboler wirkstoffe auf Kor pergewicht, Muskelkraft und Muskeltraining. *Sportarzt Sportmed.* 11:485–492, 1968.
97. **Stone, M. H., M. E. Rush, and H. Lipner.** Responses to intensive training and methandrostenolone administration: II. Hormonal, organ weights, muscle weights and body composition. *Pflugers Arch.* 375: 147–151, 1978.
98. **Strauss, R. H., H. E. Wright, G. A. M. Flnerman,and D. H. Catlin.** Side effects of anabolic steroids in weight-trained men. *Phys. Sportsmed.* 11(12):87–96, 1983.
99. **Stromeyer, F. W., D. H. Smith, and K. G. Ishak.** Anabolic steroid therapy and intrahepatic cholangiocarcinoma. *Cancer.* 43:440–443, 1979.
100. **Stromme, S. B., H. D. Meen, and A. Aakvaag.** Effects of an androgenic-anabolic steroid on strength development and plasma testosterone levels in normal males. *Med. Sci. Sports.* 6:203–208, 1974.
101. **Taylor, W., S. Snowball, C. M. Dickson, and M. Lesna.** Alterations of liver architecture in mice treated with anabolic androgens and diethylnitrosamine. *NATO Adv. Study Inst. Series, Series A.* 52:279–288, 1982
102. **Taxy, J. B.** Peliosis: a morphologic curiosity becomes an iatrogenic problem. Hum. Pathol. 9:331–340, 1978.
103. **Tepperman, J.** *Metabolic and Endocrine Physiology.* Chicago: Year Book Medical Publishers, 1973, p. 70.

104. **Thomson, D. P., D. R. Pearson, and D. L. Costill.** Use of anabolic steroids by national level athletes. *Med. Sci. Sports Exerc.* 13:111, 1981. (Abstract)
105. **Vanderwal, P.** General aspects of the effectiveness of anabolic agents in increasing protein production in farm animals, in particular in bull calves. In: *Anabolic Agents in Animal Production*, F. C. Lu and J. Rendel (Eds.). Stuttgart: Georg Thieme Publishers, 1976, pp. 60–78.
106. **Wade, N.** Anabolic steroids: doctors denounce them, but athletes aren't listening. *Science.* 176:1399–1403, 1972.
107. **Ward, P.** The effect of an anabolic steroid on strength and lean body mass. *Med. Sci. Sports.* 5:277-282, 1973.
108. **Weiss, V. and H. Muller.** Auf Frage der Beeinflussung des Krafttrainings durch Anabole Hormone. *Schweiz. Z. Sportmed.* 16:79-89, 1968.
109. **Whitelaw, M. J., T. N. Foster, and W. H. Graham.** Methandrostenolone (Diabanol): a controlled study of its anabolic and androgenic effect in children. *Pediatric Pharm. Ther.* 68:291–296, 1966.
110. **Wilson, J. D. and J. E. Griffin.** The use and misuse of androgens. *Metabolism.* 29:1278–1295, 1980.
111. **Woodard, T. L., G. A. Burghen, A. E. Kitabchi, and J. A. Wilimas.** Glucose intolerance and insulin resistance in aplastic anemia treated with oxymetholone. *J. Clin. Endocrinol. Metab.* 53:905–908, 1981.
112. **Wright, J. E.** Anabolic steroids and athletes. *Exerc. Sport Sci. Rev.* 8:149–202, 1980.
113. **Yamagishi, M., A. Hiraoka, and H. Uchino.** Silent hepatic lesions detected with computed tomography in aplastic anemia patients administered androgens for a long period. *Acta Haematol. Jpn.* 45:703–710, 1982.
114. **Young, M., H. R. Crookshank, and L. Ponder.** Effects of an anabolic steroid on selected parameters in male albino rats. *Res. Q.* 48:653–656, 1977.
115. **Zevin, D., H. Turani, A. Cohen, and J. Levi.** Androgen-associated hepatoma in a hemodialysis patient. *Nephron.* 29:274–276, 1981.

Appendix F

AMERICAN COLLEGE OF SPORTS MEDICINE POSITION STAND ON WEIGHT LOSS IN WRESTLERS*

Despite repeated admonitions by medical, educational, and athletic groups,[2,8,17,22,33] most wrestlers have been inculcated by instruction or accepted tradition to lose weight in order to be certified for a class that is lower than their preseason weight.[33] Studies[33,39] of weight losses in high school and college wrestlers indicate that from 3 to 20% of the preseason body weight is lost before certification or competition occurs. Of this weight loss, most of the decrease occurs in the final days or day before the official weigh-in[33,39] with the youngest and/or lightest members of the team losing the highest percentage of their body weight.[33] Under existing rules and practices, it is not uncommon for an individual to repeat this weight losing process many times during the season because successful wrestlers compete in 15 to 30 matches per year.[13]

Contrary to existing beliefs, most wrestlers are not "fat" before the season starts.[34] In fact, the fat content of high school and college wrestlers weighing less than 190 lb has been shown to range from 1.6 to 15.1% of their body weight with the majority possessing less than 8%.[14,28,31] It is well known and documented that wrestlers lose body weight by a combination of food restriction, fluid deprivation, and sweating induced by thermal or exercise procedures.[20,22,35,39] Of these methods, dehydration through sweating appears to be the method most frequently chosen. Careful studies on the nature of the weight being lost show that water, fats, and proteins are lost when food restriction and fluid deprivation procedures are followed.[10] Moreover, the proportionality between these constituents will change with continued restriction and deprivation. For example, if food restriction is held constant when the volume of fluid being consumed is decreased, more water will be lost from the tissues of the body than before the fluid restriction occurred. The problem becomes more acute when thermal or exercise dehydration occurs because electrolyte losses will accompany the water losses.[16] Even when 1 to 5 h are allowed for purposes of rehydration after the weigh-in, this time interval is insufficient for fluid and electrolyte homeostasis to be completely reestablished.[11,36,38,39]

* Reprint of *"Weight Loss in Wrestlers,"* ©1976 American College of Sports Medicine, *MSSE,* 8:2, 1976, pp. xi–xiii. With permission of Williams & Wilkins.

Since the "making of weight" occurs by combinations of food restriction, fluid deprivation, and dehydration, responsible officials should realize that the single or combined effects of these practices are generally associated with: (1) a reduction in muscular strength;[4,15,30] (2) a decrease in work performance times;[24,26,27,30] (3) lower plasma and blood volumes;[6,7,24,27] (4) a reduction in cardiac functioning during submaximal work conditions which are associated with higher heart rates,[1,19,23,24,27] smaller stroke volumes,[27] and reduced cardiac outputs;[27] (5) a lower oxygen consumption, especially with food restriction;[15,30] (6) an impairment of thermoregulatory processes;[3,9,24] (7) a decrease in renal blood flow[21,25] and in the volume of fluid being filtered by the kidney;[21] (8) a depletion of liver glycogen stores;[12] and (9) an increase in the amount of electrolytes being lost from the body.[6,7,16]

Since it is possible for these changes to impede normal growth and development, there is little physiological or medical justification for the use of the weight reduction methods currently followed by many wrestlers. These sentiments have been expressed in part within Rule 1, Section 3, Article I of the *Official Wrestling Rule Book*[18] published by the National Federation of State High School Associations which states, "The Rules Committee recommends that individual state high school associations develop and utilize an effective weight control program which will discourage severe weight reduction and/or wide variations in weight, because this may be harmful to the competitor..." However, until the National Federation of State High School Associations defines the meaning of the terms "severe" and "wide variations", this rule will be ineffective in reducing the abuses associated with the "making of weight".

Therefore, it is the position of the American College of Sports Medicine that the potential health hazards created by the procedures used to "make weight" by wrestlers can be eliminated if state and national organizations will

1. Assess the body composition of each wrestler several weeks in advance of the competitive season.[5,14,28,31,37] Individuals with a fat content less than 5% of their certified body weight should receive medical clearance before being allowed to compete.
2. Emphasize the fact that the daily caloric requirements of wrestlers should be obtained from a balanced diet and determined on the basis of age, body surface area, growth, and physical activity levels.[29] The minimal caloric needs of wrestlers in high schools and colleges will range from 1200 to 2400 kcal/d;[32] therefore, it is the responsibility of coaches, school officials, physicians, and parents to discourage wrestlers from securing less than their minimal needs without prior medical approval.
3. Discourage the practice of fluid deprivation and dehydration. This can be accomplished by:
   - Educating the coaches and wrestlers on the physiological consequences and medical complications that can occur as a result of these practices.

- Prohibiting the single or combined use of rubber suits, steam rooms, hot boxes, saunas, laxatives, and diuretics to "make weight".
- Scheduling weigh-ins just prior to competition.
- Scheduling more official weigh-ins between team matches.

4. Permit more participants/team to compete in those weight classes (119 to 145 lb) which have the highest percentages of wrestlers certified for competition.[35]
5. Standardize regulations concerning the eligibility rules at championship tournaments so that individuals can only participate in those weight classes in which they had the highest frequencies of matches throughout the season.
6. Encourage local and county organizations to systematically collect data on the hydration state[38,39] of wrestlers and its relationship to growth and development.

REFERENCES

1. **Alhman, K. and M.J. Karvonen.** Weight reduction by sweating in wrestlers and its effect on physical fitness. *J. Sports Med. Phys. Fit.* 1:58–62, 1961.
2. AMA Committee on the Medical Aspects of Sports, Wrestling and Weight Control. *JAMA.* 201:541–543, 1967.
3. **Bock, W.E., E.L. Fox, and R. Bowers.** The effect of acute dehydration upon cardiorespiratory endurance. *J. Sports Med. Phys. Fit.* 7:62–72, 1967.
4. **Bosco, J.S., R.L. Terjung, and J.E. Greenleaf.** Effects of progressive hypohydration of maximal isometric muscular strength. *J. Sports Med. Phys. Fit.* 8:81–86, 1968.
5. **Clarke, K.S.** Predicting certified weight of young wrestlers: a field study of the Tcheng-Tipton method. *Med. Sci. Sports.* 6: 52–57, 1974.
6. **Costill, D.L. and K. E. Sparks.** Rapid fluid replacement following thermal dehydration. *J. Appl. Physiol.* 34:299–303, 1973.
7. **Costill, D.L., R. Cote, E. Miller, T. Miller, and S. Wynder.** Water and electrolyte replacement during repeated days of work in the heat. *Aviat. Space Environ. Med.* 46:795–800, 1975.
8. **Eriksen, F.G.** Interscholastic wrestling and weight control: Current plans and their loopholes. *Proceedings of the Eighth National Conference on The Medical Aspects of Sports.* Chicago: AMA, 1967, pp. 34–39.
9. **Grande, F., J.E. Monagle, E.R. Buskirk, and H.L. Taylor.** Body temperature responses to exercise in man on restricted food and water intake. *J. Appl. Physiol.* 14:194–198, 1959.
10. **Grande, F.** Nutrition and energy balance in body composition studies. *Techniques for Measuring Body Composition*, edited by J. Brozek and A. Henschel. Washington, D.C., National Acad. Sci. & Nat. Res. Council, pp. 168–188, 1961.
11. **Herbert, W.G. and P.M. Ribisl.** Effects of dehydration upon physical work capacity of wrestlers under competitive conditions. *Res. Quart.* 43:416–422, 1972.
12. **Hultman, E. and L. Nilsson.** Liver glycogen as glucose-supplying source during exercise. *Limiting Factors of Physical Performance*, edited by J. Keul. Stuttgart Georg Thieme, pp. 179–189, 1973.
13. Iowa High School Athletic Association. 1975 Program for the 55th State Wrestling Tournament., pp. 7–9.
14. **Katch, F.I. and E.D. Michael, Jr.** Body composition of high school wrestlers according to age and wrestling weight category. *Med. Sci. Sports.* 3:190–194, 1971.

15. **Keys, A.L., J. Brozek, A. Henschel, O. Mickelsen, and H.L. Taylor.** *The Biology of Human Starvation.* Minneapolis U of Minn. Press, Vol. 1. pp 718–748, 1950.
16. **Kozlowski, S. and B. Saltin.** Effect of sweat loss on body fluids. *J. Appl. Physiol.* 19:1119–1124, 1964.
17. **Kroll, W.** Guidelines for rules and practices. *Proceedings of the Eighth National Conference on the Medical Aspects of Sports.* Chicago AMA, pp. 40–44, 1967.
18. *The National Federation 1974-75 Wrestling Rule Book.* The National Federation Publications. Elgin, Illinois, p. 6.
19. **Palmer, W.** Selected physiological responses of normal young men following dehydration and rehydration. *Res. Quart.* 39:1054–1059, 1968.
20. **Paul, W.D.** Crash diets in wrestling. *J. lowa Med. Soc.* 56:835–840, 1966.
21. **Radigan, L.R. and S. Robinson.** Effect of environmental heat stress and exercise on renal blood flow and filtration rate. *J. Appl. Physiol.* 2:185–191, 1949.
22. **Rasch, P.G. and W. Kroll.** *What Research Tells the Coach About Wrestling.* Washington: AAHPER, pp. 41–50, 1964.
23. **Ribisl, P.M. and W.G. Herbert.** Effect of rapid weight reduction and subsequent rehydration upon the physical working capacity of wrestlers. *Res. Quart.* 41:536–541, 1970.
24. **Robinson, S.** The effect of dehydration on performance. *Football Injuries.* Washington, DC: Natl. Acad. Sci., pp. 191–197, 1970.
25. **Rowell, L.B.** Human cardiovascular adjustments to exercise and thermal stress. *Physiol. Rev.* 54:75–159, 1974.
26. **Saltin, B.** Aerobic and anaerobic work capacity after dehydration. *J. Appl. Physiol.* 19:1114–1118, 1964.
27. **Saltin, B.** Circulatory response to submaximal and maximal exercise after thermal dehydration. *J. Appl. Physiol.* 19: 1125–1132, 1964.
28. **Sinning, W.E.** Body composition assessment of college wrestlers. *Med. Sci. Sports.* 6:139–145, 1974.
29. Suggested Daily Dietary Requirements. National Research Council Data, published in Oser, B.O. *Hawk's Physiological Chemistry*, 14th Edition, New York: McGraw-Hill, pp. 1370–1371, 1965.
30. **Taylor, H.L., E.R. Buskirk, J. Brozek, J.T. Anderson, and F. Grande.** Performance capacity and effects of caloric restriction with hard physical work on young men. *J. Appl. Physiol.* 10:421–429, 1957.
31. **Tcheng, T.K. and C.M. Tipton.** Iowa wrestling study: Anthropometric measurements and the prediction of a "minimal" bodyweight for high school wrestlers. *Med. Sci. Sports.* 5:1–10, 1973.
32. **Tipton, C.M.** Unpublished calculations on Iowa High School Wrestlers using a height and weight surface area nomogram. (Consalazio, C.F., R.E. Johnson and L.J. Pecora, *Physiological Measurements of Metabolic Functions in Man.* New York: McGraw-Hill, 1963, p. 27, that was constructed from the Dubois-Meech formula published in *Arch. Int. Med.* 17:863–871, 1916) plus the metabolic standards for age used by the Mayo Foundation Standards that were published by Boothby, Berkson and Dunn in *Am. J. Physiol.* 116:467–484, 1936.
33. **Tipton, C.M. and T.K. Tcheng.** Iowa Wrestling study: Weight loss in high school students. *JAMA.* 2114:1269–1274, 1970.
34. **Tipton, C.M.** Current status of the Iowa Wrestling Study. *The Predicament.* 12-30-73, p. 7.
35. **Tipton, C.M., T.K. Tcheng, and E.J. Zambraski.** Iowa Wrestling Study: Weight classification systems. *Med. Sci. Sports.* 8:101–104, 1976.
36. **Vaccaro, P., C.W. Zauner, and J.R. Cade.** Changes in body weight, hematocrit and plasma protein concentration due to dehydration and rehydration in wrestlers. *Med. Sci. Sports.* 7:76, 1975.
37. **Wilmore, J.H. and A. Behnke.** An anthropometric estimation of body density and lean body weight in young men. *J. Appl. Physiol.* 27:25–31, 1969.

38. **Zambraski, E.J., C.M. Tipton, T.K. Tcheng, H.R. Jordan, A.C. Vailas, and A.K. Callahan.** Changes in the urinary profiles of wrestlers prior to and after competition. *Med. Sci. Sports.* 7:217–220, 1975.
39. **Zambraski, E.J., D.T. Foster, P.M. Gross, and C.M. Tipton.** Iowa wrestling study: Weight loss and urinary profiles of collegiate wrestlers. *Med. Sci. Sports.* 8:105–108, 1976.

Appendix G

AMERICAN COLLEGE OF SPORTS MEDICINE POSITION STAND ON EXERCISE FOR PATIENTS WITH CORONARY ARTERY DISEASE*

SUMMARY

Exercise training improves functional capacity and reduces clinical symptoms in patients with coronary artery disease. However, such patients are at increased risk for cardiovascular complications during exercise; therefore, appropriate safeguards should be employed to minimize these risks. Based on the documented benefits and risks of exercise for patients with coronary artery disease, it is the position of the American College of Sports Medicine that most patients with coronary artery disease should engage in individually designed exercise programs to achieve optimal physical and emotional health.

INTRODUCTION

This position stand will address exercise for patients with coronary artery disease. The following points are readily recognized. Patients with coronary artery disease are not a homogeneous group and must be considered individually. They vary greatly in their clinical status including: extent of coronary artery disease, left ventricular dysfunction, potential for myocardial ischemia, and presence of cardiac arrhythmias. Some patients with coronary artery disease have had prior cardiac events (e.g., myocardial infarction, cardiac arrest) or treatments (e.g., coronary artery bypass graft surgery, percutaneous transluminal coronary angioplasty, or other coronary artery interventions). Many patients have additional medical disorders including hypertension, peripheral vascular disease, valvular heart disease, chronic obstructive pulmonary disease, and diabetes mellitus.

Exercise in the outpatient setting will be addressed in this position stand, although in-hospital, early ambulation following cardiac events is also important.

* Reprinted from *"Exercise for Patients with Coronary Artery Disease,"* ©1994 American College of Sports Medicine, *MSSE,* 26:3, 1994, pp. i–v. With permission of Williams & Wilkins.

EFFECTS OF EXERCISE TRAINING

FUNCTIONAL CAPACITY

Patients with coronary artery disease generally demonstrate reduced maximal oxygen uptake and exercise tolerance compared with their healthy contemporaries. The magnitude of the reduction varies in part with the severity of disease, and some coronary artery disease patients have normal exercise tolerance. Both a lower maximal stroke volume and heart rate may limit maximal cardiac output and oxygen uptake.[7] The magnitude of the reduction in stroke volume depends on the amount of myocardium rendered ischemic by exercise and/or the size of prior myocardial infarction. The mechanism for the reduced exercise heart rate in unmedicated patients has not been defined. Maximal exercise performance in patients with angina pectoris is limited by discomfort. In patients with classic angina pectoris, such discomfort occurs at a highly reproducible[25] rate pressure product (heart rate times systolic blood pressure) if factors such as time of day, room temperature, and body position are constant.[6] Many patients do not demonstrate this classic pattern, suggesting that coronary vasospastic changes contribute to the variation in their anginal threshold.[42]

Both the patient's behavior and the physician's recommendations may also reduce the patient's exercise capacity. Detraining occurs both from self-induced and medically required restrictions in activity. Medications such as beta-adrenergic blockers, although beneficial for symptomatic patients, may reduce exercise capacity in some patient groups, especially if these drugs are prescribed routinely or prophylactically in asymptomatic patients.

Exercise training increases functional capacity and maximal oxygen uptake ($\dot{V}O_2max$) in coronary artery disease patients by increasing the arteriovenous oxygen difference, and in some cases maximal stroke volume as well.[7] The relative contribution of these two factors to the increase in $\dot{V}O_2max$ varies with the patient population and type of training program. The increase in $\dot{V}O_2max$ in coronary artery disease patients after 3 months of training ranges from approximately 10 to 60% in published reports and averages about 20%.[16,39] Increases in maximal work capacity may underestimate the functional benefits of exercise training, because marked increases in submaximal endurance capacity can occur in healthy subjects despite modest increases in $\dot{V}O_2max$.[35]

SYMPTOMS OF MYOCARDIAL ISCHEMIA

Some of the greatest increases in effort tolerance following exercise training occur in patients with angina pectoris.[8] Exercise training reduces submaximal heart rate at any given workload or activity and delays the onset of symptoms during exercise. Some patients actually have a disappearance of anginal pain after training.[8] The reduction in anginal symptoms produced by exercise training may facilitate a decrease in drug therapy, but this benefit of exercise training has not been well quantified.

MYOCARDIAL ISCHEMIA AND PERFUSION

Despite improved exercise performance and reduced symptoms in coronary artery disease patients, there is no conclusive evidence that exercise training alone increases vessel caliber, augments collateral development, or reverses coronary narrowing.[12,39] Increased coronary diameter after exercise training has been documented in animal models of diet-induced atherosclerosis.[23] Furthermore, some exercise training studies observed increases in the rate pressure product at the onset of ischemia and reduced ST segment depression at similar rate pressure products, implying enhanced coronary flow,[10] but these improvements are not found universally. Thallium-201 scintigraphy has documented improved myocardial perfusion in some patients after training.[14] The role of reduced coronary constriction was not evaluated in these reports, and angiographic studies have failed to demonstrate changes in resting coronary caliber or collaterals.[39] Consequently, although coronary perfusion may be improved in some patients by exercise training, the mechanism remains undefined.[12]

CORONARY ARTERY DISEASE RISK FACTORS

Blood Lipids

Increased levels of low-density lipoprotein (LDL) cholesterol and depressed levels of high-density lipoprotein (HDL) cholesterol are key risk factors for the development of coronary artery disease. Recent studies also demonstrate the importance of modifying these lipoproteins in secondary coronary artery disease prevention.[20] A meta-analysis of the 8 clinical trials of cholesterol reduction in myocardial infarction survivors performed from 1965 to 1988 demonstrates a 16% reduction in fatal and a 25% reduction in nonfatal myocardial infarctions in the treated group.[34] Cholesterol treatment consisted of diet alone in three and diet plus medication in five of these studies. None of these trials, however, directly involved an exercise rehabilitation program nor, with rare exceptions,[19] have comprehensive exercise rehabilitation programs examined the relationship of lipid changes and survival. A meta-analysis of 15 reports on the effect of exercise training in postmyocardial infarction patients has shown significant reductions of total cholesterol, LDL-cholesterol, and triglycerides, and an increase in HDL-cholesterol with training.[40] These results suggest that comprehensive cardiac rehabilitation programs utilizing exercise, diet, and medication, when appropriate, would beneficially alter lipids and patient prognosis.

Cigarette Smoking

Cigarette smoking is a well-recognized, major risk factor for coronary artery disease, particularly sudden cardiac death. Furthermore, men who survive a myocardial infarction and quit smoking have a 19% mortality rate over the next 6 years, whereas the mortality rate is 30% in those who continue smoking.[36] A study of the effects of exercise training on smoking in patients recovering from acute myocardial infarction suggests that formal rehabilitation programs facilitate smoking cessation and cessation maintenance in cardiac patients,[38] but firm support for this conclusion is not available.

Hypertension Control

Uncontrolled hypertension doubles or triples the risk of cardiovascular events, and elevated blood pressure is an independent predictor of subsequent morbidity and mortality in survivors of myocardial infarction.[21] Effective control of elevated blood pressure in the myocardial infarction population reduces cardiovascular mortality by 20%.[24] Exercise training can contribute to blood pressure control,[15] but optimal blood pressure control is usually achieved by pharmacological therapy. Exercise training may contribute to hypertension management indirectly through weight reduction, but its independent contribution to blood pressure control in coronary artery disease patients has not been well documented.

Glucose Intolerance and Diabetes Mellitus

Glucose intolerance and diabetes mellitus are major risk factors for cardiovascular disease. Unfortunately, control of diabetes has not been shown to beneficially affect the development of coronary artery disease. Physical activity can help to control hyperglycemia especially when combined with weight loss.[26] Such physical activity should be of benefit to glucose control in coronary artery disease patients.

Control of Obesity

Obesity is an independent risk factor for the development of coronary artery disease.[18] Obesity is also associated with hypertension, glucose intolerance, and unfavorable lipid profiles.[27] Successful weight loss is a benefit of an exercise training program and should contribute to reduced cardiovascular morbidity and mortality.[19,28,43]

Psychological Benefits

Patients undergoing either an exercise program or an exercise and counseling program have been reported to demonstrate an improved quality of life compared with control groups.[32] Furthermore, exercise training has been documented to reduce depression in clinically depressed patients following an acute myocardial infarction.[37] Such psychological changes could be a major benefit to patients with coronary artery disease involved in exercise training programs, but two recent studies have failed to document psychological benefits.[5,31]

Cardiovascular Mortality

Published studies have documented the beneficial effects of cardiac rehabilitation programs in reducing subsequent coronary artery disease mortality.[29,30] Compared with control groups, patients assigned to exercise-based rehabilitation programs experienced a 20 to 25% reduction in fatal cardiovascular events and total mortality. These analyses did not demonstrate differences in nonfatal recurrent events. Also, the contribution of exercise training to survival of patients following coronary artery bypass graft surgery and percutaneous transluminal coronary angioplasty has not been evaluated. Nevertheless, these mortality results suggest that exercise training is one of the few interventions documented to increase survival after myocardial infarction.

Cost Benefit

The cost benefit analysis of exercise rehabilitation in patients following myocardial infarction or bypass surgery has not been well studied. Nevertheless, significant reduction in medical care costs in patients choosing to participate in an exercise-based cardiac rehabilitation program compared with nonparticipants has been reported.[1] In another study, patients undergoing cardiac rehabilitation following percutaneous transluminal coronary angioplasty experienced fewer hospital readmissions and a reduction in overall medical expenses compared with patients not receiving rehabilitation.[9] Such preliminary results suggest that the financial benefits of cardiac rehabilitation outweigh its monetary cost.

RECOMMENDATIONS

EVALUATION

Before beginning an exercise program, patients with coronary artery disease require a complete medical history, physical examination, and a graded exercise test.[4,11] The initial evaluation is directed at the patient's cardiovascular as well as general medical and orthopedic status. Further evaluation, if clinically indicated, is directed at defining any pathophysiological abnormalities, including left ventricular dysfunction, myocardial ischemia, or cardiac arrhythmias. Abnormalities identified may then be managed medically or surgically prior to beginning the exercise program.

Patients identified as high risk for cardiovascular complications during exercise include patients with unstable angina, severe aortic stenosis, uncontrolled cardiac arrhythmias, decompensated congestive heart failure, or other medical conditions that could be aggravated by exercise (e.g., acute myocarditis or infectious disease).[11] These patients should defer exercise training until the above problems are controlled.

Patients at increased risk who may be able to exercise under direct medical supervision include those with:[2,11,17] (1) Severely depressed left ventricular function; (2) resting complex ventricular arrhythmias; (3) ventricular arrhythmias appearing or increasing with exercise; (4) decrease in systolic blood pressure with exercise; (5) survivors of sudden cardiac arrest; (6) recent myocardial infarction complicated by congestive heart failure; and (7) marked exercise-induced ischemia.

It should be noted, however, that the risk-to-benefit ratio of exercise training for such patients is not defined.

The exercise prescription, especially in terms of exercise intensity and degree of monitoring and supervision, is also based on the initial clinical and exercise evaluation.

Reevaluation should be performed regularly and as clinically indicated, generally 2 to 3 months after starting a program, and then at least yearly thereafter.[11] It is important to assess the physiologic changes resulting from an exercise program as well as the possibility of disease progression.

EXERCISE PRESCRIPTION

Exercise for patients with coronary artery disease includes activities performed in formal supervised exercise programs, as well as everyday physical activities. Therefore, general daily activity is encouraged in addition to formal exercise sessions.

The exercise program for the patient with coronary artery disease is based on the traditional prescription for developing a training effect in healthy persons.[3] It is, however, modified as indicated by the patient's cardiovascular and general medical status. It involves an individually appropriate program of exercise with respect to mode, frequency, duration, intensity, and progression of exercise.[3,4,11]

Mode

Large muscle group, continuous exercise, such as walking, jogging, bicycling, swimming, group aerobics, and rowing, is appropriate for cardiovascular endurance conditioning. Upper extremity exercises performed with arm ergometers may also be utilized for those who cannot tolerate lower extremity activity for orthopedic or other reasons, and for patients whose occupational or recreational activities are dominated by arm work. Strength training is also beneficial for selected patients.[13] Resistance exercises generally are performed with a circuit training approach, up to 10 to 12 exercises using 10 to 12 repetitions of resistances that can be performed comfortably.[22] Cross-training may also help to reduce musculoskeletal problems and increase compliance.

Frequency

Minimum frequency is three nonconsecutive days per week. Some patients prefer to exercise daily. However, with increased frequency of exercise, the risk of musculoskeletal injury increases.[33]

Duration

Warm-up and cool-down periods of at least 10 min, including stretching and flexibility exercises, should precede and follow 20 to 40 min of cardiovascular exercise performed either continuously or through interval training. The latter may be especially useful for patients with peripheral vascular disease and intermittent claudication.

Intensity

Exercise in supervised programs is performed at a moderate, comfortable intensity, generally 40 to 85% of maximal functional capacity ($\dot{V}O_2max$), which correlates with 40 to 85% of maximal heart rate reserve ([maximal heart rate – resting heart rate] × 40 to 85% + resting heart rate) or 55 to 90% of maximal heart rate. Ratings of perceived exertion (RPE) may also be used to monitor exercise intensity, with the goal of keeping the intensity at a moderate level. The exercise intensity should be below a level that provokes myocardial ischemia, significant arrhythmias, or symptoms of exercise intolerance as judged clinically or by exercise testing.

The recommended intensity of exercise training varies with the degree of supervision available and the patient's level of risk. Lower exercise intensities are indicated for higher risk patients (defined above) especially when exercising outside of supervised programs or without continuous ECG monitoring.

Progression

Any exercise program for patients with coronary artery disease should involve an initial slow, gradual progression of the exercise duration and intensity.

SUPERVISION AND MONITORING

Patient supervision involves both direct patient observation and monitoring of heart rate and rhythm. Blood pressure measurement is generally performed when clinically indicated. The nature and degree of supervision and monitoring depends upon the patient's risk for exercise complications and the intensity of exercise. Supervision and monitoring should be performed most extensively when dealing with high-risk patients (defined above). Patients exercising without medical supervision and monitoring should do so at lower exercise intensities.

Risks of Exercise

Major cardiovascular complications during exercise in patients with coronary artery disease are acute myocardial infarction, cardiac arrest, and sudden death. The estimated incidence of cardiovascular complications in supervised cardiac rehabilitation programs are 1 myocardial infarction per 294,000 patient hours, 1 cardiac arrest per 112,000 patient hours, and 1 death per 784,000 patient hours.[41] Over 80% of patients who have been reported to suffer a cardiac arrest (primarily due to ventricular fibrillation or ventricular tachycardia) in supervised cardiac rehabilitation programs have been successfully resuscitated with prompt defibrillation.[41]

CONCLUSION

It is the position of the American College of Sports Medicine that most patients with coronary artery disease should engage in individually designed exercise programs to achieve optimal physical and emotional health. It is recommended that programs include a comprehensive preexercise medical evaluation, including a graded exercise test, and an individualized exercise prescription.

Appropriate exercise programs for patients with coronary artery disease have multiple documented benefits, which can be achieved with a high level of safety. These benefits include enhanced functional capacity; reductions in symptoms of myocardial ischemia, and subsequent coronary artery disease mortality; improvements in blood lipid profiles, weight and hypertension control; and, in diabetic patients, glucose tolerance. In addition, improvements in myocardial perfusion, cigarette smoking cessation, and psychological functioning may also occur.

ACKNOWLEDGMENTS

This pronouncement was written for the American College of Sports Medicine by Steven P. Van Camp, M.D., FACSM (chair); John D. Cantwell, M.D., FACSM; Gerald F. Fletcher, M.D.; L. Kent Smith, M.D.; and Paul D. Thompson, M.D., FACSM.

This pronouncement was reviewed for the American College of Sports Medicine by members-at-large, the Pronouncements Committee, and by: H.L. Brammell, M.D.; Barry A. Franklin, Ph.D., FACSM; G.R. Greenwell, M.D., FACSM; William L. Haskell, Ph.D., FACSM; Jeremy N. Morris, M.D., FACSM; and Paul Ribisl, Ph.D., FACSM.

REFERENCES

1. **Ades, P.A., D. Huang, and S.O. Weaver.** Cardiac rehabilitation and participation predicts lower rehospitalization costs. *Am. Heart J.* 123:916–921, 1992.
2. American College of Cardiology. Recommendations of the American College of Cardiology on cardiovascular rehabilitation. *J. Am. Coll. Cardiol.* 7:451–453, 1986.
3. American College of Sports Medicine. Position stand on the recommended quantity and quality of exercise for developing and maintaining cardiorespiratory and muscular fitness in healthy adults. *Med. Sci. Sports Exerc.* 22:265–274, 1990.
4. American College of Sports Medicine. Guidelines for Exercise Testing and Exercise Prescription, 4th Ed. Philadelphia: Lea & Febiger, 1991.
5. **Blumennthal, J.A., C.F. Emery, and W.J. Rejeski.** The effects of exercise training on psychosocial functioning after myocardial infarction. *J. Cardiopulmonary Rehabil.* 8:183–193, 1988.
6. **Bygdeman, S. and J. Wahren.** Influence of body position on the anginal threshold during leg exercise. *Eur. J. Clin. Invest.* 4:201–206, 1974.
7. **Clausen, J.P.** Circulatory adjustments to dynamic exercise and effects of physical training in normal subjects and in patients with coronary artery disease. In: *Exercise and Heart Disease,* E.H. Sonnenblick and M. Lesch (Eds.). New York: Grune & Stratton, 1977, pp. 39–75.
8. **Clausen, J.P. and J. Trap-Jensen.** Heart rate and arterial blood pressure during exercise in patients with angina pectoris: effects of training and of nitroglycerin. *Circulation.* 53:436–442, 1976.

9. **Edwards, W.W., B.D. Franks, Y. Iyriboz, and S.L. Dodd.** Physiological and expense implications of PTCA rehabilitation. *Med. Sci. Sports Exerc.* 22:S5, 1990.
10. **Ehsani, A.A., G.W. Heath, J.M. Hagberg, B.E. Sobel, and J.O. Holloszy.** Effects of 12 months of intense exercise training on ischemic ST-segment depression in patients with coronary artery disease. *Circulation.* 6:1116–1124, 1981.
11. **Fletcher, G.F., V.F. Froelicher, L.H. Hartley, W.L. Haskell, and M.L. Pollock.** Exercise standards: a statement for health professionals from the American Heart Association. *Circulation.* 82:2286–2322, 1990.
12. **Franklin, B.A.** Exercise training and coronary collateral circulation. *Med. Sci. Sports Exerc.* 23:648–653, 1991.
13. **Franklin, B.A., K. Bonzheim, S. Gordon, and G.C. Timmis.** Resistance training in cardiac rehabilitation. *J. Cardiopulmonary Rehabil.* 11:99–107, 1991.
14. **Froelicher, V., D. Jensen, F. Genter, et al.** A randomized trial of exercise training in patients with coronary heart disease. *JAMA.* 252:1291–1297, 1984.
15. **Hagberg, J.M. and D.R. Seals.** Exercise training and hypertension. *Acta Med. Scand.* 711:131–136, 1986.
16. **Hartung, G.H. and R. Rangel.** Exercise training in post-myocardial infarction patients: comparison of results with high risk coronary and post-bypass patients. *Arch. Phys. Med. Rehabil.* 62:147–150, 1981.
17. Health and Public Policy Committee, American College of Physicians. Cardiac rehabilitation services. *Ann. Intern. Med.* 109:671–673, 1988.
18. **Hubert, H.B., M. Feinleib, P.M. McNamara, and W.P. Castelli.** Obesity as an independent factor for cardiovascular disease: a 26-year follow-up of participants in the Framingham Heart Study. *Circulation.* 67:968–977, 1983.
19. **Kallio, V., H. Hamalainen, J. Hakkila, and O.J. Luurila.** Reduction in sudden death by a multifactorial intervention program after acute myocardial infarction. *Lancet.* 2:1091–1094, 1979.
20. **Kannel, W.B.** Contributions of the Framingham Study to the conquest of coronary artery disease. *Am. J. Cardiol.* 62:1109–1112, 1988.
21. **Kannel, W.B., P. Sorlie, W.P. Castelli, and D. McGee.** Blood pressure and survival after myocardial infarction: the Framingham Study. *Am. J. Cardiol.* 45:326–330, 1980.
22. **Kelemen, M.H.** Resistance training safety and essential guidelines for cardiac and coronary prone patients. *Med. Sci. Sports Exerc.* 21:675–677, 1989.
23. **Kramsch, D.M., A.J. Aspen, B.M. Abramowitz, T. Kreimendahl, and W.B.J. Hood.** Reduction of coronary atherosclerosis by moderate conditioning exercise in monkeys on an atherogenic diet. *N. Engl. J. Med.* 305:1483–1489, 1981.
24. **Langford, H.G., J. Stamler, Wassertheil-Smollers, and R. J. Prineas.** All-cause mortality in the Hypertensive Detection and Follow-Up Program. *Prog. Cardiovasc. Dis.* 29:29–54, 1986.
25. **Lazarus, B., E. Cullinane, and P.D. Thompson.** Comparison of the results and reproducibility of arm and leg exercise tests in men with angina pectoris. *Am. J. Cardiol.* 47:1075–1079, 1981.
26. **Leon, A.** Patients with diabetes mellitus. *Exercise in Modern Medicine,* Baltimore: Williams & Wilkins, 1989, pp. 118–145.
27. National Obesity Consensus Conference. *Ann. Intern. Med.* 100:888–900, 1985.
28. **Oberman, A., P. Cleary, J.C. Larosa, H.K. Hellerstein, and J. Naughton.** Changes in risk factors among participants in a long-term exercise rehabilitation program. *Adv. Cardiol.* 31:168–175, 1982.
29. **O'Connor, G.T., J.E. Buring, S. Yusaf, S.Z. Goldhaber, E.M. Olmstead.** An overview of randomized trials of rehabilitation with exercise after myocardial infarction. *Circulation.* 80:234–244, 1989.
30. **Oldridge, N.B., G.H. Guyait, M.E. Fischer, and A.A. Rimm.** Cardiac rehabilitation after myocardial infarction: combined experience of randomized clinical trials. *JAMA.* 260:945–950, 1988.

31. **Oldridge, N.B., G. Guyatt, N. Jones, et al.** Effects on quality of life with comprehensive rehabilitation after acute myocardial infarction. *Am. J. Cardiol.* 67:1084–1089, 1991.
32. **Ott,C.R., E.S. Sivarajan, K.M. Newton, et al.** A controlled randomized study of early cardiac rehabilitation: the Sickness Impact Profile as an assessment tool. *Heart & Lung.* 12:162–170, 1983.
33. **Pollock, M.L., L.R. Gettman, C.A. Milesis, M.D. Bah, J.L. Durstine, and R.B. Johnson.** Effects of frequency and duration of training on attrition and incidence of injury. *Med, Sci. Sports.* 9:31–36, 1977.
34. **Rossouw, J.E., B. Lewis, and B.M. Rifkind.** The value of lowering cholesterol after myocardial infarction. *N. Engl. J. Med.* 323:1112–1119, 1990.
35. **Rowell, L.B.** *Human Circulation: Regulation During Physical Stress.* New York, Oxford University Press Inc., 1986, pp. 213–286.
36. **Sparrow, D., T.R. Dawber, and T. Colton.** The influence of cigarette smoking on prognosis after a first myocardial infarction. *J. Chronic Dis.* 31:425–432, 1978.
37. **Taylor, C.B., J. Sallis, and R. Needle.** The relationship of exercise and physical activity to mental health. *Public Health Rep.* 100:195–202, 1985.
38. **Taylor, C.B., N. Houston-Miller, W.L. Haskell, and R.F. Debusk.** Smoking cessation after acute myocardial infarction: the effects of exercise training. *Addict. Behav.* 13:331–335, 1988.
39. **Thompson, P.D.** The benefits and risks of exercise training in patients with chronic coronary artery disease. *JAMA.* 259:1537–1540, 1988.
40. **Tran, Z.V. and H.L. Brammell.** Effects of exercise training on serum lipid and lipoprotein levels in post-MI patients. A meta-analysis. *J. Cardiopulmonary Rehabil.* 9:250–255, 1989.
41. **Van Camp, S.P. and R.A. Peterson.** Cardiovascular complications of outpatient cardiac rehabilitation programs. *JAMA.* 256:1160–1163, 1986.
42. **Yasue, H., S. Omote, A. Takizawa, M. Nagao, Miwak, and S. Tanaka.** Circadian variation of exercise capacity in patients with Prinzmetal's variant angina: Role of exercise-induced coronary artery spasm. *Circulation.* 59:938–948, 1979.
43. **Wilhelmsen, L., H. Sanne, D. Elmfeldt, G. Grimby, G. Tibblin, and H. Wedel.** A controlled trial of physical training after myocardial infarction. *Prev. Med.* 4:491–508, 1975.

Appendix H

THE NEW LABEL FORMAT

The new food label can be found on food packages in your supermarket. Reading the label tells more about the food and what you are getting. What you see on the food label—the nutrition and ingredient information—is required by the government.

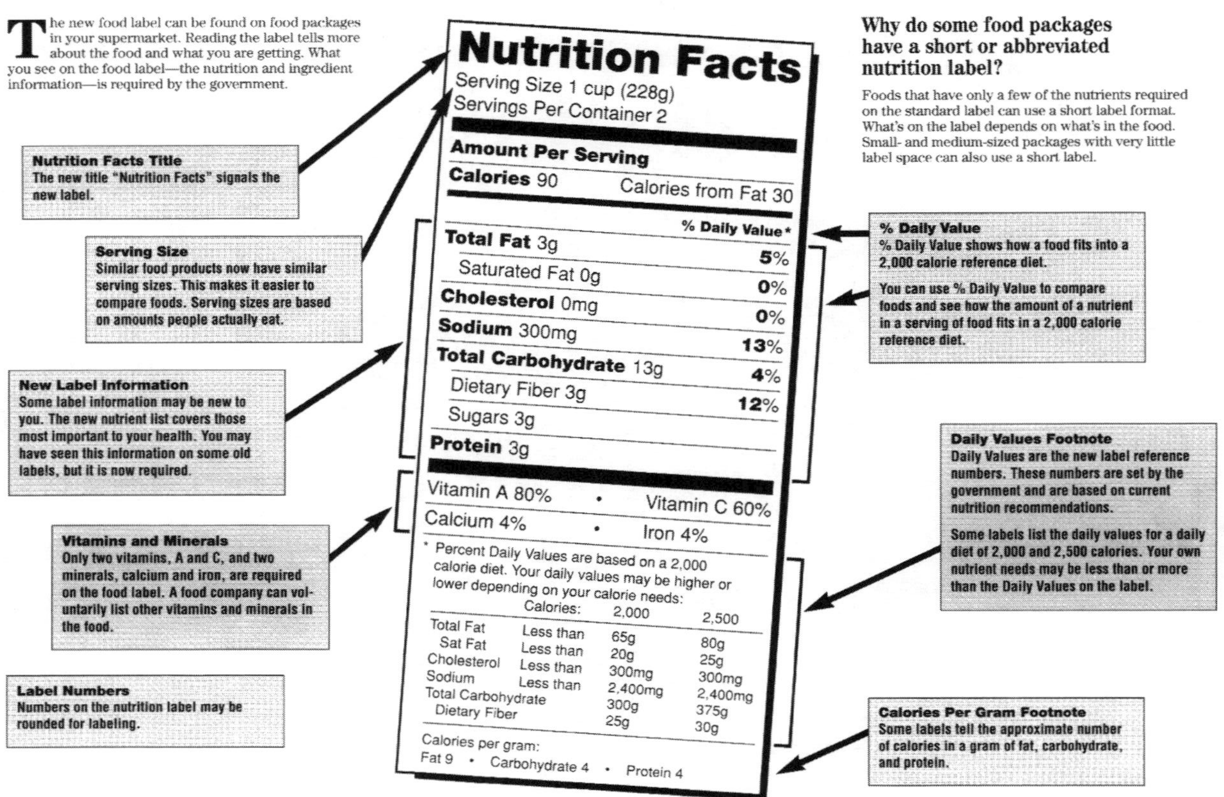

Why do some food packages have a short or abbreviated nutrition label?

Foods that have only a few of the nutrients required on the standard label can use a short label format. What's on the label depends on what's in the food. Small- and medium-sized packages with very little label space can also use a short label.

Appendix I

THE FOOD GUIDE PYRAMID ... WHAT IS A SERVING?

Food Group	Suggested Daily Servings	What Counts as Serving	Nutrients
Breads, cerals, and other grain products Whole-grain Enriched	6–11 servings from entire group (Include several servings of whole-grain products daily.)	1 slice bread 1/2 hamburger bun or English muffin a small roll, biscuit, or muffin 3 to 4 small or 2 large crackers 1/2 cup cooked cereal, rice, or pasta 1 oz ready-to-eat cereal	Enriched and whole-grain breads and cereals provide starch, thiamin, riboflavin, niacin, and iron. Whole-grains also are good sources of fiber and provide folic acid, magnesium, and zinc.
Fruits Citrus, melon, berries Other fruits	2–4 servings from entire group	A whole fruit such as medium apple, banana A grapefruit half A melon wedge 3/4 cup juice 1/2 cup berries 1/2 cup cooked or canned fruit 1/4 cup dried fruit	All fruits are good sources of potassium, folic acid, magnesium, and fiber. Citrus fruits, melons, and berries are especially good sources of vitamin C and all yellow fruits are rich in vitamin A.
Vegetables Dark-green leafy Deep-yellow Dry beans and peas (legumes) Starchy Other vegetables	3–5 servings from entire group (Include all types regularly: use dark-green leafy vegetables and dry beans and peas several times a week.)	1/2 cup cooked or chopped raw vegetables 1 cup leafy raw vegetables, such as lettuce or spinach 3/4 cup vegetable juice	Dark-green leafy vegetables are good sources of vitamins A and C, riboflavin, folic acid, calcium, magnesium, potassium, and fiber. Deep-yellow vegetables are excellent sources of vitamin A. Dry beans and peas are good sources of fiber, thiamin, folic acid, iron, phosphorus,

0-8493-7914-8/95/$0.00+$.50

Food Group	Suggested Daily Servings	What Counts as Serving	Nutrients
			zinc, potassium, protein and starch. Other vegetables contain varying amounts of vitamins, minerals, and fiber.
Meat, poultry, fish, dry beans, eggs, and nuts	2–3 servings from entire group	1 oz = 1 oz cook lean meat, poultry, fish; 1 egg; 1/2 cup cooked beans; 2 tablespoons peanut butter	Foods in this group are sources of many nutrients. These include protein, niacin, vitamins B_6 and B_{12}, iron, phosphorus, and zinc.
Milk, cheese, and yogurt	2–3 servings from entire group (3 servings for teens and women who are pregnant or breast-feeding; 4 servings for teens who are pregnant or breast-feeding)	1 cup milk; 8 oz yogurt; 1-1/2 oz natural cheese; 2 oz processed cheese	Foods in this group are good sources of calcium, protein, riboflavin, vitamin B_{12}, thiamin, and, if fortified, vitamin D. If you are unable to consume milk products, 1 cup soy milk, 1/2 cup tofu, 6 sardines with bones, and 1-1/2 cups cooked greens each provides the amount of calcium in 1 cup milk.
Fats, sweets, and alcoholic beverages	Use sparingly. Foods this group provide calories and little else nutritionally.		

Adapted from *Preparing Foods and Planning Menus Using the Dietary Guidelines,* Home & Gardening Bulletin No. 232-8, U.S. Department of Agriculture, Human Nutrition Information Service, Washington, D.C., 1989.

INDEX

C

D

E

F

G

M

N

O

T

U

V

W

Z